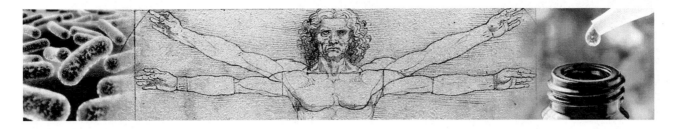

MRSA Secrets Revealed

By Michelle Moore

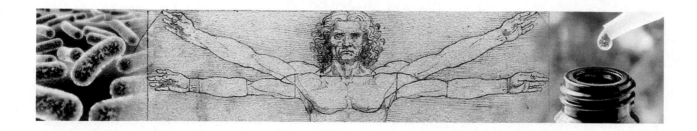

Text design and layout by Les Moore. This book was typeset in Minion Pro with Myriad Pro used as the display typeface. Cover Design: Les Moore. Cover photos: Bacteria, © iStockPhoto.com/Henrik5000; Vitruvian Man, Luc Viatour / www.lucnix.be; Oil drop © iStockPhoto.com/Synergee; Stethoscope, © iStockPhoto.com/bluestocking; Leaves, © iStockPhoto.com/robynmac; Plate, © iStockPhoto.com/Lindel; Mortar, © iStockPhoto.com/Pears2295; Michelle Moore, © Lester Moore. Front matter photos: Bacteria, © iStockPhoto.com/Henrik5000; Vitruvian Man, Luc Viatour / www.lucnix.be; Oil drop © iStockPhoto.com/Synergee.

Fifth Edition

ISBN: 978-1-939795-50-2

www.Staph-Infection-Resources.com

Dedication

This book is dedicated to those who have Staph, MRSA or other infectious diseases and to the relief of their suffering. This book is also dedicated to the Highest Light, which has been my source and inspiration for true healing and wellness.

Thanks are given to our beautiful Earth and to the amazing plants, herbs and foods that can restore and sustain our optimal health and wellbeing.

This book is written in gratitude for the gifts of wisdom, understanding and creativity that have afforded us all the blessings of both mainstream and alternative medicine.

May the words, principles and techniques in this book be accompanied by true healing for the highest good in your life.

- Michelle Moore

Contents

Introduction

Mainstream medicine has come a long way toward defeating the illnesses that have plagued mankind for thousands of years. The so-called *miracle drugs* or antibiotics are a great example. While mainstream medicine has demonstrated its great worth, its shortcomings have become much more obvious in the last few decades, especially in the area of infectious diseases. *Staph aureus* (Staph) and MRSA infections are a growing problem and even the *last resort* antibiotics are becoming less effective every year. Antibiotic resistance is also a growing issue with other superbug infections, such as tuberculosis, Typhoid (Salmonella), *C. difficile* and Enterococci.

The growing inability of mainstream medicine to successfully treat Staph and MRSA is a source frustration, disappointment, fear, and even despair for hundreds of thousands of people suffering from these potentially deadly infections. The cycle of infection, antibiotics, reinfection, more antibiotics, and so on has trapped many people in a downward spiral from which they see no escape. As a result, people's trust in the healthcare system, antibiotic drugs and mainstream medicine has wavered. At the same time, a hopeful search for alternative solutions for Staph and MRSA has been kindled.

There is Hope

The good news is that Staph and MRSA can be beat by addressing the infection from a broader perspective. By returning to the very foundation upon which mainstream medicine was originally built, natural, holistic and alternative medicine provide safe and effective avenues to overcome these infections. Furthermore, alternative medical approaches enlist the help of a very powerful weapon against infection: your own immune system.

Both mainstream medicine and alternative medicine are valuable tools. Mainstream medicine does a great job at relieving symptoms and dealing with acute health challenges. But mainstream medicine has a poor track record with chronic challenges, like recurring infections. In contrast, alternative medicine can relieve infection and also help with long-term prevention of recurring infections. Integrating both mainstream and alternative medicine provides you with more effective therapies and it greatly increases your chances of a successful outcome.

Michelle Moore's 3-Step Infection-Free Method in chapter 1 will show you how to combine the best of both mainstream and alternative medicine. The Infection-Free Method was created through years of education, research and personal experience as well as the collaborative efforts of chemists and natural medicine experts. Michelle Moore combined all this expertise and research together to create the Infection-Free Method. Whether your antibiotics have stopped working, you're looking for an alternative treatment approach, or you're taking care of someone with Staph or MRSA, this book can help you.

Infections Covered in This Book

This book applies to **all types of Staph and MRSA**. For simplicity, the terms *Staph* and *MRSA* are used throughout this book to describe several related infections. Both antibiotic resistant and antibiotic sensitive Staph infections are included (MRSA is a type of antibiotic resistant Staph).

The book applies to all antibiotic sensitive strains of Staph. *Staph aureus* (*Staphylococcus aureus*) is the most common Staph infection. This book also applies to all other Staphylococcal infections such as coagulase-negative Staph (coag-negative Staph), *Staph epidermidis* (Staph epi.) and methicillin-sensitive *Staph aureus* (MSSA). All other species of Staph bacteria (any infection with the word *Staph* in it) are also applicable.

The book also applies to all antibiotic resistant strains of Staph. The term *MRSA* used throughout this book refers to *methicillin-resistant Staphylococcus aureus*. The book also applies to *multi-drug resistant Staphylococcus aureus* and *multiple-resistant Staph aureus*. *Oxacillin resistant Staph aureus* (ORSA) and *vancomycin resistant Staph aureus* (VRSA) are also applicable to this book.

Many of the methods and techniques inside this book can be successfully applied to other types of infections, such as other bacterial, viral or fungal infections, though modifications may be needed. The topic of immune support, which is thoroughly covered in this book, also applies to any type of bacterial, viral or fungal infection.

All the ways that Staph and MRSA can cause an infection, including any type of skin, internal, bone, sinus or all other types of infections are covered in this book. The following symptoms and diagnoses also apply to this book: septicemia, endocarditis, osteomyelitis, meningitis, pneumonia, boils, folliculitis, carbuncles, impetigo, abscesses, cellulitis and furunculosis.

Making the Most of This Book

Most people have been programmed by the media, drug companies and even their doctors to expect a quick-fix cure for health problems, usually in the form of a pill. While this approach can sometimes work in the short-term, it's kind of like plugging a hole in a dam with your finger. Everything may seem OK for a while, but without warning you could be struggling to keep your head above water and wondering what went wrong.

The expectation for a simple cure that will quickly make your infection go away forever is often unrealistic. As you will learn in this book, stopping your immediate infection is important and there are multiple methods and approaches at your disposal. However, taking long-term steps so that your body can heal itself and become resistant to future infections is just as important in the long run.

Some infections can be cleared up quickly and easily, especially moderate skin infections. But many people struggle with more challenging infections that respond poorly to treatment, especially difficult internal infections and chronic recurring infections. It's also common to have other health challenges that make it more difficult to recover from an infection. So in some cases, additional steps are needed to recover beyond a simple remedy or treatment.

Restoring your long-term health is a process that may involve uncovering and treating one or more root causes and imbalances inside your body. This process can take time, and it looks a little different for each person. It may have taken you many years to arrive at the state of health that you are experiencing today. Likewise, restoring your health and enjoying long-term freedom from Staph and MRSA may also take a bit of time.

What to Do First

Because of the comprehensive nature of this book, it may be challenging to know where to start or what's most important. The Infection-Free Method in chapter 1 is broken down into three Action Steps. These three Action Steps will show you what methods are most important and what to do first.

The 3 Steps of the Infection-Free Method in chapter 1 shows the most important things to do.

Keep in mind that the three Action Steps in chapter 1 are only a short summary or guide. All the details to fully understand the Action Steps are found inside the other chapters of this book. The Action Steps will give you references to other parts of this book containing the details you need for each step, including important safety precautions and detailed step-by-step protocols.

What's Best for You?

As informative, useful and comprehensive as this book may be, it is incapable by itself of giving you the best possible results with a Staph or MRSA infection. To realize the most benefit, work with a medical professional who can help you to fine-tune what this book teaches you and develop a personalized infection recovery plan specific to your unique needs.

Everyone is different and every infection is also different. This book is not a substitute for competent and knowledgeable professional medical advice. Working with the right doctors and finding the right professional guidance will put all the pieces of the treatment puzzle together for you and give you the most benefit from whatever methods you choose to use. Because Staph and MRSA can be dangerous and can worsen quickly, working with a doctor is crucial to monitor your progress, whether you are using alternative medicine, mainstream medicine or both.

This book will help you find the best doctors and will show you how to use your doctor most effectively. While doctors are important, it is equally important to take responsibility for your health and be an active participant in crafting your own infection recovery plan.

Is Alternative Medicine Safe?

Alternative medicine can be quite safe, especially when compared to pharmaceutical drugs. Mainstream medicine relies heavily on the use of drugs that have many dangerous side effects. Even if a drug seems to work, its undesirable side effects are sanctioned and approved by the FDA on the argument that a certain amount of risk is acceptable if a large percentage of people will benefit. Such an approach negates you as an individual and is actually quite dangerous and risky compared to the personalized and holistic approach of alternative medicine.

When used knowledgeably and responsibly, the methods in this book are highly unlikely to cause any harm. Compared with the hazards of mainstream treatments and the havoc that antibiotics can cause, the potential problems associated with most natural remedies are minimal. On the other hand, the chances of achieving great benefits from natural medicine are considerable when used responsibly.

As you read about the methods in this book, you will notice that most of them are accompanied by specific statements of warning and precautions for responsible use. It is important to understand these statements and take all necessary precautions before using a remedy (the same is also true about prescription drugs). However, it is also vital that you remain confident in your own ability to use natural and alternative remedies safely and effectively and resist becoming intimidated by warnings.

Warnings and responsible precautions give you information you need to improve your ability to safely and effectively use a particular method. These warnings and precautions obviously cannot be all-encompassing or tailored to each person's unique needs. However, the precautions in this book do cover the most common issues to be aware of for the majority of people.

Taking Responsibility for Your Health

If you want to overcome MRSA, Staph or any other health challenge, it is essential to take responsibility for your health and be an active participant in crafting your own infection recovery plan. That means doing your own research and learning all you can about your infection and your health from as many trustworthy sources as possible. Be aware that every doctor, wellness program and information source has its own unique biases and pros and cons, including this book. Take everything you read with a grain of salt and make sure any information you follow is a good fit for your needs.

Ultimately, it is your task to determine the benefits and risks of the methods you are using and make your own decisions of whether to use a method or not. This is especially true of pharmaceutical drugs and antibiotics. It is also true of natural and alternative methods. Taking responsibility for your own health is perhaps the single most important step you can take to overcome your infection or any other health challenge.

Michelle Moore's Journey to Health

Michelle was always inquisitive and asked many questions from an early age. She later got her education in biology and microbiology and worked for many years as a microbiologist in the pharmaceutical industry. Michelle believed in and only used mainstream medicine. She took pain medicines to relieve pain, used prescriptions for acid-reflux and used antibiotics for infections. She did what her doctor told her to do and trusted that her doctor knew what was best.

There was just one problem with her long-cherished beliefs about modern medicine: she was getting sicker from recurring infections and the healthcare system was not helping her.

For a period of four years, Michelle suffered from recurring sinus infections that antibiotics failed to successfully treat. This was very scary for her as she didn't want bacteria *running amuck* in her head, or anywhere else for that matter. She did exactly what her doctor told her to do: she took the antibiotics prescribed to her, adding up to many different antibiotics over the years.

As her health worsened, Michelle's energy and quality of life deteriorated as all the antibiotics wreaked havoc with her digestive tract and immune system. Because of her weakened immunity, she became sick more easily and often lost time from work. She was becoming miserable and growing sick and tired of the cycle of infections, drugs, and more infections with no lasting solution in sight.

Then out of the blue something struck her. An amazing realization occurred that would never have happened if not for her health challenges. She fully realized that what her doctor was offering her was not working, nor would it magically start working any time soon. She began to wonder what other people did about their infections. Maybe someone else had gone through what she had and found a better way to deal with infections. What Michelle discovered changed her life forever.

She talked to many people, tirelessly researched medical journals on the Internet, read multiple books, attended seminars and even joined a nutritional company that focused on health through the power of whole foods. Much to her amazement, she discovered that most of today's chronic health issues are actually the result of nutritional deficiencies and a neglected immune system. And most importantly, she discovered the amazing and powerful world of plant and herbal medicine for handling infections.

Michelle discovered that therapeutic essential oils are literally the immune system of plants which are condensed down into powerful drops of life-giving, antibacterial essences. She also discovered that many of the foods she was eating weakened her immune system, making her more vulnerable to infections. She found that changing her diet and using powerful plant-based medicines made it impossible for infections to thrive in her body. She finally found the knowledge, results and hope that mainstream medicine was unable to give her.

While Michelle believes that mainstream medicine has much to offer, she now realizes that mainstream medicine also has serious limitations that must be recognized and avoided. It took her years to realize that true health is more than the absence of disease. True health is optimal and vibrant living where you wake up and greet each day with happiness, vitality and gratitude.

Michelle is now happier and healthier than ever and has not had a recurring infection since 2002. She is continually blessed to have helped thousands of people discover the natural and effective options that saved her. So now she invites you to begin your own journey along the path to optimal health and infection-free living. Michelle's hope for you is to take a leap of faith and discover the many amazing approaches that millions of other people around the world have used to regain and maintain their health.

Talk to Your Doctor

Michelle Moore is not a doctor or a healthcare practitioner. Michelle is someone who overcame many health obstacles that traditional medicine could not solve. The information in this book is based upon Michelle's research, education and personal experience and is for educational purposes only. This information is not intended as a substitute for advice provided by your physician or other healthcare professional or any information contained on or in any product label or packaging.

The information in this book and any associated resources is not intended to treat, cure, prevent, or diagnose disease or medical conditions, nor is it intended to prescribe forms of medical treatment. The author and Embrace Health, Inc. do not distribute medical advice and are not responsible for use or application of the information contained herein. Do not disregard professional medical advice or delay in seeking professional advice because of something you have read in this book.

Issues concerning health should be referred to your physician or a qualified health professional. If you have a health condition, or if you are pregnant, nursing, on medication(s), or have allergies, please consult with your physician before starting any new wellness, diet or exercise program, and any new treatment or herbal, homeopathic or nutritional supplement. When choosing a healthcare provider, do you own research and check the validity of their professional qualifications to ensure they are right for you.

The author of this book has used her best efforts in preparing this information. The author and Embrace Health, Inc. make no representation or warranties with respect to the accuracy or completeness of this book. Because there are always risks involved, the author and Embrace Health, Inc. are not responsible or liable for any adverse consequences resulting from the use or misuse of any of the information contained within this book or associated resources. Unless otherwise noted, information in this book and statements regarding dietary supplements have not been evaluated by the Food and Drug Administration.

1

Michelle's 3 Step Infection-Free Method

For every kind of Staph and MRSA infection, there are several common actions that can speed recovery and reduce the risk of future outbreaks. This chapter contains Michelle Moore's 3 Step Infection-Free Method for stopping stubborn infections, accelerating the healing process and avoiding recurring infections. Because there's a lot of information in this book, refer back to chapter 1 often to keep yourself focused on the most important actions to take.

Three Action Steps to Recovery

Staph and MRSA are hardy, stubborn and clever bacteria that can grow quickly into huge numbers. MRSA has learned to resist most standard treatments and can be hard to stop with even the newest *last resort* antibiotics. These bacteria learn by sharing resistance information with each other and even with other species of bacteria. They also work together in a coordinated way to form protected colonies in your body to shield themselves, repel treatments and cause recurring infections.

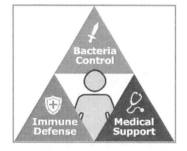

Bacteria Control, Medical Support and Immune Defense are the 3 Action Steps of Michelle Moore's Infection-Free Method.

Fighting such a dangerous, organized and resourceful enemy requires a powerful and strategic plan of attack. Michelle Moore's Infection-Free Method is broken down into three Action Steps. The Action Steps will show you how to control MRSA and Staph on multiple fronts and win the battle against these infections.

The three Action Steps of Michelle's Infection-Free Method are: 1) bacteria control, 2) medical support and 3) immune defense. These steps are coordinated to work together, providing strong offensive, defensive and support strategies for your body's immune system army. All three Action Steps should be followed at the same time for the best possible outcome with a stubborn infection.

Action Step 1 is about controlling the bacteria that are causing the infection. If you've been struggling with antibiotics that don't work, then the remedies and methods in Step 1 could literally save your life. Action Step 2 is about avoiding common medical mistakes that delay your recovery and make your infection worse. Finally, Action Step 3 is about speeding your recovery, rooting out hidden bacteria, regaining your health and making your body resistant to future infections.

Personalizing the Infection-Free Method

There are different kinds of Staph and MRSA and every infection sufferer has unique health challenges and needs. For example, children may need different remedies or lower usage amounts than adults. Skin infections, internal infections and sinus infections can all require different remedies or approaches. People who are caregivers for a hospitalized parent may need specific support on working within the healthcare system and preventing hospital infections and medical mistakes. The three Action Steps that make up the Infection-Free Method can be customized to fit different types of infections, people and circumstances.

The chapter references in the tables below show you where to find the details to personalize and customize each of the three Action Steps to best suit your own particular needs. The references will show you where to find important details about usage amounts, safety precautions, step-by-step protocols and important background information for each of the Action Steps.

How to Follow the Action Steps

NOTE: The Action Steps are only a summary of the *whats*, not the *hows*. Refer to the chapter references shown in the tables below for important details on how to follow each step.

The Action Steps are not meant to be used by themselves. For the required details to understand and follow each step, read the chapters or sections referenced in the last (far right) column of the tables labeled *Details*. Please use the references and read the necessary details before following each Action Step. As you read this book, refer back to the Action Steps to keep yourself on track and focused on the most important things. Keep the following tips in mind to get the most benefit from the three Action Steps:

- **Follow as much of the Action Steps as possible** for maximum results or for challenging infections. That means using Steps 1, 2 and 3 together at the same time. Action Step 1 is most important if you have an active infection.

- **You may not need every type of support** listed in the Action Steps, especially for mild infections. The types of support toward the top of each table are generally the most important.

- **Individual needs and results vary.** Consulting with a qualified healthcare practitioner familiar with the protocols in the Action Steps is highly recommended.

- Some parts of the Action Steps include nutritional supplements designed to support your body to heal itself. **Consult with your doctor before starting any new supplement or health program.**

MRSA and Staph infections deserve respect. These infections can worsen quickly, can be very difficult to treat and can be life-threatening. No matter what treatments, remedies or methods you choose to use, always work with a qualified healthcare professional to monitor your progress and provide additional medical support if needed. The Action Steps are for informational purposes only and are not a substitute for medical advice. The statements below have not been evaluated by the Food and Drug Administration (FDA). The products, protocols and methods in the Action Steps are not intended to diagnose, treat, cure or prevent any disease.

◇◇

NOTE: Enlist the help of a medical professional to monitor your progress regardless of what methods or remedies you choose to use.

◇◇

Action Step 1: Bacteria Control

One of the biggest mistakes people make is relying solely on just one single remedy or treatment. MRSA and Staph are formidable bacteria with a knack for infiltrating the body in multiple ways. If you have a skin infection, the bacteria probably go much deeper than your skin. You want to control the bacteria on multiple fronts for best results. That means bacteria control at the site of the infection, internally (systemically) and in your surrounding environment.

In, On and Around

The core principle of Action Step 1 is called *In, On and Around*:

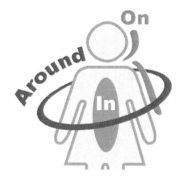

- **In** stands for internal or systemic support to control the infection from the inside out.

- **On** stands for control of bacteria on the skin using topical skin remedies.

- **Around** stands for controlling bacteria in the environment around you.

Your best choice of remedy depends on what type of MRSA or Staph infection you're dealing with. Find the subsection below that best matches the type of infection you have. For example, if you have an internal infection, then skip ahead to the subsection titled "For Internal Infections" on page 12.

If your infection is mild, you may not need to follow every *Type of Support* listed in the tables below. However, following all types of support (*In, On and Around*) can provide the strongest bacterial control. Likewise, some of the actions in the *Action Summary* column may not apply to you or may not be crucial, depending on your unique needs. For the information required to follow each action, refer to the *Details* column in each table.

Different Types of Infections

The vast majority of MRSA and Staph infections are addressed in the tables below. However, if you don't see the specific type of infection that you have listed in the tables, you can find the details you need later in this book. For example, for MRSA or Staph urinary tract infections (UTIs), there are additional details listed in "MRSA Bladder and Urinary Tract Infections" on page 195.

Children and Elderly

Many of the protocols and methods detailed in Action Step 1 may need to be adjusted for children and the elderly. Also, some of the methods may not be appropriate for children or the elderly. Be sure to follow the detailed usage instructions and precautions for any methods you choose to use.

For Skin Infections

Skin infections include boils, folliculitis, impetigo, furunculosis and carbuncles. Skin infections can be also be infected wounds, burns, cuts or abrasions, or anywhere on the skin that is infected with MRSA or Staph. For deep abscesses, cellulitis and deep surgical site infections, refer to the section on internal infections later in Acton Step 1.

The following table will show you the *In, On and Around* actions to take for skin infections. For best results, all three types of support (in, on and around) are followed together at the same time. **Skip over this section if you have a sinus or internal type of infection with no skin symptoms.**

Skin Infections

Type of Support	Action Summary	Details
In: internal or systemic	• The Botanical Blend protocol provides broad-spectrum internal support and is safe, well-tolerated and easy to use. Other options include: • The Antibacterial Blend essential oil. • The essential oil Broad-Spectrum Internal Protocol. • Stabilized allicin liquid. For any of the above, beginning at the low or moderate usage amount is generally suitable, depending on infection severity.	• "Botanical Blend Protocol" on page 106 • "The Antibacterial Blend" on page 145 • "Broad-Spectrum Internal Protocol for Adults" on page 156 • "Stabilized Allicin" on page 95
On: external, at site of infection on skin	• Tea tree essential oil is excellent for infection support on sensitive skin areas. It's also a good choice for children and elderly. • The Antibacterial Blend oil is suitable for general skin use. Other options include: • Genuine Manuka honey. • Stabilized allicin gel. Apply the above several times per day or when changing dressings.	• "Tea Tree Oil" on page 140 • "The Antibacterial Blend" on page 145 • "Manuka Honey" on page 97 • "Stabilized Allicin" on page 95
Around: home and environmental	• Control airborne bacteria by air diffusing tea tree and/or eucalyptus essential oils. • Add either tea tree or the Antibacterial Blend essential oil to your bath water or body wash for skin decolonization support. • Follow proper cleaning, laundry, disinfecting and personal hygiene practices. Use natural, non-toxic products to support your immune system whenever possible.	• "How to Air Diffuse Essential Oils" on page 132 • "Bathing With Essential Oils" on page 134 • "Sanitizer and Personal Care Recipes" on page 272 • Cleaning on page 276 • Hygiene on page 267 • Laundry on page 285

For Nose and Sinus Infections

The table below applies to nose and sinus Staph and MRSA infections. For best result, all three types of support (in, on and around) are followed together at the same time. **Skip over this section if you have a skin or an internal infection with no nose or sinus symptoms.**

11

Nose and Sinus Infections

Type of Support	Action Summary	Details
In: internal or systemic	• The Botanical Blend protocol provides broad-spectrum internal support and is safe, well-tolerated and easy to use. Other options include: • The Antibacterial Blend essential oil. • The essential oil Broad-Spectrum Internal Protocol. • Stabilized allicin liquid. Beginning at either the low or moderate level usage amount is generally suitable, depending on infection severity.	• "Botanical Blend Protocol" on page 106 • "The Antibacterial Blend" on page 145 • "Broad-Spectrum Internal Protocol for Adults" on page 156 • "Stabilized Allicin" on page 95
On: external, at site of infection on skin	• For nose or sinus infections, dilute tea tree essential oil for topical application in the nose. Rosemary and lavender oil can also be added for extra support. • For sinus infections, daily neti pot sinus rinses with tea tree oil added to the rinse water. Other options include: • Add genuine Manuka honey or stabilized allicin gel to neti pot rinse water.	• "Tea Tree Oil" on page 140 • "Sinus Rinsing Technique" on page 133 • "Manuka Honey" on page 97 • "Stabilized Allicin" on page 95
Around: home and environmental	• Control airborne Staph and MRSA by air diffusing tea tree and/or eucalyptus oils. • Add either tea tree or the Antibacterial Blend essential oil to your bath water or body wash for skin decolonization support. • Follow effective and safe cleaning, disinfecting and personal hygiene practices. Use natural, non-toxic products to support your immune system whenever possible.	• "How to Air Diffuse Essential Oils" on page 132 • "Bathing With Essential Oils" on page 134 • "Sanitizer and Personal Care Recipes" on page 272 • Cleaning on page 276 • Hygiene on page 267

For Internal Infections

The table below applies to internal infections, including deep abscesses, cellulitis, deep surgical site infections and infections of the bone, blood and lungs. This applies to any type of internal Staph or MRSA infection. For best result, all three types of support (in, on and around) are followed together at the same time. **Skip over this section if you have a skin infection or a nose or sinus infection.**

Internal infections are often more severe than other types of MRSA and Staph. If you have a critical or life-threatening infection, then there's a good chance you're already admitted to a hospital. Using alternative remedies can be restrictive or more challenging in hospitals and other healthcare settings (see "Action Step 2: Medical Support" on page 13 for more on this topic).

Internal Infections

Type of Support	Action Summary	Details
In: internal or systemic	• The Botanical Blend protocol provides broad-spectrum internal support and is safe, well-tolerated and easy to use. Other options include: • The Antibacterial Blend essential oil. • The essential oil Broad-Spectrum Internal Protocol. • Stabilized allicin liquid. The highest usage amount of the remedies above may be needed, or a combination of remedies, depending on infection severity. • High level intravenous (IV) vitamin C can be very helpful for systemic infections and can usually be administered in hospitals and some doctor offices with a little diligence and planning.	• "Botanical Blend Protocol" on page 106 • "The Antibacterial Blend" on page 145 • "Broad-Spectrum Internal Protocol for Adults" on page 156 • "Stabilized Allicin" on page 95 • "Using IV Vitamin C Therapy" on page 101
On: external, at site of infection on skin	Apply tea tree or Antibacterial Blend essential oil topically as close as possible to the infection's internal location, such as the chest for a lung infection, on the skin above a bone infection, or on the skin over an abscess. Apply the oil several times per day. • For extra support, you can increase the skin absorption of essential oils which helps push the oil deeper into the body.	• "Tea Tree Oil" on page 140 • "The Antibacterial Blend" on page 145 • "How to Increase Skin Absorption" on page 129

Internal Infections		
Type of Support	**Action Summary**	**Details**
Around: home, hospital room or surroundings	• Control airborne Staph and MRSA by air diffusing tea tree and/or eucalyptus oils. • Add tea tree or the Antibacterial Blend essential oil to your bath water or body wash for skin decolonization support. • Follow preventative measures for healthcare infections (details in Action Step 2 below).	• "How to Air Diffuse Essential Oils" on page 132 • "Bathing With Essential Oils" on page 134 • "Sanitizer and Personal Care Recipes" on page 272 • Cleaning on page 276 • Hygiene on page 267

Action Step 2: Medical Support

 For many Staph and MRSA sufferers, the single biggest obstacle that delays recovery is the healthcare and medical support they receive. One of the best ways to speed your recovery is to recognize and avoid the most common healthcare pitfalls and medical mistakes. Getting proper medical support is crucial, regardless of which treatment approach you choose to use. It's important to be under the care of a knowledgeable doctor and be proactive in your treatment for the best results.

Another important part of controlling an infection is using methods to ease the secondary symptoms that often accompany Staph and MRSA. In addition, there are several techniques that complement natural remedies which can enhance the healing process. The table below will show you the most important ways to ensure good medical support and effective infection management.

If your infection is mild, you may not need to follow every *Type of Support* listed in the table below. However, following all the types of support can provide the most benefit, especially if you've had challenges with your doctor or hospital. Likewise, some of the actions in the *Action Summary* column may not apply to you or may not be crucial, depending on your unique needs.

Type of Support	**Action Summary**	**Details**
Getting the right tests	• If you think you have MRSA or Staph, get a bacterial culture test from your doctor. This test will identify what's causing the infection and will help in getting the right antibiotic. • If your antibiotics are not working, ask your doctor for an antibiotic susceptibility test. This test will determine which antibiotics will work for your specific infection.	• "Testing for MRSA and Staph" on page 45

Type of Support	Action Summary	Details
Finding the right doctors	• Know the 10 key questions to ask your doctor. • If needed, find a doctor who is knowledgeable about Staph and MRSA, or get a second opinion. • Consider seeing an Infectious Disease (ID) specialist. ID doctors are more likely to have MRSA and Staph experience and better treatment success rates. • Consider seeing a Functional Medicine or Naturopathic doctor with alternative medicine experience.	• See the guidebook *Top 10 Questions to Ask Your Doctor About MRSA* • "How to Get Better Medical Care" on page 42
Reducing antibiotic side effects	• Ask your doctor to explain all the side effects and contraindications of any prescribed antibiotics. • Take the full course of antibiotics unless directed otherwise by your doctor. This helps prevent antibiotic resistance and reinfections. • Control antibiotic side effects, including daily probiotics to reduce antibiotic dysbiosis.	• "Antibiotic Side Effects" on page 77 • "Antibiotic Resistance" on page 67 • "Reducing Antibiotic Side Effects" on page 173
Infection management techniques	Use specific infection control techniques (as applicable): • Wound dressing, caring for boils and abscesses. • Skin and nose decolonization and sinus rinsing. • Children's remedy tips and pet remedies. • Bladder infection treatments and airborne MRSA.	• "Infection Management Techniques" on page 189
Symptom relief	Take remedies for specific symptoms as needed: • Pain, scars, fever, and secondary infections.	• "Secondary Conditions and Challenges" on page 173
Protection from hospital infections	Take specific actions before, during and after any hospital stay to reduce the risk of catching hospital infections or getting reinfected.	• "How to Avoid Hospital Infections" on page 56
Using alternatives in hospitals	If you choose to use alternative remedies in a healthcare facility, be sure to take the steps needed to maximize your health freedom with supplements.	• "Using Supplements in Hospitals" on page 58
Avoiding medical mistakes	Learn how to spot the most common medical errors and mistakes and take steps to avoid them.	• "Avoiding Medical Mistakes" on page 55
Being proactive in you healthcare	Get in the drivers seat of your healthcare and become informed and proactive.	• "Taking Control of Your Healthcare" on page 48

As stated earlier, follow Action Step 2 concurrently with Action Steps 1 and 3 for best results.

Action Step 3: Immune Defense

 The most powerful and effective weapon you have against Staph and MRSA is your body's immune system. Surprisingly, some antibiotics only stop bacteria from reproducing without actually killing the bacteria themselves. It's up to your immune system to find and kill off the remaining bacteria left behind.

Even more surprising, choosing the right foods to eat is the fastest and most effective way to boost the defensive powers of your immune system. This crucial fact is the key to speeding your recovery. Proper nutrition is even more critical for prevention of recurring outbreaks in the future. The table below shows the most important ways to boost your immune system and support your body's natural defenses.

If your infection is mild, you may not need to follow every *Type of Support* listed in the table below. However, following all the types of support below can provide the strongest immune defense. Likewise, some of the actions in the *Action Summary* column may not apply to you or may not be crucial, depending on your unique needs.

Type of Support	Action Summary	Details
Sugar and carb elimination or reduction	• Sugar feeds bacterial infections. Shut down the infection's *supply lines* by eliminating sugar and processed foods during an active infection. • Some carbohydrates and sugars may be added back after the infection is gone.	• "Choose Your Sugars Wisely" on page 238
Probiotic support	• Antibiotic treatments and harsh decolonization protocols kill healthy bacteria that protect against invading bacteria. Use probiotics to help re-establish protective flora.	• "Probiotics: The Good Bacteria" on page 209
Daily green smoothie	• Eat one green smoothie per day to boost your body's nutrient intake, preferably organic.	• See smoothies on page 253
Vitamin D	• Many people are deficient in this antimicrobial vitamin. Get tested and supplement if needed.	• "Vitamin D, the Antibiotic Vitamin" on page 167
Biofilm and L-form bacteria support	• Support body to eliminate Staph and MRSA stealth bacteria to reduce chronic, recurring infections.	• "Biofilm and L-Form Support" on page 186
Stress control	• Stress has an immediate negative impact on your immune system. Take simple steps to reduce and control stress, especially during an infection.	• "Stress Management" on page 233

Type of Support	Action Summary	Details
Detoxification	• Reduce or avoid common food and environmental toxins, including glyphosate. • Antibiotics tax your liver. Some herbal remedies and essential oils may also tax the liver. Support your liver and lymphatic system. • After the infection has cleared, periodically detoxify your colon, liver or other bodily systems if well tolerated.	• "Healing Crisis and Detoxification Support" on page 217 • "Liver Support" on page 176
Reducing secondary infections	Address secondary infections if applicable: • *C. difficile* associated diarrhea. • Candida, yeast and fungal infections. • Urinary tract infections caused by *E. coli* or Klebsiella.	• "Co-Infections and Secondary Infections" on page 181
Long-term maintenance	• Take low level daily amounts of specific infection support remedies to control recurring MRSA and Staph infections.	• "Maintenance and Preventative Remedies" on page 207

Frequently Asked Questions

Below are answers to the most frequently asked questions about Michelle Moore's Infection-Free Method and its three Action Steps. This section will let you know what to expect when following the Action Steps.

What Should You Do First?

If you have an active infection, then Action Step 1 is most focused on stopping the infection. However, Action Steps 2 and 3 are important too. While all the methods in each step are important, the actions toward the top of each table are generally the most crucial for the majority of people.

Should You Do Everything in the Action Steps?

If you have a challenging or recurring infection that has been difficult to control, then following as much of the three Action Steps as possible can provide the maximum benefit. That means using Action Steps 1, 2 and 3 together at the same time. That also means following as many of the *Types of Support* as possible, as listed in the Action Step tables.

If your infection is mild or you've had good success with your treatments, then you may not need every *Type of Support* listed in the tables above. Within each table, the *Types of Support* toward the top are generally more important than the ones toward the bottom. Likewise, some of the actions in the *Action Summary* column of the tables may not apply to you or may not be crucial, depending on your unique needs.

Should You Follow Every Method In This Book?

This book contains many methods, remedies and techniques for controlling infections and supporting the immune system. At first glance, it can be hard to know which methods are most important. Fortunately, the most important methods for the average person with MRSA or Staph are summarized in the Action Steps in this chapter. Focusing your efforts on the three Action Steps is the best place to start for most people.

If you are already following most of the methods in the Action Steps, then adding other methods in this book according to your needs may provide further benefit. If for some reason you are unable to use a particular method listed in the Action Steps, then finding a substitute method elsewhere in this book may be very helpful, as detailed below.

What About Methods Not Listed in the Action Steps?

The Action Steps include Michelle's preferred methods and protocols. However, this book details many other helpful protocols, remedies and options that are not part of the Action Steps. These other options can be used as alternatives to the protocols listed in the Action Steps if needed or appropriate.

For example, if you have an allergy to olive leave extract, then consider using one of the other infection remedies listed in the Alternative Remedies chapter instead. Likewise, your doctor may have preferred remedies or protocols not listed in the Action Steps which you may choose to use.

Remember that everyone is different. While the Action Steps may be helpful for the majority of people, you may need to adjust the steps somewhat to achieve ideal results. Armed with the knowledge inside this book, along with the guidance of a medical professional, you can adjust and adapt the Action Steps to best suit your needs.

How Long Will it Take?

The effectiveness, optimal usage amount, and time to achieve results vary from person to person and from remedy to remedy. Supplement quality is a very important factor. However, as a general rule, people often start seeing results within a few days to a few weeks. Be aware that other health challenges, such as chronic disease conditions or other infections, typically make MRSA and Staph harder to get rid of, slowing the time it takes to see results. Advanced age, very young age or the inability to follow the Action Steps completely can also lengthen the time to see results. Because some people occasionally experience less benefit than others from a particular remedy or approach, switching to a more effective remedy can speed up the recovery process.

How Effective are the Action Steps?

There are countless remedies, supplements and treatment approaches available for MRSA and Staph infection support, all with varying degrees of safety and effectiveness. The remedies in Action Step 1 were chosen for their strong activity against Staph bacteria and from direct experience in using them successfully. These remedies also have activity against bacterial biofilms, which are linked with recurring infections which are largely unaffected by antibiotic treatments.

The key to unlocking the full effectiveness of the Action Steps is to attack the infection on multiple fronts at the same time. The remedies in Action Step 1 are often not enough by themselves, especially for long-standing infections. Following Action Steps 1, 2 and 3 together usually provides the fastest and most complete results.

The Action Steps were created based on years of research and personal experience and they have helped many people recover from Staph and MRSA. However, the Action Steps should not be considered a cure-all because results can vary from person to person. For the most effectiveness, customize the Action Steps to best fit your own unique needs with the help of a medical professional who has experience using the methods inside the Action Steps.

Are These Remedies and Protocols Safe?

The remedies in the Action Steps were chosen because they are non-toxic when used appropriately and contain herbal ingredients with a long track record of safety. When used according to the usage amounts, precautions and protocols specified in this book under the supervision of a medical professional, the remedies are very well tolerated by the vast majority of people. If any remedy is not well tolerated, it should be discontinued or replaced immediately.

Be aware that when starting any new healing program for the first time, you may start to feel tired, sluggish or get a headache. This can happen when you start eating healthier foods, start a probiotic or take infection remedies. While you may consider this response a negative reaction, it's caused by an excess of old toxins and/or dead bacteria being flushed out of the body resulting in a temporary detoxification reaction. Be sure to read "Healing Crisis and Detoxification Support" on page 217 so you know what symptoms can occur and what steps to take to minimize detox symptoms.

What if You're Already Taking Antibiotics?

Many of the protocols in the Action Steps can work along with antibiotic drugs safely and effectively. However, because some antibiotics can be rendered less effective when combined with some supplements, it's best to take any supplements at least two hours apart from antibiotics. This is a general rule of thumb for all supplements or remedies, including the ones in this book. Be sure to ask your doctor about combining herbal supplements with the specific antibiotics you are taking if you have further concerns.

You'll also find a chapter devoted to antibiotics for Staph and MRSA called "Antibiotic Treatments, Resistance and Limitations" on page 67. Follow Action Step 2 above to help ensure that your antibiotics are appropriate and will work for your infection. Because many antibiotics are not effective and some have debilitating and dangerous side-effects, many people are turning to safer, non-antibiotic approaches, as detailed in this book.

What If Your Doctor Won't Support You?

Most doctors have no training or experience with complementary, holistic, alternative or natural medicine. Ask your doctor how much knowledge, training and personal experience she has with any alternative remedies that she either recommends or discourages. Many people find that getting a second opinion or finding a new doctor who is supportive is extremely helpful. Being proactive with your health and taking an active role in your healthcare is very important, especially if you've been struggling with stubborn or recurring infections.

Many people have good results seeing an ID doctor if their family doctor or GP is unfamiliar with MRSA or Staph, or if they are not getting good results with their GP. However, most ID doctors are still firmly rooted in mainstream medicine and are unfamiliar with alternatives. If you are happy with your GP and the results you are getting, seeing an ID doctor may be less important to you. Seeing a Naturopathic Doctor (ND) or an MD certified in Functional Medicine can provide a high level of support for using the methods in this book.

2 Understanding Staph and MRSA

In September of 2013, the Centers for Disease Control and Prevention (CDC) released a report highlighting the top 18 antibiotic resistant superbug infections threatening the United States. In the report, MRSA was second only to *Clostridium difficile* as the superbug killing the greatest number of people each year[1]. In a recent study, drug resistant *Staph aureus* (including MRSA) was found to be responsible for approximately 1.2 million hospital infections each year. While resistant MRSA and Staph infections were once predominantly hospital related infections, they are now commonplace in communities around the world.

With the increasing number of antibiotic resistant infections, the CDC has warned that the age of antibiotics may soon be drawing to an end, returning the world to a pre-antibiotic era. Antibiotics can no longer be relied upon exclusively to stop MRSA, Staph and other infections. The more antibiotics are used, the more resistant bacteria become to them.

The good news is that there are other effective ways to handle MRSA besides antibiotics. Antibiotics may certainly be necessary and they can be life-saving, but over-reliance and misuse of these drugs has been a recipe for disaster. As you will learn later in this book, there are many alternatives to antibiotics, some of which are simple, inexpensive and have the potential to provide immediate results.

What is MRSA?

MRSA stands for Methicillin Resistant *Staphylococcus aureus* and is pronounced as *mer-sah* or as *mersa*. MRSA is a microscopic life form called a bacterium that has learned to resist the effects of penicillin-type antibiotics (including the antibiotic methicillin). This resistance to penicillin and other antibiotics is why MRSA is called a *superbug*. The problem of resistance is why MRSA is often difficult to treat with antibiotics.

MRSA can cause infections nearly anyplace on or inside the human body. The most common types of MRSA are skin and surgical site infections. The severity of an infection can range from mild to severe and the condition can become life-threatening.

MRSA was first discovered in the United Kingdom in 1961. Since the late 1990's, cases of MRSA have significantly increased in North America and Europe. MRSA now spans the globe with infections found in many countries. MRSA is most prevalent in the United States, the UK, and Australia. The UK has the highest incidence of MRSA and the Netherlands has the lowest incidence. MRSA is also common in Mexico, Canada, India, areas of South East Asia and in Northern Africa. Some studies show that MRSA is especially prevalent in warmer parts of the United States, including Atlanta, Texas, Los Angeles and Florida.

Staph Versus MRSA

Staph, which is short for *Staphylococcus*, is a group of bacteria that are often found on the skin, in the nose and in the upper respiratory tract of people. *Coagulase-negative Staph* species generically means the bacterium is a type of Staph, but not the more virulent *Staph aureus*.

Staphylococcus aureus (*Staph aureus* for short) is a particular Staph species that causes the most infections. MRSA is simply an antibiotic resistant strain or form of *Staph aureus*. In fact, there are many different strains of *Staph aureus* and MRSA bacteria.

The main difference between MRSA and Staph is that MRSA is often harder to treat with antibiotics. MRSA infections can also have more serious symptoms than Staph infections. While *Staph aureus* bacteria are quite common on people and in communities, MRSA bacteria are less common.

Most natural infection remedies are broad-spectrum and can be used for controlling both Staph or MRSA. In contrast, only certain antibiotics that Staph or MRSA are not resistant to will be effective. In addition, many antibiotics are only useful under certain specific conditions. Therefore, the list of antibiotics that are effective against MRSA is short and growing shorter each year.

VRSA, ORSA, MSSA, and Mercer

There are several other names and abbreviations sometimes used to refer to MRSA and Staph infections. MRSA is sometimes called Multi-drug Resistant *Staphylococcus aureus* or Multiple-resistant *Staph aureus*. These two terms mean a strain of *Staph aureus* that is resistant to multiple types of antibiotics. ORSA stands for Oxacillin Resistant *Staph aureus* where oxacillin is another penicillin-type antibiotic. Sometimes the term *mercer* is used incorrectly to refer to MRSA.

VRSA stands for vancomycin Resistant *Staph aureus*. Currently vancomycin is one of the antibiotics of last resort for highly resistant infections. Unfortunately, some *Staph aureus* strains have become resistant to vancomycin, leaving few effective antibiotics for doctors to prescribe. Staph bacteria are even starting to become resistant to newer antibiotics such as Zyvox.

MSSA stands for Methicillin Sensitive *Staphylococcus aureus*, which is a strain of *Staph aureus* which is still sensitive or treatable using methicillin type antibiotics.

MRSA is Not a Virus

The term *MRSA virus* is an misnomer. The term is sometimes seen on the Internet in articles and in the media. MRSA and Staph are not viruses: they are bacteria. Viruses are sub-microscopic infectious agents that are responsible for diseases such as smallpox, rabies, the flu, bird flu and common colds. Viruses are immune to antibiotics. A contributing factor to antibiotic resistance is the improper use of antibiotics for viral infections like the common cold and flu. Oftentimes patients want to feel better and take home a bottle of pills and doctors often comply. Antibiotics may make people feel better, at least mentally, but at what cost?

What are Bacteria?

Bacteria are microscopic, single celled organisms that are much smaller than the cells that make up the human body. In fact, it takes approximately 1000 bacteria to span the width of a pin head. They can range in length from about 0.5 micrometers to as large as 50 micrometers (1 micrometer is 1/1000 of a millimeter). Bacteria do not have a cellular nucleus like human cells do.

Bacteria come in different shapes and sizes. Bacteria can be rod or cigar shaped, spiral shaped and round (like Staph and MRSA). The names of bacteria actually come from how they look under a microscope. The term *coccus*, which is part of the name *Staphylococcus*, means round or oval in shape. The *staphylo* part of the name *Staphylococcus* signifies that the bacteria prefer to clump together in irregular clusters as opposed to chains or geometrically shaped groupings common to other bacterial species.

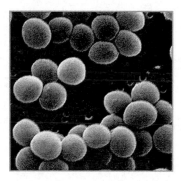

Bacteria are microscopic lifeforms that come in many shapes, sizes and species.

Bacteria live in virtually every environment on Earth and make up a large portion of the Earth's biomass. Bacteria rapidly reproduce by dividing in half and making copies of themselves, often in a matter of minutes. Bacteria of all kinds are an unseen but significant part of the natural environment.

In the human body, there are close to ten times the number of bacterial cells as compared to human cells, with most bacteria populating the skin and digestive tract. They are required to break down nutrients that the body cannot. In fact, your body would not survive without the beneficial bacteria living on and inside you.

As mentioned earlier, bacteria are different from viruses, fungi and parasites. Infections caused by viruses (such as the cold and flu) require very different treatment methods than bacteria.

Good and Bad Bacteria

It's very important to understand that not all bacteria are *bad*. In fact, your life depends upon bacteria. Many different species of *good* bacteria are a natural and necessary part of your body, performing critical functions that your body could never do on its own. For example, without the three to four pounds of bacteria living in your intestines, you would not be able to digest food or absorb important vitamins and nutrients.

One of the most important roles of good bacteria is to help protect you from bad bacteria. For example, the good bacteria that naturally live all over your skin keep bad bacteria from gaining a foothold and starting an infection. But even bad bacteria are not truly bad. Most bacteria serve valuable purposes in nature, such as breaking down wastes or serving as a food source for small organisms. Bacteria only become bad when they get out of balance with good bacteria or when they get somewhere they are not supposed to be, like on an implanted medical device or inside of a surgical wound.

L-form Stealth Bacteria

Bacteria have been around for a long time and are very clever when it comes to survival. Research performed by Dr. Lida Mattman has scientifically proven that some bacteria (including Staph) have learned how to change form and go into hiding inside the human body for long periods of time[2]. These mutated *L-form* bacteria are extremely small and very hard to detect using standard tests.

L-forms are also highly resistant to antibiotics and are virtually invisible to the body's immune system. L-forms may also form biofilms or hide inside the body's own red or white blood cells. Like wolves in sheep's clothing, L-form bacteria can lie in wait for an opportunity and can be a key cause of reinfections. Certain types of antibiotics can trigger the formation of these mutated L-forms. L-forms are further discussed in the chapter "Antibiotic Treatments, Resistance and Limitations" on page 67.

Biofilms and Chronic Infections

Another bacterial survival strategy is called a *biofilm*. Staph, MRSA and many other bacteria build biofilms as a way to protect themselves. Biofilms are clusters of bacteria that are hidden within a tough slime layer that sticks to bodily tissues or medical implants. Biofilms protect the bacteria inside from treatments and from your own immune system.

As with L-form bacteria, biofilms are another antibiotic resistance mechanism that should be considered for anyone struggling with chronic, recurring infections. To understand biofilms, refer to the chapter "Antibiotic Treatments, Resistance and Limitations" on page 67. Refer to "Biofilm and L-Form Support" on page 186 for details on how to handle biofilms.

The Root Cause of MRSA and Staph

Simply coming into contact with bacteria may not be the root cause of an infection. Likewise, simply killing the bacteria associated with an infection may not be the best tactic for achieving a lasting recovery.

People come into contact with all kinds of bacteria every day without any problems. Most of these bacterial encounters don't lead to an infection because your body is designed to protect you from such things. Most bad bacterial exposures are brought back into balance by your body's good bacteria and your immune system before an infection has a chance to develop.

If some bad bacteria do gain a foothold, your body's immune system normally squashes the emerging infection quickly before dangerous symptoms develop. However, if your immune system is compromised, or if you are exposed to too many bacteria all at once and your body can't adequately protect itself, an infection can develop. This often happens during hospital stays, where you can be exposed to many different bacteria when your immune system is most stressed.

Sometimes your body needs a little extra help to get rid of an infection and get back to normal health. Without such help, the infection can easily get out of control, leading to serious illness or even death. In mainstream medicine, this is when antibiotics are prescribed. These drugs work by either killing or slowing down the infection. Natural methods and remedies can also provide your body with extra help to get over an infection.

However, it's your body's own immune system that works on many levels to finish up and completely wipe the infection out. For your long-term success you need to address your immune system and incorporate supportive strategies into your plan to root out any remaining bacteria. In the following chapters, you'll learn about mainstream and alternative treatment options as well as methods to boost your body's natural defenses.

Complete Elimination of Staph and MRSA

Staph bacteria are a normal part of the community of microorganisms that make up a good and healthy skin *flora*. They naturally can live on your skin and don't normally cause any harm. There are at least thirty different types of Staph that live cooperatively on other organisms and are found in the soil. Because Staph bacteria live on people, you'll find them wherever people live and spend time. Nowadays, there is no way to avoid coming into contact with Staph or MRSA bacteria during the course of normal life. As described above, casual community exposure usually poses no problem unless the bacteria get where they shouldn't be, and/or your natural defenses are out of balance.

There are people who have eradicated MRSA from their body using mainstream or alternative methods, so it is possible to get rid of these bacteria. It's also possible to remain a *carrier* of these bacteria without ever becoming infected. You can get better if you have MRSA and be free from recurring infections, but total elimination of all bacteria, or all Staph or MRSA is not the best goal. A better goal is maintaining a proper balance of beneficial bacteria and supporting your body's resistance to infections by strengthening your immune system.

Infections Linked to Chronic Diseases

Bacterial infections are now being linked to many different chronic diseases. In 2006, the CDC released a paper stating, "Infectious agents have emerged as notable determinants, not just complications, of chronic diseases. Not infrequently, infection may simply represent the first misstep along a continuum from health to long-term illness and disability. To capitalize on these opportunities, clinicians, public health practitioners, and policymakers must recognize that many chronic diseases may indeed have infectious origins."[3]

In other words, infections are very likely linked to many modern-day chronic diseases. In 2005, 133 million Americans, or nearly half of all adults, had at least one chronic illness, such as cancer, arthritis and Inflammatory Bowel Disease[5]. Also, 70% of all American deaths are due to chronic disease[4]. What if bacterial infections were one of the causative agents of these diseases?

Dave Relman, Ph.D., assistant professor of medicine and microbiology and immunology at Stanford University in California argues, "The list of chronic inflammatory diseases with possible microbial etiologies is extensive; it includes sarcoidosis, various forms of inflammatory bowel disease, rheumatoid arthritis, systemic lupus erythematosus, Wegener granulomatosis, diabetes mellitus, primary biliary cirrhosis, tropical sprue, and Kawasaki disease… the concept of pathogenic mechanism should be viewed broadly."[6]

Perhaps this is the reason why the second leading cause of death in the U.S., behind lung cancer, is now cancer caused by bacteria, viruses and fungi.

As mentioned above, according to the CDC, infectious agents likely cause more cancers, immune-mediated syndromes, neurodevelopmental disorders, and other chronic conditions than currently thought. In fact, they argue that the potential to avoid or minimize chronic disease by preventing or treating infections is substantially underestimated by the medical community. Therefore, understanding how to prevent and control infections may help control and prevent potential chronic diseases as well.

3

Symptoms, Risk Factors and Carriers

Because MRSA and Staph share many of the same symptoms, it can be hard to tell the difference between the two. While being familiar with the symptoms is important, laboratory testing at your doctor's office is the only way to know for sure what you are infected with. The risk factors for catching MRSA and Staph are very similar, but with a few key differences.

This chapter will show you the most common signs and symptoms of both Staph and MRSA, plus key differences between healthcare-associated and community-acquired infections. You'll also learn important facts about carriers and how to avoid getting infected.

Staph and MRSA Carriers

Staph aureus bacteria are a normal part of many people's bodily flora. The bacteria prefer moist, warm areas including the nose, throat, armpits and groin. People who have the bacteria on their skin but don't have an infection or any symptoms are called *carriers*. Staph carriers account for about 20 to 30% of the population in the United States. A person can be a Staph carrier without ever becoming infected. However, a Staph carrier can spread the bacteria to someone else who may then become infected. People can be carriers without ever knowing it.

The above facts about Staph carriers also holds true for MRSA carriers, however only 1 to 5% of the population are MRSA carriers. Like Staph carriers, a MRSA carrier may never get an infection or show any symptoms, but they can pass the bacteria on to others who may then become infected.

Of note, being a MRSA carrier increases your chance of infection. Recent studies have shown that persistent MRSA carriers do have an increased risk of infection over those who are not carriers. Those who are at greater risk, such as the young, elderly and immune-compromised, are often put on decolonization procedures to try and eliminate MRSA from their skin and nose.

How People Catch Staph and MRSA

Staph and MRSA bacteria are spread by contact with other people or objects. People with active infections are more contagious, but carriers can also spread the bacteria to others. You can pick up these bacteria through direct skin-to-skin contact, by touching contaminated surfaces or objects, and to a lesser extent from coughing and other forms of airborne transmission.

Fortunately, exposure alone doesn't mean you'll get infected. The bacteria need to get inside you in order to cause an infection. The skin and mucous membranes are the body's first line of defense, however, abrasions and cuts allow an easy route for MRSA to enter the body.

While the majority of MRSA infections used to occur in hospitals, MRSA is now spreading rapidly through communities around the world. There are two main kinds of MRSA depending on how people get an infection: Healthcare-Associated MRSA (HA-MRSA) and Community-Associated MRSA (CA-MRSA). Both types of MRSA, their symptoms and how people catch them are discussed in more detail later in this chapter.

Not All Exposures Lead to Infections

Being near or touching someone who has an active Staph or MRSA infection doesn't mean you will get infected yourself. The bacteria must get into your body in sufficient numbers and gain a foothold against your immune system to cause an infection. The key factor that determines whether or not you get infected is your predisposition to infection and how many bacteria you're exposed to. Factors that put people at higher risk of infection are detailed in the Risk Factors sections below.

Because people are exposed to disease-causing bacteria more often than they realize, one of the best ways to reduce your risk of infection is to strengthen your body's natural defenses. The more healthy, balanced and well maintained your immune system, the lower your risk of infection. The chapter "Boosting Your Immune System" on page 223 will provide techniques and methods for restoring and maintaining a strong immune system.

Airborne MRSA

Until recently, it was believed that MRSA and Staph bacteria could only spread through direct contact with an infected person or by touching a contaminated object. But recent studies have confirmed that airborne transmission is responsible for a significant number of MRSA infections.

MRSA bacteria can get into the air in at least two ways. First, the bacteria often inhabit the upper respiratory system in people. Therefore, the simple act of coughing or sneezing can create a MRSA or Staph airborne aerosol. Second, the human body naturally sheds millions of tiny skin particles every day which become airborne as dust particles. These tiny airborne particles offer an easy ride for MRSA, Staph and other disease-causing microorganisms to spread through the air.

Breathing in these particles or getting them on your skin provides a convenient route for the bacteria to potentially colonize or live on your body. Fortunately, your body has many defenses against invading bacteria from the air. Yet airborne transmission can be significant for people with a weakened immune system or those in close quarters with others, such as a hospital.

A recent study showed that MRSA can spread to both medical staff and patients through airborne transmission in hospitals[7]. The study was conducted in a hospital ward and found MRSA recirculating in the air, among the patients and on inanimate objects in the area, especially when there was movement in the patient's rooms.

Airborne MRSA is an important consideration in hospitals because they can have considerable amounts of MRSA in them. Some hospitals are getting better at maintaining air filtration systems that can filter out MRSA, but this is not widely performed. There are ways to help protect yourself from airborne MRSA, as detailed in "Controlling Airborne Bacteria" on page 206.

Risk Factors and Activities

Many factors can increase your risk of developing a Staph or MRSA infection. It's important to know which activities increase your risk and how to be proactive in prevention. However, it's also important to understand that your immune system's strength plays a bigger role in infection control than your involvement in increased-risk activities. Below are common factors that can increase the risk of getting a Staph or MRSA infection.

- A history of Staph or MRSA infections.
- A history of skin infections or open, slow-healing wounds.
- Living in close proximity to a carrier or an infected person.
- Crowded living or working conditions, including military barracks, day care centers, schools, sports team facilities, dormitories, prisons and correctional facilities.
- Poor hygiene and inadequate hand washing, especially in crowded environments and public places.
- Recently visiting, being admitted to or working in a hospital or healthcare facility.
- IV drug users.
- Nursing home caregivers.
- Anyone with a compromised immune system due to any of the following reasons:
  » Illness or underlying medical condition
  » Stress (a major factor)
  » Recent antibiotic use
  » Poor nutrition or diet
  » Very young or old age

Childbirth Risks

A common concern for MRSA or Staph carriers who are pregnant is the risk of passing the bacteria onto their newborn during childbirth. Fortunately, this risk appears to be fairly low. However, in a 2012 study of 500 pregnant women, it was found that MRSA was not passed at birth but was likely to pass to the baby a few months later[8]. Fortunately, the babies in the study rarely became infected with the bacteria even though they became carriers. The researchers plan to do further studies to see if newborns carrying the bacteria may have greater protection against getting infected with MRSA later in life.

HA-MRSA

MRSA first appeared in U.S. hospitals in the 1970s, resulting in what's known as Healthcare-Associated MRSA (HA-MRSA). Conditions in hospitals make them the ideal breeding ground for antibiotic resistant superbugs. Hospital patients and staff have a much higher risk of infection than the general public. Hospital staff that do not follow proper sanitary procedures, which unfortunately is quite common, transfer bacteria from patient to patient throughout the day. The combination of many sick patients with weakened immune systems, close quarters, and medical workers moving from patient to patient makes hospitals the ideal environment for contagious infections to spread, including MRSA and Staph.

People entering hospitals for routine care or even simply visiting can catch HA-MRSA. According to a nationwide survey of 1200 U.S. hospitals and health-care facilities, up to 1.2 million people are infected with drug resistant Staph (which include HA-MRSA) at healthcare facilities each year[9].

HA-MRSA Risk Factors

The following HA-MRSA risk factors increase the chances of getting Staph or MRSA in hospitals, medical clinics, doctor's offices, nursing homes and other healthcare facilities:

- Recent hospitalization, especially if over 14 days in duration.

- Weakened immune system or chronic health condition treated in a hospital.

- Multiple hospital visits or being admitted to a hospital multiple times.

- A stay in an intensive care unit.

- Treatment for burns or any surgical wounds.

- Living in a long term care facility.

- The use of invasive medical devices such as catheters, IV's, dialysis machines, feeding tubes, stents, artificial hips and knees and other implanted devices.

- Recent antibiotic use. Antibiotics can increase the chances of acquiring MRSA.

- Anyone who works in a hospital, nursing home or other healthcare facility.

- Anyone who visits someone inside a hospital or healthcare facility or who has close contact with someone recently discharged from a hospital.

HA-MRSA Symptoms

HA-MRSA can manifest as skin infections, surgical site infections, and notably more serious internal infections like septicemia (blood infection), osteomyelitis (bone infection), catheter associated urinary tract infections (bladder infection) or pneumonia (lung infection). HA-MRSA is resistant to more types of antibiotics than other kinds of MRSA.

Preventing HA-MRSA

For step-by-step details on how you can minimize your chances of getting HA-MRSA when visiting or being admitted to a hospital or other healthcare environment, be sure to read "Staying in Hospitals: What You Need to Know" on page 51.

CA-MRSA

In the last two decades MRSA has become much more common outside of healthcare and hospital environments, resulting in what's known as Community-Associated MRSA (CA-MRSA). CA-MRSA occurs in otherwise healthy people who have not been recently hospitalized within the past year, or have not had a medical procedure, such as dialysis, catheterization, or surgery.

According to the Journal of the American Medical Association (JAMA), CA-MRSA has become the most frequent cause of skin and soft tissue infections presented to emergency rooms in the United States.

CA-MRSA often causes a more virulent infection than HA-MRSA, making it faster spreading, more invasive and more serious. What is concerning about CA-MRSA is that clinical syndromes not previously associated with CA-MRSA are becoming more common. One syndrome in particular is necrotizing fasciitis, a rapidly progressive and life-threatening condition that kills cells of the skin, soft tissue, and deep fascia and is often called a *flesh eating* infection.

Some strains of CA-MRSA carry the PVL gene which allows the bacteria to create a toxin that attacks macrophages (immune system cells in your body). PVL MRSA causes enhanced tissue necrosis and PVL's presence in CA-MRSA has been associated with lethal necrotizing pneumonia, cellulitis, abscesses, and furuncles. Fortunately, not all strains of CA-MRSA are strongly virulent. However, it's a good idea to be extra diligent and proactive if you suspect CA-MRSA.

CA-MRSA Risk Factors

Some of the more common risk factors and high-risk groups for catching a CA-MRSA infection are listed below.

- Children and neonatal babies. Because CA-MRSA can enter the body through a cut or scrape and can quickly cause a widespread infection, it is more problematic in young children. Young children may be more susceptible to CA-MRSA because their immune systems aren't fully developed. They are also more likely to acquire dangerous forms of pneumonia. Neonates are also more susceptible as their skin (their first line of defense against invading bacteria) is not quite fully developed. It can take 2-4 weeks to fully develop, and up to 8 weeks in extremely premature neonates.

- Players of contact sports. Many sports teams, school teams and even the NFL, have been affected by CA-MRSA. Because of frequent skin-to-skin contact, shared locker rooms, shared spas and common gym equipment, CA-MRSA can spread from person to person easily.

- Users of needles for injecting medications or drugs. Insulin dependent diabetics, IV drug users and any other group that injects themselves regularly is at a higher risk of infection.

- Health club, gym and athletic club members. CA-MRSA can be spread among people who share gym equipment, floor mats, hot tubs, towels, uniforms or any sports or exercise equipment.

- Anyone with a weakened immune system. People taking immune-suppressive drugs or who have HIV/AIDS are more likely to get CA-MRSA or have more severe symptoms.

- Living in crowded or unsanitary conditions. Anyone living in close quarters, such as military training camps, prisons, dormitories and long-term care facilities, has an increased risk of infection.

- Having a family member with a MRSA infection or who is a MRSA carrier. Bacteria and/or infections can spread through direct casual contact, sharing of personal items like towels or razors, and through a couple's sexual contact.

- Being in crowded public places, such as grocery stores, subway stations and amusement parks.

- Touching objects frequently handled by other people. Objects like shopping cart handles, door knobs, food sampling spoons, waiting room magazines, elevator buttons, remote controls, toys and most other commonly touched surfaces can harbor CA-MRSA and many other pathogens.

- Getting a tattoo or any other procedure that penetrates the skin.

CA-MRSA Symptoms

CA-MRSA has important distinctions that set it apart from HA-MRSA. CA-MRSA is usually confined to the skin and soft tissues. In 75% of cases, CA-MRSA causes skin infections, such as boils or abscesses. Deeper infections, such as cellulites or pneumonia, are less common. CA-MRSA is often confused and mis-diagnosed as a spider bite. CA-MRSA is more susceptible to a wider range of antibiotics than HA-MRSA. However, CA-MRSA is more virulent than HA-MRSA and can progress into serious infections quickly.

Note: MRSA and Staph infections are often misdiagnosed by doctors as spider bites, especially brown recluse spider bites. If you have infection symptoms but can't remember being bitten by a spider, you may have a Staph or MRSA infection.

Signs and Symptoms

Because of the recent increase in CA-MRSA in communities, strains of CA-MRSA are now showing up in hospitals and HA-MRSA can be found in the community. Therefore, the distinction between these two types of MRSA can get blurred. Both community and hospital MRSA and Staph can share similar symptoms. These symptoms can also be caused by other types of infections or even other unrelated medical conditions. The following sections show what different kinds of Staph and MRSA can look like and what symptoms they can manifest.

Note: Not all infections are caused by Staph or MRSA. The symptoms below may be caused by another type of infection or a health condition unrelated to an infection. If you have any concerns about any symptoms you have, be sure to contact a healthcare professional.

Where Infections Appear on the Body

MRSA and Staph infections can show up anywhere on or inside the body. However, there are areas where these bacteria have an easier time surviving, or where these infections most often appear. The list below shows the most common parts of the body where Staph and MRSA cause infections.

- Areas where clothing can cause friction or skin irritation offering an opening to infection, such as the legs, buttocks and shaving areas.

- Sweaty, moist or warm areas such as the armpits, neck, face, nose, buttocks, groin and feet.

- Deep infections like cellulitis are most common on the arms, hands, lower legs and face.

An Overview of MRSA and Staph Symptoms

Skin Infections

- Skin infections are the most common type of Staph and MRSA and are typically CA-MRSA.

- Lumps, pimple-like bumps, blisters or boils are common. Skin infections are often accompanied by swelling and reddening of the surrounding skin area. The center of the lump often has a white or yellow pus filled head, which sometimes drains on its own.

- Lumps are often tender, itchy and warm to the touch and can become deep sores with increasing pain and swelling if left unchecked.

Deep Tissue Infections

- Deeper skin infections such as cellulites are serious and can cause significant swelling and tenderness and often are deep red in color and can be large. Sometimes red streaks on the skin may radiate out from the center of the cellulitis. Bumps and blisters may or may not be present.

- Deeper skin infections, such as pus-filled abscesses, often require surgical incision and draining by a medical professional. Never try to squeeze or lance abscesses or boils yourself. Doing so can push the bacteria deeper inside your body and cause a much more serious or potentially life threatening infection. Recent research has indicated that biofilms can hide inside of boils and abscesses.

Bladder Infections

Staph or MRSA can cause a bladder or urinary tract infection (UTI) if the bacteria travel up into the urethra and then into the bladder where urine is stored. Staph and MRSA may also form a biofilm inside the bladder. Risk factors for UTIs include recent hospitalization, catheter use, being elderly, living in a nursing home or other long-term care facility and repeated antibiotic use.

The main symptoms of a UTI can include the following, however, elderly people can get UTIs and may not exhibit some of most of these symptoms:

- Painful burning sensation when urinating.

- Frequent urination and a desire to keep going, even after you've emptied your bladder.

- Lower abdomen pain, discomfort or pressure.

- Lower back or pelvic pain.

- Urinary incontinence.

- Bloody or cloudy urine.

- Fever, chills and nausea are often signs of severe or complicated infections.

Sinus infections

Community acquired MRSA can cause sinus infections which are challenging to address because the sinuses are encompassed in bone making this a deeper type of infection. It may take lengthy treatment times to reach all the bacteria present in the sinuses. These infections commonly are biofilm infections, which can further complicate treatment. Neti pot sinus rinses can be a very helpful way to control these infections.

Surgical Site Infections (SSI)

Surgical incision sites can become infected, usually by HA-MRSA or a number of other pathogens. Staph and MRSA surgical site infections usually involve red or swollen areas around the surgical incision site and the site can be slow to heal.

Symptoms of More Serious Infections

Most MRSA and Staph infections are limited to the skin. However, infections can also enter the bloodstream and spread to internal organs. Infected surgical sites may also lead to serious infections. The following symptoms may indicate an internal infection.

- Fever
- Chills
- Weakness or fatigue
- Nausea
- Shortness of breath
- Rashes
- Headache
- Muscle aches
- Joint pain
- Acute pain

Internal Medical Conditions Caused by Staph and MRSA

Internal infections are serious and require immediate medical care. Internal infections can cause extreme pain in the muscles and joints as well as other more severe symptoms. Staph and MRSA internal infections can lead to the follow medical conditions:

- **Septicemia.** An infection of the blood, septicemia can lead to shock, circulatory collapse and death. People with large areas of severe burns are particularly susceptible.

- **Endocarditis** is an infection of the heart valves that can lead to heart failure.

- **Meningitis** is an infection in the brain or spinal column.

- **Pneumonia** is a lung infection often involving abscess formation in the lungs. An underlying lung disease is the usual precursor.

- **Osteomyelitis** is an infection of the bone. Bone infections can also cause inflammation in the tissues nearby.

Skin-Related Medical Conditions Caused by Staph and MRSA

Skin infections can present themselves in several different ways. All of the conditions listed below can be caused by MRSA and Staph infections. However, these conditions may be caused by other types of infections, or by a medical condition unrelated to an infection. Getting tested by your doctor is the only way to know for sure if you have Staph, MRSA or another type of infection.

- **Boils.** Boils are bumps with a pus filled head that are usually small and superficial near the surface of the skin. If boils enlarge and grow together, they can form a multi-headed lump called a **carbuncle**. Do not try to squeeze, lance or drain these on your own as you can push the infection deeper inside your body. Boils are often treated by lancing and draining by a doctor and may include a course of antibiotics.

- **Folliculitis.** Similar to boils, folliculitis is an infection of a hair follicle, forming bumps usually less than a quarter inch in diameter, often surrounded by an area of inflamed red or pink skin. Folliculitis usually forms white heads and they can occur anywhere on the skin. The areas affected are often itchy and sometimes painful.

- **Impetigo.** Impetigo looks like crusty oozing bumps, blisters or lesions, usually yellow to red in color, that break open easily. These crusty scabs are made of dried blood serum and are most common on the face, legs and arms. Impetigo can spread easily to other parts of the body. Impetigo is more common in children than adults.

- **Abscess.** Abscesses are pus filled cavities that form deep under the skin that rarely have a head or drain on their own. You can sometimes feel the fluid inside of an abscess if you press on it with your fingers. It is important that you do not try to lance or drain these on your own as you can push the infection deeper into your body. A boil is a small, shallow abscess.

- **Cellulitis.** Cellulitis is a deeper and more serious infection with significant swelling and tenderness. It has a deep red color and often increases in size as the infection grows. Doctors often draw a line on the skin around a cellulitis infection to determine if it's growing or shrinking over time. Sometimes red streaks may radiate out from the center. Bumps and blisters may or may not be present. Cellulitis is most common on the lower legs, but can also be on the arms, hands and face. The elderly and people with compromised immune systems are at a higher risk for this condition.

- **Furunculosis.** Furunculosis occurs when hair follicles become infected deeper in the tissues, with swelling and red skin (also called boils). If the abscesses are larger than boils, or if there are multiple boils, the condition is usually called a carbuncle.

Photos of MRSA Progression

The following series of photographs shows how a MRSA surgical site infection (SSI) slowly progressed over a 14 month period. All five photos are from the same female patient after plastic surgery for a tummy tuck. The scarring around the belly button is the result of the man-made navel. The patient's wounds did not heal for 2 years.

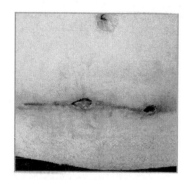

Image # 1. Initial image taken 2 years after surgery.

After 14 months of mainstream medical care, no conventional treatments worked to heal the open wound. The patient did not respond to any antibiotics or medications. After extensive testing, doctors could not come up with an underlying cause for this infection.

◇◇

Note: The photos shown here depict what one person's MRSA infection looked like. For a more complete picture of what MRSA and Staph can look like, please view Michelle Moore's MRSA Staph photo web page at: www.staph-infection-resources.com/info/mrsa-pictures/

◇◇

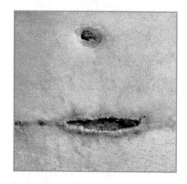

Image # 2. One month after the initial image.

Image # 1 is of a wound infected with MRSA. This infection occurred as a complication 2 years after cosmetic plastic surgery was performed for a breast reduction. The patient's wounds did not heal and eventually got infected with MRSA.

Image # 2 shows the scars around the man-made navel, visible at the top. Between the wounds a hollow tunnel of infection is visible under the skin, to be opened at a later date. This patient was being treated at the Mayo Clinic in Minnesota. At the time of this photo, no treatments had been successful in closing the open wounds. This photo was taken one month after Image # 1 and the doctors could not identify the infection's cause.

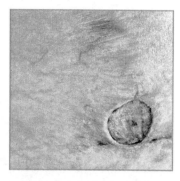

Image # 3. Two months after the initial image.

Image # 3 was taken two months after the original image. The belly button is at the top. The wound opened up below the belly button.

Image # 4 was taken nearly a year after the preceding image. The infection was still active and the wounds were not healed. As in the prior images, the infection is visible toward the bottom and a man-made navel is visible toward the top of the photo. The infection still had not responded to medications.

Image # 5 was taken fourteen months after the initial image. This is a closeup view of the infection site and the man-made navel visible in the previous 4 images is not visible as it is outside the top frame of the image. No treatment had yet been found to heal the wound completely.

As the images show, MRSA can be a very long struggle for some infection sufferers. Mainstream medicine is often unsuccessful at treating MRSA and at a loss for what causes recurring infections. The following chapter on mainstream medicine will help you get the most benefit from mainstream medicine while avoiding its most common pitfalls and drawbacks.

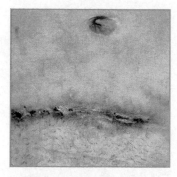

Image # 4. One year later.

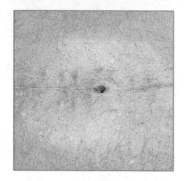

Image # 5. Fourteen months after the initial image.

How to Know if You are Infected

Symptoms alone are not enough to tell if you have Staph or MRSA. Only a medical test can confirm if you have a MRSA or Staph infection. Therefore, risk factors, symptoms and photos can be a helpful guide, but they are not a substitute for getting tested by your doctor. For details about testing, see the section "Testing for MRSA and Staph" on page 45.

If you think you are infected, consider seeing your doctor as soon as possible. Be aware that MRSA and Staph are commonly misdiagnosed as bug or spider bites. Avoid puncturing or squeezing any pus filled heads yourself. Incising and draining should only be performed by a healthcare professional to prevent the infection from spreading or getting worse.

4   Doctors and Mainstream Medicine

Mainstream medicine, also called conventional, allopathic, western, or orthodox medicine, is a very recent development in human history. For thousands of years, highly successful traditional medical techniques have been practiced and refined. To this day, in many modern first-world countries such as France and Japan, traditional or holistic medicine (what is now called *alternative* in the U.S.) is practiced side-by-side with mainstream medicine.

Mainstream medicine is the core practice of the healthcare system of the United States and much of the western world, including most hospitals, doctors and other healthcare providers. Mainstream medicine has many advantages and has saved many people's lives. Mainstream medicine also has significant disadvantages and it works better for some things than for others.

In mainstream medicine, a disease condition is usually viewed as an isolated event, confined to the area in which it manifests itself (an inflamed colon, skin infection, lung cancer, etc.). A solution is usually sought through mechanical (surgical) and chemical (pharmaceutical) means. Seeking to understand *why* the infection or disease appeared in the first place is usually not explored. The focus of mainstream medicine is usually on the symptoms of a disease rather than the root cause.

Mainstream and alternative medicines are complementary and both play an important role in attaining and maintaining optimal health. Alternative medicine will be covered in detail in the chapter "What is Alternative Medicine?" on page 83.

The FDA, Drugs and Doctors

The Food and Drug Administration (FDA) was originally formed to protect the public from unsafe drugs and unhealthy food processing that was widespread in the early part of the 20th century. The FDA was given broad powers to oversee all aspects of the drug industry, serving as the gatekeeper for approval of all drugs marketed and sold in the United States.

Only FDA approved drugs can claim to diagnose, cure, prevent or treat a disease. The FDA requires that pharmaceutical companies perform multiple animal and human clinical studies to prove the safety, set the proper dosage, and prove the effectiveness of a new drug. These studies are also used to support any claims that are made about a drug for marketing. Clinical studies are extremely expensive, often lasting for years and requiring extensive resources to design, conduct, monitor, and to generate a study report. On top of this, the FDA also requires extensive and labor intensive systems to be developed and maintained by drug manufacturers to control, monitor and thoroughly document every aspect of drug development, characterization, testing, shelf life determination, manufacture, distribution, and post-market safety monitoring.

Pharmaceutical companies only choose to develop novel man-made drugs that can be patented and thus generate large profits

The FDA's requirements make it extremely expensive, challenging and time consuming to develop new drugs and get them to market. As a result, pharmaceutical companies only pursue new patentable drugs which allow the company to enjoy a legal monopoly on the drug for a number of years. This monopoly enables the pharmaceutical company that develops a new drug to set its own price with no competition for a period of time. The monopoly allows the company to make enough money to pay for the drug's long and expensive development. Once the drug's patent expires, low-priced generic forms of the drug typically flood the market, sometimes overnight, quickly and significantly reducing the innovator company's profits.

Since natural remedies and traditional therapies are natural and cannot be patented, there's no monetary incentive for pharmaceutical companies to go through the long and expensive FDA approval process to develop such products.

Therefore, natural remedies, no matter how effective, are disfavored, discounted and marginalized by drug companies and the medical system they are part of. Beyond that, pharmaceutical companies have a vested interest in minimizing the use of natural remedies because such remedies are in direct competition with their patented money-making drugs.

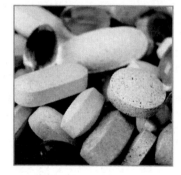

While some drugs are necessary and save lives, mainstream medicine relies too heavily on them.

To insure continued financial growth, drug companies strive to get as many health conditions as possible to be labeled as a *disease*. You've probably seen the commercials on TV for all kinds of new drugs to treat medical conditions that were unheard of a few years ago. Remember that the FDA requires that only approved drug products can claim to diagnose, mitigate, cure, prevent or treat a disease. By labeling a medical condition as a disease, a drug company can develop a new patented drug to treat it, ensuring a continued pipeline of new drugs and money to sustain the company's future.

As an example, even obesity is now categorized as a disease. In truth, obesity is not a disease at all. You don't catch obesity, nor is it usually the result of something broken in the body that must then be fixed by a special drug. Obesity is developed, pound by pound, as a result of super-sized and poor nutrition, neglected emotional health, toxic build-up or unwired metabolic processes and inflammation resulting from lack of nutrients and toxins used in processed foods. The real *cures* for obesity are a diet of unprocessed foods that are rich in micro-nutrients, high quality nutritional supplements, emotional or spiritual therapy and other non-pharmaceutical approaches. At best, mainstream medicine can artificially decrease the appetite and staple the stomach to address the symptoms of obesity, but these measures do not address the root cause. In the end, the very things that would help people the most are marginalized and discounted by the same medical system that people rely on to help them.

Alternative Remedies Kept From the Public

An unfortunate consequence of the FDA and the mainstream medical system is that legitimate, safe and effective natural therapies that actually help people are constantly at risk of being labeled as an *unapproved drug product* by the FDA. Even raw foods such as cherries have been targeted by the FDA as unapproved drugs for simply claiming that cherries have health benefits. Such FDA bullying can result in the recall and seizure of products, often resulting in financial disaster for the maker of the product. Because of how the system works, highly effective alternative therapies are kept from reaching a significant level of public awareness.

While there are drugs that are necessary and that save lives, mainstream medicine often relies too heavily on them. Drugs like antibiotics have certainly saved many lives and are often required for serious infections. However, for most people, alternative therapies and methods that are often much safer with less side-effects are never made available and are often put down by their doctors. Your doctor can only offer you what she knows from her mainstream medical schooling and years of heavy marketing and influence from the drug companies. Most medical doctors only know about mainstream therapies and have very little if any knowledge about alternatives.

> Mainstream medicine is the only option
> that you will likely get from your doctor

Because there are so many forces keeping alternative therapies from reaching you, it's crucial that you be proactive, learn what your options are, and take charge of your own health. Use your doctor as an important resource, but understand that your doctor can't be familiar with every option that exists. If you want to include alternative therapies, you can ask for a second opinion or find an integrative, functional medicine or Naturopathic doctor. Your options for handling infections include both mainstream and alternative medical approaches. You can start taking charge of your health by learning how to use your doctor and the mainstream medical system as important resources without over-relying on them.

NOTE: It is not suggested that you should ignore your doctor or that your doctor is *bad*. It is up to you to take charge of your health and find out about all options available to you. Use your doctor(s) as an important resource, but in the end, you get to make your own informed treatment decisions.

How to Get Better Medical Care

With an understanding of its pros, cons and limitations, the mainstream medical system can be used to your best advantage. If you choose to, you can successfully combine mainstream and alternative approaches together to address your specific needs. In the end, you'll gain the most benefit from using both approaches together.

Do You Have the Right Doctor?

Your doctor is one of the most valuable and important resources you have in treating your infection. However, each doctor has her own unique strengths, weaknesses, biases, and level of experience treating MRSA and Staph infections. There are also some doctors who are simply better than others. Regardless of whether you are using a medical doctor or a Naturopathic doctor, you must understand the limitations of your doctor to get the best possible treatments and experience the fastest recovery.

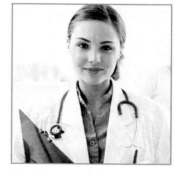

Many doctors have little or no experience with MRSA and Staph diagnosis or treatment.

It is very important to interview any new or prospective doctor to make sure she is the best match to help you with your infection. Choosing a doctor is a personal decision, and nobody can make that decision like you can. Some of the important considerations to take into account when choosing a doctor include her experience and success in treating infections, her treatment styles and approach to medicine and how open she is to alternative methods if you choose to use such methods while under her supervision.

Your Doctor's Hands May Be Tied

There are several limitations imposed on doctors that often prevent you from receiving the best medical care. Doctors are increasingly being forced into a bureaucratic mode of practicing medicine. This is particularly true of mainstream medical doctors. Doctors are under constant pressure from insurance companies to cut costs and get patients in and out of their offices quickly. That means that you get less personalized treatment attention in favor of faster, one-size-fits-all *standard protocol* treatments.

The FDA, American Medical Association (AMA) and drug companies put pressure on doctors to favor mainstream allopathic medicine and prevent the use of alternative medicine. The AMA 's oversight and the risk of medical malpractice lawsuits puts heavy pressure on doctors to use standard protocol treatments in their practice. Even if your doctor knows of more effective tests and treatment options, she will often not offer them because they are not part of the *standard protocol*.

How to Find a Good Doctor

An important part of taking charge of your health is finding a doctor who values the patient's healthcare choices and encourages patient participation in healthcare. It's also important that your doctor is a good personal fit for you and your healthcare needs. Be sure to interview your doctor and consider asking her the important questions below:

- Does your doctor have knowledge and experience treating patients with MRSA and Staph infections? Ask about your doctor's success rate and how many MRSA patients she has successfully treated.

- Will your doctor support your choice to use natural, holistic or alternative medicine, in whole or in combination with mainstream medicine? Is your doctor willing to monitor your progress while you use alternatives?

- Is your doctor open to communicating the pros, cons and level of need for any prescribed treatments, tests or medical screening? This includes covering potential drug side-effects. Will she prescribe the least number of drugs possible?

- Will your doctor include the patient as part of the decision process and be respectful of the patient's desires and wishes?

- Is your doctor willing to describe the patient's health challenges and treatment options clearly, thoroughly, and patiently and also to answer patient questions?

- Is your doctor (or hospital) proactive in reducing the risk of healthcare associated infections, including the use of any kind of antibiotic stewardship program?

- Is your doctor familiar with herbal remedies, probiotics and other key alternative therapies described in this book? Preferably she already uses alternative medicine and provides alternatives to her patients.

Infectious Disease (ID) Doctors

Family doctors and primary or general care physicians often have limited experience and knowledge of Staph and MRSA. Misdiagnoses and ineffective treatments are unfortunately very common. Such blunders waste your time and money and expose you to treatments that don't even help you.

What's worse, a mis-diagnosis will delay you from getting proper treatment, often leading to more severe symptoms.

An Infectious Disease (ID) doctor is a medical doctor who specializes in infections like MRSA. They have more knowledge and experience treating infections than general physicians. ID doctors are not immune to making mistakes, but they are more likely to identify your infection correctly and get you on the appropriate treatment path more quickly. Most ID doctors follow mainstream treatment methodology.

- You can find an ID doctor near you by searching online or by asking your regular doctor or a healthcare facility for suggestions. Wellness.com has a large number of ID doctor listings on their website: www.wellness.com/find/doctor

- To help evaluate a new doctor, you can read reviews of over 720,000 doctors at the following website: www.vitals.com

- Depending on your insurance, you can get a referral to an ID doctor from you're primary physician, or you can locate one yourself. The following AMA website allows you to search by physician specialty in a given state. This free website will list doctors who are AMA members only: https://apps.ama-assn.org/doctorfinder/html/patient.jsp

- Use the following website to view a disciplinary history report for any doctor you are considering seeing. There is a $9.95 fee for each doctor's report: www.docinfo.org

Partnerships Between MDs and Naturopathic Doctors (NDs)

A Naturopathic Doctor (ND) is trained in natural and holistic medicine at accredited medical colleges. An ND can write prescriptions and perform the same functions as most medical doctors, however, they focus on the body as a whole, addressing the root cause of illness and they use alternative therapies. An ID/ND partnership can provide you with fully integrative healthcare, giving you the best combination of mainstream and alternative options. Ask your ID doctor if she is open to integrative medicine or willing to partner with a ND to support you.

Like any other type of doctor, be aware that not all NDs are the same. Be sure to read the chapter titled "Naturopathic Medicine: Safe & Effective Healthcare" on page 61 for more information on how to find an ND, and how they can help you with your infection treatment.

Ask your doctor to be open to communication and adopting a team approach with other medical doctors and any specialists, including a naturopathic doctor. Cooperation between a general physician, medical specialists and a naturopathic or alternative healthcare provider is uncommon unless you are proactive about creating such a partnership. It's up to you to ask for your doctor's cooperation in teaming up with your other doctors to provide you with the best care.

MDs Certified in Functional Medicine

Functional Medicine is a personalized approach to healthcare that focuses on prevention and treating underlying causes in addition to treating symptoms. Any medical doctor can choose to become a practitioner of functional medicine by getting certified with The Institute for Functional Medicine (IFM). Functional Medicine practitioners have a greater understanding of overall health, wellness and the underlying cause of infection and disease. The website below can help you to locate a medical doctor in your area who is a certified Functional Medicine practitioner: www.functional-medicine.org/practitioner_search.aspx

Testing for MRSA and Staph

Staph and MRSA can have identical symptoms, but they require very different antibiotic treatments. The symptoms of Staph and MRSA can also look like other kinds of medical conditions, or even spider bites. Therefore, the best way to get the right antibiotics is to get tested first.

The only way to know what's causing your infection is to get tested. Taking the wrong antibiotics can delay your recovery, waste your money and expose you to negative side effects with no benefits. Taking the wrong antibiotic can also increase bacterial resistance.

The standard protocol used by many doctors is to prescribe a broad-spectrum or general-purpose antibiotic for anything that looks like an infection. Doctors often use a trial and error approach with antibiotics, hoping to eventually find one that works. The trouble is, MRSA is immune to these broad-spectrum antibiotics.

That's why MRSA testing is so important. Getting a MRSA test will help your doctor to prescribe antibiotics that have a better chance of working. Because MRSA testing is not always the standard protocol, you may have to ask your doctor to be tested. Some hospitals actually perform testing to screen all newly admitted patients for MRSA. This kind of screening helps hospitals to manage and reduce the prevalence of infections.

Testing for MRSA and Staph is simple and inexpensive and can easily be done by your doctor in just a few minutes. However, it may take several days for the test results to come back from the lab, depending on the type of test and the laboratory. There are two main categories of testing that are important, as detailed in the sections below.

Culture Tests

The simplest test for Staph is called a *bacterial culture test*, sometimes called a *culture test* or simply a *culture* for short. Getting a culture test if easy and can be arranged through your doctor. The test is usually carried out in the following steps:

- **Taking the sample.** Nose or throat swabs are most common. For skin infections, your doctor may take a swab sample directly from the infected area. Pus or fluid may also be collected from weeping wounds, abscesses or other types of skin infections. Sputum may be collected for lung infections. For bladder or urinary infections, urine can be collected.

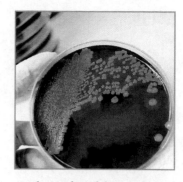

A culture of Staph bacteria growing on an agar plate.

- **Lab testing.** The swab (or other sample) is sent to a laboratory for testing. The sample is transferred to a round *agar plate* containing bacteria growth medium and food. The plate is stored under controlled environmental conditions that make the bacteria grow quickly (incubation). Once enough bacteria have been cultured on the plate (usually 1 - 3 days), the bacteria are viewed under a microscope and tests are performed to confirm the exact species of the bacteria.

- **Getting results.** The test results are sent back to your doctor, identifying what type of bacteria is causing your infection.

Most culture tests require two to five days to get results back from the lab. However, some newer tests can be done much faster. Two examples of fast tests are the *BD GeneOhm StaphSR Assay* and the *IDI-MRSA* test. These two tests only take 1 to 2 hours to perform, require no laboratory and can tell the difference between MRSA and less dangerous Staph bacteria. Since these are new tests based on new technology, many doctors do not use them yet. Ask your doctor if she can provide these tests for you as an alternative to standard culture testing.

Susceptibility Testing

There are many different strains or variations of MRSA and Staph bacteria, all within the same bacterial species. An antibiotic that kills one strain of MRSA can be less effective on another strain. Study results show that one third of MRSA patients initially receive the wrong treatment, nearly doubling their risk of death[10]. *Antibiotic susceptibility testing*, also called *sensitivity testing*, identifies which antibiotic will work best for a person's specific infection.

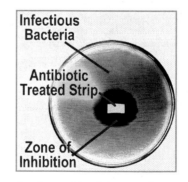

A culture of Staph bacteria being tested against an antibiotic.

Susceptibility testing is especially helpful if your antibiotics have stopped working or you have a history of recurring infections. Ideally your doctor will perform both a culture and susceptibility test from the beginning. Susceptibility testing starts the same way as a culture test, but the methods used at the laboratory and the type of results they provide are quite different. Below are the main components of susceptibility testing:

- **Taking the sample.** This is the same as the culture test above.

- **Lab testing.** The bacteria causing your infection are grown on multiple agar plates, like the one shown in the image at right. Tiny paper disks, each laced with a different antibiotic drug, are placed on each plate. If an antibiotic kills the bacteria, a zone of no growth will form around the paper disk. The larger this *zone of inhibition*, the more effective the antibiotic is at killing the bacteria causing your infection.

- **Getting results.** The results are sent to your doctor, identifying the most promising antibiotic to treat your particular infection.

For additional details on how to work with your doctor and a ready-made list of questions to ask about your infection, treatment and testing, be sure to read the companion guide *10 Questions to Ask Your Doctor about MRSA* by Michelle Moore.

Make the Most of Your Health Insurance

When you factor in the rising cost of prescription drugs, the growing expense of inpatient and outpatient care, loss of time from work, and incomplete health insurance coverage, the cost of handling a prolonged infection can be overwhelming. And the cost of fighting these infections is growing every year. In fact, half of all U.S. bankruptcies are caused by medical bills. Surprisingly, most people in debt due to illness are middle-class workers that do have health insurance.

There are several steps you can take to lower your healthcare costs and get the maximum reimbursement from your insurance company:

- **Use alternatives.** Alternative medicine is much more economical in the long run than mainstream medicine. This is especially true if you do not have medical insurance. Many alternative treatment methods cost very little compared to using expensive pharmaceutical drugs. Because alternative medicine addresses the underlying root cause of your infection, the high cost of dealing with recurring infections is reduced.

- **Know your insurance coverage.** Find out what your insurance will cover and what it won't before going to the doctor or hospital. Contact your insurance provider and check your policy to ensure that it covers your doctor visits, referrals and any medications you may need. Also check on coverage for naturopathic doctors as many will take insurance.

- **Fill out insurance claims properly.** Get assistance in filling out any insurance claims so you know the proper coding to use for your treatments to get maximum reimbursement of your costs. This is especially true if you use alternative medicine. Many alternative methods are covered by insurance companies if you code the expenses properly on the insurance claim forms.

- **Choose a good healthcare plan.** If possible, consider finding an insurance company that will cover more of your medical expenses. With the recent Affordable Care Act, the Silver and Gold plans may offer lower out-of-pocket expenses and may cover more of your infection related bills.

- **Alternative healthcare plans.** Historically, several insurance companies have had the best record for coverage of alternative therapies. Oxford Health Plans is a major healthcare plan that provides comprehensive coverage for many alternative services, including Naturopathic medicine, acupuncture, chiropractic, and other specialties, such as nutrition, yoga, and massage therapy. Plans that offer limited coverage to some subscribers include American Western Life Insurance Company, Blue Cross/Blue Shield, Kaiser Permanente, Mutual of Omaha, and Prudential. Many of these plans cover chiropractic care while others include herbal remedies, acupuncture, and/or other forms of alternative medicine.

Taking Control of Your Healthcare

Your biggest asset in treating a Staph or MRSA infection is knowledge. Reading this book is a great first step, combined with what you can learn from your doctor, other infection sufferers and your own research.

The second step is to take responsibility for your own health, be proactive, take control and implement what you learn. This second step requires self-confidence and the realization that you know yourself better than anybody else. Your doctor and your research can provide you with valuable advice and direction, but in the end, you get to decide what is best for you.

Getting Better Medical Support

Mainstream and alternative medicine have two different views about healing. If you mention *alternative remedies* to your doctor, or ask about boosting your immune system, your doctor will probably look at you like you're crazy. And, you may hear your doctor say something like "just take this prescription and you'll be fine", or "all that alternative stuff probably won't hurt, but it probably won't help either".

Alternative methods are not taught in mainstream medical schools (at least not in the U.S.), so most medical doctors are not familiar with them. Alternative medicine is also swept under the rug by the very system that your doctor is a part of. If your doctor does not know about or understand alternative medicine, she will not offer you any alternative options for Staph and MRSA.

If your doctor won't support you, there are several actions you can take to get the medical support you need. You can ask your doctor for her support using alternative methods. Fortunately more medical doctors are learning about and supporting the use of alternatives. You can also find a doctor familiar with alternative medicine, such as a Functional Medicine doctor or a naturopathic doctor. Working with both an MD and ND can give you the best of both worlds. Above all, it's important to take responsibility for your health, know how the medical system works and how to side-step it's pitfalls. It's also important that you work as a partner with your doctor, and be proactive to ensure that you get the personalized healthcare you deserve.

Work as a Partner With Your Doctor

Work with your doctor as a partner in managing your infection. Don't be afraid to question your doctor's suggestions or get a second opinion. Your doctor works for you. Regardless of what treatment approach you use, be open with your doctor and ask for her support and guidance.

One of the most important things to discuss with your doctor are the pros and cons of antibiotics before taking them. For most mainstream medical doctors, antibiotics are the default treatment for Staph and MRSA. Although the right antibiotic can quickly halt the growth of infection, these powerful drugs have many undesirable side effects. Antibiotics can make you prone to other dangerous infections and they can make you more vulnerable to reinfection. There is more information about antibiotics in the chapter "Antibiotic Treatments, Resistance and Limitations" on page 67.

For infections that are not eminently serious or life threatening, consult with your doctor about alternative options before resorting to antibiotics. Alternative methods can work as well or even better than antibiotics and many also enhance your immune system. A supportive doctor should monitor your condition while you use alternative methods. Your doctor should also be willing to team up with an alternative doctor if you choose to enlist one. In many cases, such a collaborative approach can allow you to successfully treat your infection without using antibiotics.

5 Staying in Hospitals: What You Need to Know

People go to hospitals to get well. People expect modern-day hospitals to be safe places to heal and recover from diseases. While hospital care is certainly life-saving for many people, staying in a hospital also has significant health risks. Unfortunately, many people leave a hospital with more medical problems than they had beforehand, including Healthcare-Associated Infections (HAIs) like MRSA, Staph, *C. difficle* and others.

For much of human history, hospitals were places to avoid. Unfortunately, many of the same problems that plagued hospitals for centuries are still present. Hospitals are the number one breeding ground for dangerous infections, including antibiotic-resistant superbugs. Hospital staff can make mistakes that can threaten your health and even your life. And if you choose to use integrative or natural medicine or deviate from *standard protocol* treatments, getting a hospital to support you can be an uphill battle.

If you or a family member are currently in a hospital or if you have an upcoming medical procedure, this chapter will show how to reduce your chances of medical mistakes and infections during your hospital visit. You'll also learn tips for successfully using supplements and alternative remedies in hospitals if you choose to. Hospital care provides many benefits, but it's important to take charge of your hospital stay and your healthcare to make your visit as safe and as short as possible.

The Dangers of Healthcare-Associated Staph and MRSA

People enter hospitals for a variety of different reasons. Bacteria are everywhere, and each type of medical intervention, whether it be open-heart surgery, hip replacement, child birth, or traumatic wound or burn care, carries specific risks of infection and methods for avoiding infection.

A 2007 APIC study (Association for Professionals in Infection and Epidemiology) showed that drug resistant Staph infections (which include Healthcare-Associated MRSA) affect an estimated 1.2 million healthcare patients each year. And HA-MRSA accounts for as many as 50-70% of these *Staph aureus* infections. Of these, serious or invasive HA-MRSA infections occur in 94,000 people each year, resulting in at least 19,000 deaths.

The 2007 CDC (Centers for Disease Control and Prevention) Surveillance Summary found that 64% of the Staphylococcus aureus (Staph) strains in American hospitals are MRSA.

51

75% of hospital rooms in the United States have MRSA in them

The CDC has reported that the proportion of HA-MRSA infections has been increasing: 2% of Staph infections in U.S. intensive-care units were MRSA in 1974, 22% in 1995, and 64% in 2004. While these numbers reflect the incidence of infection while undergoing hospitalization, HA-MRSA can be acquired while simply visiting a healthcare facility. No matter what the reason is for entering a hospital, you need to know the risks and how to best protect yourself.

Are You at Risk?

Whether you have MRSA, Staph or another medical condition, anyone going to a hospital should have the right mindset, knowledge and tools to help protect themselves. If any of the following describes you, be sure to review the steps outlined in this chapter to help ensure your stay is a healthy one:

- You or a family member are currently admitted to a hospital.

- You have an upcoming surgery or other medical procedure in a hospital.

- You are visiting someone in a hospital or you work in a hospital.

Be sure to review healthcare MRSA risks and symptoms as detailed in "HA-MRSA" on page 30.

Insurance Limited on Preventable Infections

Fighting MRSA and Staph infections can be a complicated, laborious and expensive process, especially for people who are older or immune compromised. The average HA-MRSA hospital infection adds $35,000 to a patient's bill and an 10 extra days to their hospital stay. The cost typically is passed on to the patient and Medicare.

Unfortunately, insurance is starting to curtail payments to cover hospital errors and may eventually stop paying to treat infections that could have been prevented. As of 2008, the Centers for Medicare and Medicaid Services (CMS) no longer reimburses hospitals for costs related to treating certain hospital associated infections. This change is creating a needed urgency for healthcare facilities to eliminate these infections as hospitals are often held liable for costs not covered by insurance companies. It's crucial to your health and your pocketbook that you be proactive about protecting your health when entering these facilities.

Taking Charge of Your Hospital Stay

When you visit a hospital for medical care, you are paying the hospital to provide you with a service. As a paying customer, you have every right to look out for your interests and to find the best hospital that provides the services you need. Below are tips to help you take charge of your hospital stay, be proactive and ensure that you get the best care possible.

- **Understand how the system works.** Hospitals are profit driven and they exist to make money. Most people think that hospitals are driven solely by the noble purpose of caring for people and making them healthy. But most hospital decisions that affect your health are driven as much by profit motive and legal protection as they are by a desire to help you. It is therefore important to stand up for yourself, be attentive to what happens to you and be on the lookout for medical mistakes and other pitfalls to avoid.

- **Know your rights.** A doctor's power to make decisions for you is based solely on how much power you give the doctor. Ultimately, it's your decision to take a medication or not, or to have a procedure performed or not. Taking charge of your own health decisions is even more important if those decisions hold risks. If you are unable to make your own decisions, then in most cases your family holds the power to make medical decisions.

- **Meet with your hospital doctor.** For medical procedures referred to a hospital, you probably won't know the doctor who will be treating you. Be sure to meet with your hospital doctor and ensure she understands your needs prior to your hospital stay. You will see important questions to ask your surgeon or hospital doctor in a following section.

Choosing a Good Hospital

Not all hospitals are the same. Some hospitals have more modern equipment, better trained staff and better management than others. Some hospitals have advanced systems to track medications and monitor patient care in order to minimize medical errors. In particular, some hospitals have much better infection control programs than others.

Choosing a good hospital is crucial before you set foot inside the front door. The following tips will help you gauge how good a hospital is at providing medical care and protecting its patients:

- If possible, **choose a top tier, 4 or 5 star hospital** and/or Joint Commission Accredited Hospital. Using a lower rated hospital may increase your chances of getting a healthcare-associated infection. See the *Find Hospitals* page on the website www.HealthGrades.com for hospital ratings. Also see the website www.QualityCheck.org from the Joint Commission for a listing of accredited hospitals.

- **Find a high-tech hospital if possible.** Look for hospitals that use computerized systems for tracking patient information and history, prescriptions and procedures. Such hospitals often use a bar-coding system for tracking patients and medications. The number of medical mistakes often drops dramatically after instituting such systems. These improvements help ensure that medications and procedures are proper and appropriate for you.

- Look for hospitals that use a **Checklist Protocol** for procedures. This simple listing is just like a recipe that nurses or doctors should follow when performing any procedure. Checklists help eliminate mistakes and can reduce infections resulting from inserting IV's, catheters or other routine procedures.

Questions to Ask Your Hospital Doctor Before a Procedure

If you need a specialized medical procedure, your primary care physician or specialist will refer you to a hospital that has its own doctors and medical staff. As such, the doctor who will be treating you will be a hospital doctor, not your primary doctor.

Because you don't know your hospital doctor and they don't know you, it's very important to meet with them before your hospital stay so you understand exactly what's going to happen to you in the hospital. Below are important questions to ask your hospital doctor before any medical procedures or operations are performed.

- Healthcare-Associated Infections (HAIs) such as *S. aureus*, MRSA, coagulase-negative Staph and many others are a major risk with any invasive medical procedure. If you need surgery, ask the surgeon what their rate of infection is for the procedures they preform. Be assertive and don't be afraid to ask for this information. Choose a surgeon with a low infection rate.

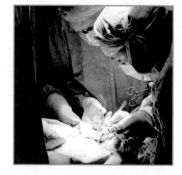

Invasive medical procedures are a common way to catch MRSA.

- Ask how many people catch HAIs in the hospital and what measures are taken to reduce such infections.

- If you're having an operation, ask your doctor about the need for a pre-operative antibiotic. Taking an antibiotic one hour before the first incision is sometimes prescribed to prevent surgical site infections. If you have a history of C. *difficile* or other resistant infections, this option needs to be considered very carefully.

- Ask your doctor about keeping you warm during surgery. Patients who are warm tend to resist infections better than cold patients.

- Ask that staff do not shave the surgical site. If hair must be removed before surgery, ask that clippers be used instead of a razor. Razors leave behind small nicks in the skin which can allow bacteria to enter your body and cause a skin infection.

- Ask your doctor about monitoring your glucose (sugar) levels continuously during and after surgery, especially if you are having cardiac surgery. When blood glucose levels are tightly controlled, heart patients resist infection better.

- Find out exactly what will be happening during your stay, including all procedures, protocols and medications, so you know what to expect.

- Find out what measures are taken to reduce the risk of blood clots and other post-surgery risks after being discharged from the hospital.

- Find out how much communication and cooperation there will be between the hospital doctor and your regular doctor, your natural doctor or any specialists you may be seeing.

- Ask if the doctor will support you in using alternatives, either with or without a prescription.

Avoiding Medical Mistakes

Doctors, nurses and other hospital staff are not perfect. They can make mistakes and they don't always follow proper procedures like hand washing between patients. Some of these mistakes are minor while others can be very hazardous to your health. Mistakes can happen easily given how busy hospitals get and how many different procedures and patients hospital staff have to keep track of. Below are tips to help you avoid medical errors during your hospital stay.

- **Be observant and proactive.** Be aware of everything that's done to you during your stay. Question all medications and procedures to ensure they are correct for you. Question anything that doesn't seem right and stand up for yourself.

- **Get a health advocate.** If possible, ask a family member or friend to assist you during your hospital stay. A health advocate will help you understand what's going on, communicate with and question hospital staff, perform personal tasks you're unable to do yourself and in general *watch your back*. A health advocate is essential if you cannot communicate well or be assertive.

- **Avoid unnecessary tests.** Doctors rely heavily on testing to make important medical decisions about your health. Unfortunately, many medical tests are highly inaccurate and prone to false or misleading results. Unneeded diagnostic tests can lead to misdiagnoses and improper treatments. Some tests can even be dangerous to your health. As a rule of thumb, avoid medical tests unless one or more of the following is true:

  » There is strong reason to believe you have the disease, either based on your medical history or symptoms.

  » The risk to your health is very high if you do have the disease.

  » If you are in a high-risk group for the disease.

  » The test is very accurate. Accuracy has two important parts: 1) the likelihood of a positive result for someone who has the disease and 2) the likelihood of a negative result for someone who is disease-free. Many tests are prone to false positive results, often leading to unnecessary treatments and medical procedures.

How to Avoid Hospital Infections

Staying in a hospital is the number one way to catch a superbug infection, including MRSA, Staph, *C. difficile*, Carbapenem-resistant Enterobacteriaceae (CRE) and many others. Even hospital visitors have ended up with MRSA or other infections. Healthcare-Associated Infections (HAIs) are serious problems that are widespread in hospitals, nursing homes, MRI facilities and other healthcare settings. The risk is higher for people receiving invasive medical care or surgery, getting catheters or PICC lines, or giving birth. Infection risks are also higher for the elderly, babies and people with compromised immune systems.

Steps to Take Before a Hospital Stay

Taking steps to prepare your body before a hospital stay is an important part of reducing the risk of healthcare infections, especially if you are having surgery. The chapters on "Boosting Your Immune System" on page 223, "Probiotics: The Good Bacteria" on page 209 and "Foods and Your Immune System" on page 237 provide more details about some of the tips below.

- Start eating immune boosting foods and herbs, raw foods and alkalizing foods at least a few weeks before your hospital stay. These steps help bolster your immune system for HAI risks. Be sure to find out if any specific foods or supplements are contra-indicated before surgery.

- Take probiotics before, during and after your visit. Probiotics are important to reestablish healthy gut bacteria that get diminished with antibiotic use.

- 3 to 5 days before surgery, start bathing in natural antimicrobial washes. This is especially helpful if your immune system is weak. Essential oils are an excellent natural antimicrobial choice for bathing and are detailed inside the section "Bathing With Essential Oils" on page 134.

- If you have a history of any kind of infection, ask your surgeon to have you tested or examined for signs of infection at least one week before you go into the hospital. If you have an active infection, extra precautions can be taken to protect you and others from further infection.

- Stop smoking well in advance of a surgical procedure. If you smoke, consider getting help to stop because smoking can make you more prone to HAIs and other diseases.

Steps to Take While In the Hospital

Below are tips and techniques to help reduce the risk of infection during your hospital stay. Many are also important considerations if you are visiting someone:

- **Request that all staff wash their hands** before treating you or touching you. Ask visitors to wash their hands too. Better yet, have them put on new gloves before touching you.

- **Run a cold-air essential oil diffuser** in your room. This is one of the easiest and most cost effective ways to reduce airborne bacteria. Visitor, patient and hospital staff activity in rooms increases the number of particles with bacteria floating in the air.

- **Continue taking probiotics** and eating as many whole, unprocessed foods as you can. Alkalizing foods like greens can help maintain your immune system.

- **Cover your TV remote control with a latex glove.** Remote controls can become heavily contaminated with bacteria. Covering the remote with a glove protects your hands from contamination while allowing the buttons to be pressed.

- **Leave your jewelry at home.** Jewelry can harbor bacteria and promote infections.

- **Wash your hands frequently** with natural soap and water. Bring your own soap from home if possible. Avoid antibacterial soaps and sanitizers that are used everywhere. Antimicrobial soaps can weaken your immune system and contribute to antibiotic resistance, as detailed in the chapter "Hand Washing and Hygiene" on page 269.

- **Make sure your doctor is not wearing a tie.** Ties are rarely washed and they brush across many patients, transferring bacteria from one person to another. If your doctor is wearing a tie, ask them to tuck it into their shirt. Doctor's gowns with long sleeves and dangling cuffs present a similar hazard.

- Before your doctor uses a **stethoscope**, ask that the diaphragm (the flat surface) be wiped with alcohol. This applies to all physical objects shared with others, including blood pressure cuffs. Doctors rarely remember to sanitize these items before visiting their next patient.

- Make sure that **high-touch surfaces** are sanitized often. This includes: doorknobs, bed rails, phones, light switches, wall areas around the toilet, restroom surfaces and faucets, toilet handles, sinks and dispensers and the edges of privacy curtains.

- **Avoid touching your hands to your mouth**, and do not set food or utensils on furniture or bed sheets. Bacteria like *C. difficile* and viruses can live for days to months on surfaces and can cause infections if they get onto your body or in your mouth.

- When getting an MRI, request that all **MRI pads** and contact surfaces be cleaned before entering the scanner. MRI scanners are often heavily contaminated with bacteria and inadequately cleaned between patients, especially mobile MRI units.

- **Avoid a urinary tract catheter** if possible. Catheters increase your chances for a bladder infection. If you do require one, have it removed as soon as possible.

- If you need an IV, make sure it's inserted under clean conditions and changed every 3 to 4 four days. Hospital staff should wear masks and gloves when inserting or changing your IV and your skin should be sanitized. Staff should follow a protocol checklist to ensure all safety precautions are being performed.

Using Supplements in Hospitals

An important part of taking charge of your health is knowing how to use supplements in healthcare facilities. Taking supplements to support your body is especially important when you are staying in a hospital and dealing with a health challenge. Unfortunately, getting support to use supplements, herbal remedies and natural products in a healthcare facility can be a big challenge.

Most hospitals frown on patients using supplements. Many facilities forbid supplement use without a doctor's prescription. On the other hand, some facilities allow patients to use any dietary supplements they choose. While some health centers have formal policies about supplements, many others have inconsistent and confusing policies or no policy at all. Some facilities hand over the responsibility for supplement decisions to the doctor, pharmacist or another practitioner.

Why Supplements Can Be Challenging

There are many reasons why your rights to use supplements and alternative remedies can be limited in healthcare centers. There are official guidelines for the use of supplements and alternative medicine in healthcare facilities. As you might expect, these guidelines were written by organizations within the mainstream medical system which are skeptical of natural health, namely the Joint Commission and American Society of Health-System Pharmacists (ASHP).

Some facilities try to compromise between the official guidelines and the patient's wishes to use supplements. But there are legal reasons that discourage such a compromise.

Formal studies on the effectiveness and safety of supplements are often lacking. And information on the possible interactions between supplements and pharmaceutical drugs is limited. Therefore, doctors, hospitals and health centers run the risk of lawsuits if they are too lenient with supplements.

Most doctors and health centers lack knowledge, experience or training in supplements and alternative medicine. Even if a facility is open to the use of supplements and herbal remedies, doctors and other practitioners are likely to stick with the standard mainstream protocols that they know best, just to be safe.

What You Can Do

If you want to use supplements or natural products in a hospital or nursing home, you may need to be a bit creative. Below are tips for using supplements in a health care center:

- **Safety first.** Talk with your doctor about possible side effects and drug interactions with your supplements. While most natural products are very safe on their own, some herbs and alternative remedies may reduce the effectiveness of certain medications, including antibiotics. Some supplements may need to be taken apart from certain medications. And some natural remedies are best avoided if you are pregnant or taking drugs with contraindications to those remedies.

- **Get a prescription.** If possible, get a prescription for the supplements you want to take. Many healthcare facilities will only allow supplements that a doctor prescribes. For example, some doctors are prescribing probiotics along with antibiotics. Keep in mind that some facilities require supplements to be ordered, administered and stored in a controlled manner. Therefore, you may not be able to bring your own supplements from home.

- **Foods to replace supplements.** Many health care facilities allow outside foods and snacks to be brought in. Fortunately, some foods can serve as replacements for common supplements. For example, antioxidant supplements can be replaced by eating foods such as raw blueberries that are rich in natural antioxidants. An excellent substitute for probiotic supplements are fermented foods such as raw sauerkraut, kefir, miso and kombucha tea.

- **Cosmetic uses.** Some natural products have both cosmetic uses and health benefits. You may be able to use such products openly for their cosmetic effects while benefiting quietly from their medicinal properties. For example, lavender essential oil is commonly used for a calming foot massage, as an air freshener and to scent hand soaps and shampoos. But lavender oil can also provide support for infection healing, stress reduction and the immune system support. Tea tree essential oil can be added as a natural antibacterial to personal care products and liquid soaps while also helping prevent healthcare associated infections.

- **Food additives.** Many people are creative and hide some supplements inside foods, such as putting essential oils into a protein shake or a green smoothie. Manuka honey can be added to hot tea. However, care must be taken because some natural remedies may not mix well with certain drugs. As mentioned above, it is best to have your doctor's support when using supplements in the hospital, nursing home or other healthcare facility.

Common Supplement Myths

If you ask your hospital doctor about supplements, you will probably hear one of the common myths perpetuated by mainstream medicine. You may hear that vitamins interfere with medications or test results. You may also hear that supplements are dangerous after surgery.

Most supplement myths are based on ignorance rather than hard scientific data or clinical experience. However, there are times when a supplement might interfere with a medication or a medical procedure. The following tips can help you sidestep vitamin myths and avoid potential interference between supplements and your medications:

- Most doctors and hospital staff automatically discourage the use of any vitamins or supplements for all procedures and medications. If this happens to you, be sure to **ask which specific vitamins or supplements interfere with your specific medications, tests or procedures.**

- Do your own research and check your supplements for **contraindications and precautions**.

- **Review your supplements and medications with your doctor.** A functional medicine MD or Naturopathic Doctor (ND) will have much more knowledge and experience with supplements than most MDs.

- As a general rule of thumb, **take supplements or vitamins a few hours apart from your medications**. Avoiding using supplements and medications at the same time can help reduce the risk of any unknown supplement-medication interactions.

6 Naturopathic Medicine: Safe & Effective Healthcare

There are many safe, effective and well established methods for handling infections and other illnesses beyond the limited scope of mainstream medicine. Progressive medical doctors have begun to adopt these alternative therapies for treating and preventing infections, often with great success. Sadly, alternative methods are not part of the curriculum in most medical schools and as a result, most medical doctors have no knowledge or experience with them.

Because of the limitations of mainstream medicine and its sky-rocketing costs, millions of people have started seeking non-toxic, effective and affordable natural healthcare. Naturopathic medicine has grown rapidly to meet this rising demand. Its focus is on disease prevention and natural therapeutics, such as botanical medicine, lifestyle counseling and nutrition.

Due to naturopathic medicine's growth in recent decades, partnerships between naturopathic doctors (NDs) and conventional medical doctors have become more readily available. This collaboration has made more effective therapies available and it has increased consumer satisfaction with healthcare providers. The best news is that more people are recovering their health by adding naturopathic medicine to their healthcare options.

What is Naturopathic Medicine?

The core principle of naturopathic medicine (also called naturopathy) is that the human body is a self-healing mechanism. If your body is given the proper raw materials and support it needs, it is naturally able to heal itself of nearly any disease, including chronic infections like Staph and MRSA.

The primary focus of naturopathy is addressing the root cause of a disease, not in masking the symptoms. Naturopathic medicine views your body as an interconnected system that must be considered as a whole when treating or preventing disease. The significant impact that your mind and emotional state have on your health is also recognized and taken into account.

Naturopathic medicine stresses the prevention of illness before it takes place. In fact, naturopathic approaches are far more successful for preventing reinfections than mainstream medical approaches. If you have an existing health problem, non-invasive natural therapies are used if at all possible. These methods may include herbal medicine, nutrition, aromatherapy, homeopathy, nutritional supplementation, IV therapy, traditional Chinese medicine, acupuncture, hydrotherapy and counseling to name just a few.

Pharmaceuticals like antibiotics may be prescribed, but typically only in combination with natural remedies or other supportive therapies. Most people are surprised to find that natural methods are often just as effective as pharmaceuticals, without the toxicity or negative side effects.

"Naturopathic medicine is a distinct primary healthcare profession that emphasizes prevention, treatment, and optimal health through the use of therapeutic methods and substances that encourage individuals' inherent self-healing process. The practice of naturopathic medicine includes modern and traditional, scientific, and empirical methods." The American Association of Naturopathic Physicians, www.naturopathic.org

What is a Naturopathic Doctor?

A licensed naturopathic doctor (or naturopath) is a medical professional trained just as thoroughly as a medical doctor. They can serve as primary care practitioners and are trained in diagnosis, prevention, management and the treatment of both acute and chronic health conditions.

Licensed NDs complete a rigorous four-year program at a naturopathic medical college and must pass professional board exams. Accredited naturopathic colleges include standard medical curriculum but also include additional study in clinical nutrition, botanical medicine, and other holistic therapies. In some states, an ND can prescribe pharmaceutical drugs, although natural non-pharmaceutical methods are usually preferred.

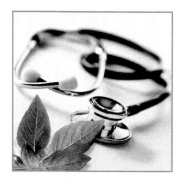

Naturopaths are trained in both holistic and mainstream medicine at accredited medical schools.

Just like any doctor, each naturopath has an area of expertise. Some NDs have specific knowledge and experience in treating infections while others may lack any MRSA experience.

Naturopaths Compared to Medical Doctors

Mainstream medical doctors usually target their treatments to the specific organ or part of your body in which symptoms appear. Doctors are therefore divided into specialties based on specific body parts or systems, such as infectious disease doctors specializing in infections or cardiac physicians specializing in the heart. For details about mainstream medicine, see the chapter "Doctors and Mainstream Medicine" on page 39.

Mainstream medical treatments typically bring quick relief but by and large they do not address the underlying cause of the health issue. The power of the body to heal itself is usually underestimated and downplayed by most mainstream medical doctors.

Mainstream medicine is highly effective at treating acute injury, trauma and emergencies. However, mainstream medicine often fails with chronic and degenerative disease conditions because it ignores the underlying cause of the disease. Mainstream medicine has a poor track record for keeping people healthy and preventing them from getting sick in the first place because of its reactive approach toward disease.

In contrast, naturopathic medicine is very successful at treating chronic and degenerative disease conditions because it addresses the root cause of the disease. Naturopathy is also effective at prevention because of its proactive approach focused on bolstering your underlying health. In addition, naturopathic methods are generally safe, natural and non-invasive.

As an example, taking the right antibiotic might bring swift relief from the symptoms of an infection. But this therapy does not fix what either contributed to, or caused the infection in the first place. Antibiotics also weaken your immune system, leaving you more prone to reinfections. A list of the pros and cons of alternative medicine versus alternative medicine can be found in the section "Natural Approaches: Pros and Cons" on page 85.

How to Find a Good Naturopath

Ensure that a prospective naturopathic doctor is well educated. One way to gauge education is where an ND went to school. There are several accredited naturopathic schools in the United States and Canada that are highly respected:

- Bastyr University, Seattle, Washington and San Diego, California

- Southwest College of Naturopathic Medicine, Scottsdale, Arizona

- National University of Health Sciences, Lombard, Illinois

- National College of Naturopathic Medicine, Portland, Oregon

- University of Bridgeport College of Naturopathic Medicine, Bridgeport, Connecticut

- Canadian College of Naturopathic Medicine, Ontario, Canada

- Boucher Institute of Naturopathic Medicine, Vancouver, British Columbia, Canada

Visit the website of the Association of Accredited Naturopathic Medical Colleges (AANMC) for more information about these schools at www.aanmc.org. Another beneficial gauge of education and professionalism is membership in the American Association of Naturopathic Physicians (AANP). The AANP web site at www.naturopathic.org will give you a listing of member NDs in your area.

It is possible to become a naturopathic doctor through completion of an online course, which can lack the level of education available at one of the accredited naturopathic schools listed above. Even if an ND successfully graduated from an accredited naturopathic college, she still needs to pass board exams to receive a valid license to practice naturopathic medicine. Ask a prospective naturopathic doctor if they have both a graduation diploma and a current license to practice naturopathic medicine.

A good ND should take the time to gather extensive information from you about any health issues, diet, physical condition, lifestyle, stress level and emotional health before initiating any action. She should use this information in combination with blood work or other diagnostic tests to customize a recovery and prevention plan specific to your needs. Your approach toward handling MRSA or Staph should be geared toward long-term restoration and maintenance of your health in addition to alleviating your immediate symptoms.

Make sure that your naturopath has a balanced and integrative view of medicine. Naturopathic medicine is outstanding when practiced correctly. Likewise, mainstream medicine can also be outstanding when practiced correctly. Your ND should be open to both kinds of medicine and understand the dictum *use the right tool for the right job*. Mainstream medicine has its pros and cons, just like naturopathy, and both approaches can be valid and beneficial when used properly.

Not All Naturopaths Are the Same

Like any other doctor, each naturopath has her own specialties, level of experience with treating infections and their own unique treatment approaches. Every naturopath also has her own unique personality, treatment biases, strengths and weaknesses. You want to find a naturopath that you have confidence in and who is a good match for your own personality, medical philosophy and the treatment approaches you want to use.

Medical philosophy, or paradigm of treatment, can vary widely from one ND to another. For example, some naturopaths are more allopathic (aligned with mainstream medicine) or *evidence based* in their practice. Other naturopaths are more alternative and intuitive in their methods of diagnosis and treatment. For example, Bastyr University for naturopathic medicine stresses research, evidence-based medicine and is relatively allopathic in its approach to medicine. An ND from Bastyr is therefore more likely to favor integrative or mainstream medicine in their treatment approach. In contrast, other schools of naturopathic medicine tend to be more alternative, intuitive and natural in their medical paradigm, providing a broader and more alternative curriculum to their naturopathic students.

In addition to philosophy of treatment, most naturopathic doctors will also favor particular treatment approaches and remedies with which they are most familiar and experienced. For example, one naturopathic doctor may use homeopathic medicine exclusively and know very little about essential oils or IV vitamin C therapy. Another ND may only use botanical remedies and Chinese herbal medicine. Yet another naturopath who specializes in essential oil therapy may have limited experience with homeopathy. It is important to understand both the medical philosophy and the treatment approach of any naturopath you intend to work with in treating your infection.

Tips for Choosing an ND

- Look for an ND with specific experience in treating and handling chronic infections, especially Staph or MRSA.

- If possible, find an ND who is in partnership with a knowledgeable medical doctor.

- Verify that she has a diploma from an accredited naturopathic college.

- Verify that she has a current active license to practice naturopathic medicine.

- Be very open and ask for her success rate in treating Staph or MRSA infections.

- Ask how much she charges and how frequently she suggests seeing you.

- Ask if your medical insurance is accepted and what services and products are covered.

- Ask if help will be provided filling out insurance forms to maximize reimbursements.

- If you cannot find a naturopathic doctor in your area, try to find one that will do phone consultations. A long-distance phone consultation can be a great complementary addition to your medical doctor's treatments and help you with long term recovery and prevention.

Getting the Most Benefit From a Naturopath

As with any doctor, it's important that you feel comfortable with your ND and have confidence with her professionalism, experience and training. The nature of holistic and integrative medicine requires that you be proactive in your health. An ND will direct and guide you in natural ways to improve your infection, but it's your responsibility to make the required changes. Making beneficial lifestyle changes can take some time and effort on your part. To get the most value from integrative medicine, be a partner with your ND.

Many people use naturopathic physicians as their primary care physicians. Naturopathic medicine is very successful at treating most conditions that don't involve trauma or emergencies. A naturopathic doctor can determine when mainstream medical care is necessary to supplement your naturopathic care and can help you find the best medical doctor if needed.

To get the most benefit from seeing an ND, adopt a long-term mindset instead of seeking a quick-fix. If you are willing to make changes in your lifestyle and put some effort into your long-term success, naturopathic medicine may be your answer to achieving optimal health.

7 Antibiotic Treatments, Resistance and Limitations

Antibiotics are the standard mainstream treatment for infections like MRSA and Staph. Antibiotics were embraced as *miracle drugs* soon after their discovery in the 1930s and have saved countless lives in the years since then. Today there are many different classes and types of antibiotics, each one optimized and best suited for treating different types of infections. Antibiotics are heavily used in medicine as the preferred treatment for all sorts of infections. These powerful drugs are also used extensively in the animal farming industry, largely for disease prevention purposes.

Antibiotics can make the difference between life and death, especially for serious and advanced infections. The proper antibiotic often turns the course of an infection in a short amount of time. Despite the benefits of these drugs, the growing problem of antibiotic resistance is rendering them less effective every year.

What are Antibiotics?

An antibiotic is a drug that inhibits or stops the growth of bacteria. Antibiotics are used to treat bacterial infections and are not effective against yeast, fungus or viral infections (viruses are the agents that cause a cold or the flu). The choice of antibiotic varies depending on the type of bacteria and the location and ability to reach the infection. If the bacteria are resistant to a particular type of antibiotic, it is excluded from use for that particular infection. Antibiotics are used orally, topically and intravenously (IV). IV antibiotics are used in more serious cases, such as septicemia or other internal infections like osteomyelitis. In mainstream medicine, antibiotics are the first line of defense against infections like Staph, MRSA and other superbugs.

Antibiotic Resistance

The Archives for Internal Medicine estimates that between 40% and 60% of hospital MRSA infections are resistant to *first-line* antibiotics. In other words, the standard protocol antibiotics or the first-choice antibiotics are no longer working against MRSA. The percentage of resistant MRSA is increasing, based on an examination of records from seven million hospital stays at one-fifth of

U.S. hospitals. To better understand what's fueling antibiotic resistance, a brief look at the history of the first antibiotics is helpful.

The first man-made antibiotic called penicillin was introduced in the early 1940's. Staph bacterial quickly developed penicillin resistance. By 1950, 40% of hospital *Staph aureus* isolates had become penicillin resistant, and by 1960 this number had risen to 80%. Some strains of Staph have become resistant to most if not all of the penicillin-related antibiotics, as well as other types of antibiotics.

Although a properly chosen antibiotic can be very successful at halting an infection quickly, the more these powerful drugs are used the less effective they become. Bacteria have an amazing ability to quickly adapt to the drugs people invent to kill them. An antibiotic that works well at treating someone's infection the first time may be useless the next time.

Antibiotic resistance occurs for four main reasons as listed below. These four topics will be described in more detail in subsequent sections:

1. Bacteria reproduce very quickly.

2. Bacteria communicate and share information with each other.

3. Antibiotics are often misused and/or overused by doctors, hospitals and the livestock industry.

4. Antibiotics are misused by patients.

Bacterial Reproduction

Bacteria, like all living things, change over time in response to their environment. Because bacteria reproduce very quickly (sometimes in mere minutes), they evolve and change on a very fast time scale, adapting to their surroundings in order to survive. This process of evolution or mutation happens in people, too, but much slower and over periods of thousands of years.

For example, natives of the high Andes Mountains of South America have larger lungs and bigger chests than people anywhere else on earth. These natives adapted to the low oxygen high mountain environment over thousands of years in order to survive in their environment.

When people first began living in the high Andes, most had normal sized lungs. But because each person is unique and random DNA mutations naturally occur, a small percentage of early Andeans happened to have slightly more lung capacity than normal. Because of the low oxygen environment, these particular Andeans tended to survive longer and reproduce more efficiently. As a result, the few people that happened to have more lung capacity had slightly more opportunity than others to pass on their genes to the next generation of Andeans. In this way, each new generation had slightly more people with the genes that caused larger lungs. Over thousands of years, this natural selection process caused high mountain Andean natives to have larger lungs than people native to other parts of the world.

Bacteria evolve by random mutation using the same natural selection process that people do, but in a matter of days, months or years instead of millennia. In fact, *Staph aureus* bacteria can reproduce every half hour and can create 50 generations in a single day.

Consider a hypothetical antibiotic (antibiotic A) used to treat an infection. Although most of the infecting bacteria may die when exposed to antibiotic A, the few that happen to be immune to antibiotic A survive to pass on their genetic material to the next generation. Because of their rapid reproduction rate, generations pass by very quickly, each more resistant than the generation before. In this way, the bacteria species as a whole mutates and becomes resistant to antibiotic A in a relatively short amount of time.

Bacterial Communication

Bacteria communicate with each other using chemical mechanisms that allow them to share information about how to survive. One type of communication is called quorum sensing. Quorum sensing allows bacteria to change their behavior based which other bacteria are present and what those other bacteria are doing.

Another type of communication is a swap of genetic material called plasmid exchange and it can even occur between different species of bacteria (i.e. between a Staph and E. coli bacteria). For example, when one bacterial species becomes resistant to antibiotic A, it can transfer its resistance genes to other species of bacteria. This allows the other bacteria to become resistant to antibiotic A as well, even though they may never have encountered antibiotic A. This exchange of resistant genes provides a quick shortcut to the usual natural selection process caused by random mutations.

Plasmid exchange is encouraged by stressing the bacteria, which is exactly what happens when they are exposed to antibiotics. This means that the use of antibiotics can hasten the development of antibiotic resistance.

Misuse and Overuse of Antibiotics

Antibiotics are relied upon heavily by mainstream medicine and are also widely used in the animal farming industry. Because these drugs can be highly effective at stopping infections, they are often over-prescribed, over-used and outright abused and misused by doctors and animal farmers alike. Oftentimes, instead of being reserved for serious infections, antibiotics are routinely prescribed as a general prevention measure just in case an infection develops.

As an example, 60% of kids are treated with antibiotics for a common cold[11]. It is a known fact that colds are viral infections, not bacterial infections, and antibiotics are not effective against viral infections.

Recently the United Kingdom's health secretary called upon UK doctors to stop prescribing antibiotics for minor health problems like coughs, colds and sore throats. This is part of a government initiative to prevent the spread of antibiotic-resistant superbugs. As mentioned previously, over-prescribing of antibiotics is one reason antibiotic resistance has become such a big problem.

Additionally, antibiotics are routinely fed to livestock as a preventative against diseases caused by unsanitary and unhealthy crowded living conditions. Antibiotics also help fatten livestock quicker, decreasing the amount of time it takes to go to the market. Amazingly, more than 80% of the antibiotics used in the U.S. are given to feed animals that have no disease! Antibiotics used in farming get into your food supply in the form of meat and also into groundwater supplies from farm runoff, further increasing your exposure to these drugs. Water treatment processes do not remove antibiotics from the water supply, unless you have a special water treatment process in your home.

New research is indicating that the widespread use of glyphosate (used in Roundup) and other herbicides used on food crops is also contributing to the problem of antibiotic resistance. The same resistance mechanisms that bacteria develop to resist pesticides help the bacteria to resist other chemical toxins, including antibiotic drugs. For more details see the chapter "GMO Foods, Glyphosate & Immune System Stress" on page 259.

Constant low-level environmental exposure to antibiotics stresses bacteria and they become more resistant more quickly. As a result, many antibiotics that worked just a few years ago are no longer effective. Today, many kinds of bacteria have learned to resist multiple antibiotics, resulting in multi-drug resistant superbug infections.

Misuse of Antibiotics by Patients

Another common way antibiotics get misused is caused by patients. Antibiotic resistance is quickened when people stop taking their antibiotics before they have finished the full course of prescribed pills. Stopping your prescription early leaves behind bacteria that were able to survive the antibiotic and allows them to pass on their genes to other bacteria. These resistance genes result in new strains of bacteria that are more immune to the antibiotic. Unless directed by your doctor to stop, be sure to finish all antibiotic pills your doctor gives you, even if you feel better.

Curbing Antibiotic Resistance

There are ways to slow and even reverse the problem of antibiotic resistance. But the only way to turn the problem around is to implement a multi-faceted approach. Such an approach must include the medical industry, farmers, government, and the people who use antibiotic drugs. You can do your part by using antibiotics properly, knowledgeably and only when really needed. For details on what you can do to help, see the section "How You Can Help Reverse Resistance" on page 80.

Biofilms and Chronic Infections

Biofilms are a powerful way bacteria can resist antibiotics. Staph, MRSA build biofilm structures in order to protect themselves. Biofilms are a tough polysaccharide slime-layer that houses clusters of embedded bacteria. Biofilms can stick to bodily tissues as well as implanted medical devices in the body.

Biofilms form a barrier against antibiotic treatments and your own immune system, creating an effective hiding place for bacteria. Biofilms also provide a home base from which bacteria are released into your body to seed more biofilms or cause infections. After an antibiotic treatment is complete, bacteria can leave the protection of the biofilm and cause infections elsewhere. Examples of biofilms you're likely familiar with include the slime layer coating the inside of your pet's water dish and the dental plaque on your teeth.

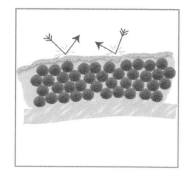

Biofilms: Bacteria cluster together on bodily tissues or implanted medical devices and exude a protective covering that repels antibiotics and hides the bacteria from the immune system.

According to the National Institute for Health (NIH), biofilm infections are implicated in 65-80% of all chronic bacterial infections[12]. The NIH also states that nearly all healthcare-associated infections involving medical devices (prosthetics, bone implants, catheters and pacemakers) are biofilm infections. Aside from device infections, biofilms are also implicated in chronic wounds, abscesses, chronic sinus infections, and most stubborn recurring infections, including Staph and MRSA.

Because biofilms are an emerging area in research, there are limited studies on effective treatments. Until recently, antibiotic research and natural remedy studies have been performed using only free-floating bacteria, not bacteria encased within biofilms. Emerging research shows that very high concentrations of antibiotics are needed to kill biofilms, up to 1000 times higher than the amount needed to kill free-floating bacteria[13]. Antibiotic use at this level would be toxic to people.

Biofilm Treatment

Researchers are now looking at ways to break down biofilms or stop biofilm production so the bacteria inside can be exposed to tolerable levels of antibiotic treatments. Some newer studies have shown specific herbal, enzymatic and plant substances help break down the biofilm structure. A few potent herbal remedies have been successful at stopping serious chronic and recurring infections. While these products have not been tested against biofilms *per se*, emerging research and clinical evidence suggests that some herbal treatments have activity against biofilms, including manuka honey, garlic extracts and some essential oils. Refer to "Biofilm and L-Form Support" on page 186 for more details.

Hidden L-form Bacteria

Another bacterial survival strategy is the creation of *L-form* bacteria. Research has shown that bacteria living in your body can exist in an altered state called L-forms. These mutated bacteria are also known as Cell Wall Deficient (CWD) bacteria and sometimes *stealth bacteria*. At least 50 different kinds of bacteria, including Staph and MRSA species, can form L-forms[14]. Much of the L-form research has been performed by Dr. Lida Mattman who was nominated in 1997 for the Nobel Prize for Medicine for her work in this area.

L-forms are not limited to bacteria. Yeast species such as Candida can also create L-forms, which can complicate recovery from an infection. Candida and yeast infections are secondary infections that often occur after taking antibiotics.

To become an L-form, bacteria shed their cell walls and become smaller and harder to detect. L-forms often clump together in the body to hide more easily. They can actually hide undetected within your body's own immune system cells (white blood cells) and red blood cells. L-forms have also been documented around cancerous tumors.

What Causes L-forms?

Bacteria transform into the L-form state when they become stressed. Bacteria can get stressed by most anything that can change their living environment, including the following:

- Antibiotics (penicillin-class antibiotics have been documented to cause Staph L-forms).

- Nutrient-deficient diets (processed foods, diets high in sugar).

- Mental or emotional stress.

- Prescription drug use or other factors that create acidic conditions inside the body.

Because L-forms are a new area of research, most doctors have never even heard of them. It will take a while before the medical community recognizes and accepts this area of research. Specific research on MRSA L-forms is sparse and the implications on recurring infections have not been studied fully. Fortunately some research is being done. Understanding more about L-forms will likely have a positive impact on many of today's chronic health issues, especially for those suffering from recurrent infections.

Diagnosis and Treatment of L-forms

Diagnosis of L-forms is very difficult because they can lay dormant for years within your body and are very hard to find due to their mutated nature. L-form bacteria cannot be cultured or detected by standard laboratory tests. Most L-form testing is being done in the research field, not in the clinical arena.

One treatment sometimes used for difficult resistant infections is the prescription of multiple antibiotics at once, in an attempt to attack the infection on multiple fronts. Another approach that has been used to treat L-forms is called the Marshall Protocol. This protocol uses low doses of antibiotics over a long period of time in combination with special supplements and diet changes. This protocol is on the fringe of mainstream medicine but has gained some level of recognition by the FDA. The protocol is detailed on the following website www.marshallprotocol.com.

Since antibiotics are one way L-form bacteria can be created, antibiotics may not be the best treatment option. Antibiotics also create additional stress on the body by indiscriminately killing other types of bacteria, including the healthy bacteria in your gut.

A good way to help guard against L-forms is to bolster your immune defenses and use remedies that target the bacteria. A combination of antibiotics and alternative approaches that target biofilms may also be helpful. A strong immune system may lessen or even eliminate the need for antibiotics for many infections, thus putting less stress on your body and causing fewer L-forms. For more details about addressing L-forms see the section "Biofilm and L-Form Support" on page 186.

Antibiotics for Staph Infections

There are quite a few antibiotics that work for treating non-antibiotic resistant Staph infections. The type, location and severity of the infection all help determine which antibiotic is prescribed. Other factors considered include pregnancy, drug allergies, other health conditions and medications being taken.

The best way to prescribe an antibiotic that will work for your particular strain of Staph is to get a susceptibility test first. This will verify that the antibiotic will work against the Staph bacteria causing your infection. Commonly prescribed antibiotics include, but are not limited to, the following:

- B-lactams such as Oxacillin and Flucloxacillin.

- First generation Cephalosporins, including Cefazolin, Cephalothin and Cephalexin.

- Lincosamides such as Clindamycin and Lincomycin.

- Macrolides such as Erythromycin.

- Tetracyclines, including Doxycycline and Minocycline.

- Sulfa drugs.

- Mupirocin cream (for nose infections).

- Vancomycin (IV) and Linezolid are generally reserved for severe or resistant MRSA strains.

Most of the above antibiotics are for less severe Staph infections. MRSA is resistant to B-lactam antibiotics and to many of the above antibiotics as well.

Fortunately, Staph is typically easy to treat and the antibiotics prescribed will generally work. If you have a mild Staph infection, antibiotics may not be required and treatment may instead include wound incision, drainage or warm compresses. However, for serious infections, your doctor will likely prescribe an antibiotic. Staph infections can sometimes turn into MRSA, which requires special antibiotics as described in the section below.

Antibiotics for MRSA

Antibiotics are the standard medical therapy for skin and internal MRSA infections. Antibiotic therapy is often prescribed for:

- Skin infections such as boils or abscesses that do not respond to incision and drainage.

- Systemic or internal infections such as bone, implant or lung infections.

- Severe local symptoms.

- Severe internal infections that require surgery to remove infected areas.

- Immune-suppressed or immune-compromised people.

Because MRSA is resistant to most broad-spectrum and standard protocol antibiotics, newer antibiotics such as the *glycopeptides* Vancomycin and Zyvox may be prescribed. Unfortunately, there are strains of MRSA that are becoming resistant to these two drugs. When it comes to antibiotics, the list of what works for some strains of MRSA is growing shorter each year.

As with normal Staph infections, the type and severity of infection play an important role in choosing the best antibiotic. There are also several types of antibiotics that are best avoided due to problematic side effects, or because MRSA is resistant to the drugs.

Antibiotics to Avoid

Several classes of antibiotic drugs no longer work against MRSA and should be avoided if you have MRSA. Taking such drugs will do nothing to help your infection or they have too many drawbacks. Taking ineffective antibiotics delays you from receiving proper treatments, allowing time for the infection to grow worse. Ineffective antibiotics also weaken your immune system unnecessarily and can cost a lot of money, depending on your insurance coverage. The following drugs are best avoided because MRSA is resistant to them or because they have high risks of dangerous side effects:

- **Penicillin class antibiotics**, including methicillin, penicillin, and amoxicillin. MRSA is resistant to these drugs.

- **First generation cephalosporins** such as cefazolin, cephalothin and cephalexin. These are a penicillin-like class of antibiotics that may still be used for non-resistant *Staph aureus* infections or some mild cases of MRSA.

- **Fluoroquinolone class antibiotics** such as ciprofloxacin (cipro for short) and levofloxacin. Per the CDC, MRSA can quickly become resistant to these drugs. Fluoroquinolones can also have very severe side effects and have been associated with myelosuppression, temporary and permanent neuropathy (tingling and numbness) and lactic acidosis during prolonged therapy. Fluoroquinolones also have a high risk of causing MRSA or *C. difficile* colonization. The 2012 antibiotic guidelines from the Infectious Diseases Society of America (IDSA) has recommended avoiding fluoroquinolone antibiotics because of the many side effects.

- **Macrolide class antibiotics** such as erythromycin, clarithromycin and azithromycine. MRSA can quickly develop resistance to these drug.

MRSA Antibiotics for Skin Infections

Below are the most commonly prescribed antibiotics for MRSA skin infections, which are commonly picked up in the community as CA-MRSA. The side-effects and precautions below are not all-inclusive. Be sure to read the drug product insert and talk with your doctor for a complete listing.

- **Clindamycin.** This drug has been successfully and widely used for the treatment of soft tissue and skin infections as well as bone and joint infections and abscesses caused by Staph and MRSA.

    Resistance: MRSA is becoming increasingly resistant to clindamycin in the United States.

    Side effects and precautions: Clindamycin's most common side effect is diarrhea. This drug can also cause *C. difficile* overgrowth infections in the colon. Other side-effects are pseudomembranous colitis, nausea, vomiting, abdominal cramps, skin rashes and more.

- **Linezolid** (brand names: **Zyvox**, Zyvoxid or Zyvoxam). Approved by the FDA in 2000, Linezolid is often prescribed for soft tissue and skin infections. It is also prescribed for MRSA pneumonia, especially HA-MRSA pneumonia. It's commonly prescribed to people of all ages and is one of the most expensive treatment options. A single course can cost $1,000 - $2,000 for 20 tablets.

    Resistance: To minimize MRSA resistance, linezolid is often a *last resort antibiotic* which is not prescribed unless Vancomycin or other antibiotics don't work. Cases of MRSA resistance have been reported.

    Side effects and precautions: Linezolid's most common adverse events when used for short durations include diarrhea, vomiting, headache, dizziness, and nausea. Long-term use has led to serious effects including bone marrow suppression, myelosupression, low platelet counts, peripheral neuropathy, optic nerve damage and lactic acidosis. Linezolid is also associated with causing *C. difficile* secondary infections in the colon.

- **Mupirocin** (brand name: **Bactroban**). Mupirocin is commonly prescribed as a topical cream for minor skin infections and lesions for *Staph aureus*, MRSA and Streptococcus infections. This drug is often prescribed to reduce or eliminate MRSA colonization in the nose. Mupirocin is often prescribed before surgical procedures to help prevent the surgical site from becoming infected with MRSA. The drug is prescribed for children and adults and there is limited safety data for pregnant and nursing mothers.

    Resistance: MRSA resistance to mupirocin is occurring in some communities.

Side effects and precautions: Possible side effects of mupirocin include headache, rashes and nausea as well as burning, dizziness and secondary wound infection. Like other antibiotics, prolonged use may result in overgrowth of bacteria that are not susceptible to it, as well as an overgrowth of fungal organisms (such as secondary yeast infections).

- **Trimethoprim-sulfamethoxazole** (brand name: **Bactrim and Septra**). Bactrim is not FDA-approved for the treatment of Staphylococcal infections, including MRSA. However, laboratory tests have shown most CA-MRSA strains are susceptible so this drug, making it a treatment option for Staph and MRSA. It is commonly used for skin and wound infections, urinary tract infections, lung infections, ear infections, septicemia, and other types of infections.

  Side effects and precautions: Bactrim is not recommended for women in their third trimester of pregnancy or infants less than 2 months old. Side effects can include mild allergic reactions, fever, sore throat, skin rashes, cough, diarrhea, and serious adverse effects can include myelo-supression, acute renal failure, severe liver damage and more.

- **Tetracyclines** (**Doxycycline** and Minocycline). These drugs are often effective in the treatment of soft tissue and skin infections, but not for deep or more severe infections.

  Side effects and precautions: Tetracyclines are not recommended during pregnancy or breast feeding. They are not recommended for children under 8 years of age because of potential decreased bone growth and tooth discoloration. Doxycycline side effects can include an increased risk of sunburn when exposed to sunlight, diarrhea, and allergic reactions. Minocycline side effects can include risk of sunburn, upset stomach, diarrhea, dizziness, headache, tinnitus, vomiting and allergic reactions. Serious but rare side effects for minocycline can include fever, yellowing of the eyes or skin and vision changes.

MRSA Antibiotics for Internal and Severe Infections

Hospitalized patients with complicated, severe or internal infections are often prescribed one of the following antibiotics. These infections can include deep soft-tissue infections, surgical site infections, major abscesses, wound infections and infected burn patients.

Oftentimes a broad-spectrum antibiotic is used in conjunction with the following antibiotics. Most options below use intravenous methods of delivering the drug into the body. A picc line may be used for prolonged treatment. Please note that the side-effects and precautions below are not all-inclusive. Be sure to read the drug product insert and talk with your doctor for a complete listing.

- **Intravenous (IV) Vancomycin.** Vancomycin is often called an antibiotic of last resort for MRSA, though resistance against it has been growing. Vancomycin requires IV administration into a vein and can occasionally have severe side effects. Duration of treatment can last weeks to months. Tissue penetration is variable and vancomycin has limited penetration into bone. It's often prescribed for pneumonia (both HA-MRSA and CA-MRSA strains).

Resistance: Some strains of MRSA are now becoming resistant to Vancomycin, with one strain called VRSA (Vancomycin resistant *Staph aureus*).

Side effects and precautions: Serious side effects of vancomycin can include ringing in ears, diarrhea, and hearing problems. Like most antibiotics, it can cause secondary infections like thrush or yeast infections. Because this medication is eliminated through the kidneys, it could cause kidney problems in the elderly or those with impaired kidney function.

- **Oral or intravenous (IV) linezolid (Zyvox).** See the skin infection section above for more information about linezolid.

- **IV Daptomycin.** Daptomycin is FDA approved for adults with *Staph aureus* bacteremia (blood infections), some forms of endocarditis (heart valve infections) and some skin and soft tissue infections. The safety and efficacy of daptomycin in children has not yet been established.

- **Oral or Intravenous (IV) clindamycin.** See the skin and soft tissue infection section above for more information on clindamycin.

When to Use Antibiotics

For mild and even moderate infections, using antibiotics only as a last resort (with the support of your doctor) may be the best course of action. Using antibiotics only when really needed spares you from potential and sometimes dangerous side effects of these drugs. Plus it helps slow the problem of antibiotic resistance.

There are viable alternatives to antibiotics, including many natural remedies. These alternatives can be especially important if antibiotics have been unsuccessful, or if you have experienced severe antibiotic side effects. Natural and alternative remedies definitely have benefits over antibiotic drugs, which you'll learn more about in the chapter "What is Alternative Medicine?" on page 83.

Antibiotics can literally save your life if they successfully stop a severe infection. But it is important to understand how these potent drugs work, what their limitations and side effects are, and how to make the best use of them.

Antibiotic Side Effects

Antibiotics can have significant and undesirable side effects, many of which can actually cause your body to be more prone to reinfections once your antibiotic treatment is complete. Even if antibiotics stop your MRSA infection, these drugs often cause secondary yeast, viral and bacterial infections.

Each antibiotic has its own list of undesirable side effects (be sure to read the product insert), but there are some effects that are common to most of these drugs. Some of the main side effects are listed below, along with suggestions on how to counteract them.

Dehydration

Staying properly hydrated is crucial when taking antibiotics because many of these drugs cause you to become dehydrated. See the section "Water, Water Everywhere" on page 247 for details on how to stay properly hydrated.

Allergic Reactions

Many people have experienced mild and even severe allergic reactions to antibiotics. Mild allergic reactions consist of an itchy rash or slight wheezing. Severe allergic reactions (anaphylaxis) can be life threatening and usually includes swelling of the throat, inability to breathe, and low blood pressure. If you experience any of these severe symptoms, immediately contact your local emergency services. See the section "Reducing Antibiotic Side Effects" on page 173 for methods to relieve moderate skin rashes and itchiness associated with antibiotics.

Organ Dysfunction

Some side effects are more severe and, depending on the antibiotic, may disrupt the function of the kidneys, liver, bone marrow, or other bodily systems or organs. Blood tests are usually performed to monitor for such reactions.

Weakened Immune System

Most antibiotics weaken you immune system, leaving you more prone to reinfections and secondary infections. The killing off of your friendly bacterial flora is a major way antibiotics weaken your natural defenses. See the chapter "Boosting Your Immune System" on page 223 and the section "Secondary Infections" on page 79 for details.

Gastrointestinal Upset

Many antibiotics cause nausea and/or diarrhea. Many of the same methods used to boost your immune system will also ease your gastrointestinal symptoms. See the section "Reducing Antibiotic Side Effects" on page 173 for methods to relieve moderate stomach upset.

Antibiotic Resistance, Biofilms and L-forms

As you've read above, the overuse of antibiotics is creating problems for the future of these drugs. Many doctors fall into the trap of over prescribing antibiotics and patients commonly stop taking antibiotics before their prescription is done. Therefore, it's partially up to you to help control antibiotic resistance by using antibiotics properly and only using them when really needed

Antibiotic use also puts stress on bacteria and as a result they can form biofilms and mutated L-form stealth bacteria. As detailed previously, stealth bacteria have been implicated in causing recurring infections and secondary infections. For details about controlling stealth bacteria, see the section "Biofilm and L-Form Support" on page 186.

Secondary Infections

A common side effect of taking antibiotics is surprisingly *more infections*. All too often, a fungal, viral or bacterial infection will strike days, weeks or even months after a Staph or MRSA infection has cleared. The loss of friendly and protective bacteria in your gut from antibiotic use can allow for bad organisms like yeast or *C. difficile* to overgrow and cause infections. These so-called *secondary infections* can sometimes be more dangerous and problematic than the original infection. Yeast, candida and *C. difficile* are three common secondary infections after having Staph or MRSA. The section "Co-Infections and Secondary Infections" on page 181 will detail these three infections and other common secondary infections.

www.RxISK.org is an independent drug safety website where you can research your antibiotic for all side effects that people are experiencing. You can also report drug side-effects at this website.

The Future of Antibiotics

How long will people be able to depend upon antibiotics to treat infections? Every year, more strains of bacteria become resistant to more types of antibiotics. More outbreaks of resistant bacteria are popping up in hospitals and communities all around the world. Resistant infections become more common and more difficult to treat as time passes on.

Mankind is in a neck-and-neck race to develop new antibiotics faster than bacteria can become resistant to them. Unfortunately, it takes years to develop new antibiotics, get FDA approval and finally make them available for use. There is a very real possibility that antibiotics will soon be useless and other methods for handling infections will have to be used.

Hope for The Future

There may be a ray of hope for the continued effectiveness of antibiotic drugs. As long as there are antibiotics, bacteria will learn to resist them. However, there are ways to slow down and even reverse the problem of resistance. The current war against superbugs can only be won if everyone begins to use these powerful drugs conservatively, knowledgeably and with respect.

Hospitals that adopt initiatives and have a dedicated infection prevention and control plan have reduced the incidence of superbugs in their hospitals. These antibiotic stewardship hospital programs require training and buy-in by the doctors and all hospital staff and include revised protocols, patient screenings and intensive monitoring.

Studies show that superbugs living in hospitals can slowly lose their antibiotic resistance and evolve back into less dangerous and more normal bacteria. This reversal of bacterial resistance can happen over time if the hospital closely monitors and cuts back on the use of antibiotics through rigorous programs. Such antimicrobial stewardship programs require knowledgeable pharmacists, infectious-disease specialists and microbiologists working together in order for the program to be effective. A prime goal of such initiatives is to restrict prescriptions of specific antibiotics when they become less effective at fighting infections.

⬦⬦

By managing the type of antibiotics that are prescribed and only using antibiotics when needed, hospitals can actually reverse antibiotic resistance.

⬦⬦

Antibiotic drugs may yet have a future as a valuable tool in treating infections for many years to come. The medical community has the power to slow down the growth of superbugs and reserve antibiotics for use only when necessary. But bacteria will only slow down their war of survival against antibiotics if humans are willing to use antibiotics more wisely and more discriminatingly. The good news for humanity is that there are safe and effective natural remedies that are inherently free of the threat of antibiotic resistance. Using alternative treatments whenever possible can help keep antibiotics working and available for when they are most needed.

How You Can Help Reverse Resistance

Below are actions you can take to reduce the problem of antibiotic resistance. They will also help preserve the effectiveness of antibiotics for future generations to come. Taking the steps below can also reduce your personal risk of encountering antibiotic resistant superbugs and can help your treatments work better.

- Partner with your doctor to reduce or replace antibiotics with alternative treatments if possible, reserving antibiotics as a last resort. Naturopathic doctors and other holistic medical professionals are experienced in alternatives and can support you while using such treatments.

- Insist that your doctor confirm what type of infection you have before prescribing any antibiotics, especially if you suspect you have MRSA.

- If you have a cold, flu or ear infection, do not ask your doctor to prescribe antibiotics, as they are not effective against viral infections.

- If you do take antibiotics, take the *full course*, even if you feel better before the prescribed course is complete.

- Avoid the common antibacterial soaps and personal care products that can contribute to the growth of antibiotic resistant bacteria.

- Eat foods that are not tainted with antibiotic residues or superbugs by buying antibiotic free meats. Request that your supermarket carry these foods and/or buy meat from a local farm not using antibiotics. See more about antibiotic free foods and organic foods in the chapter "Foods and Your Immune System" on page 237.

- Buy organic produce, avoid GMO foods and limit your use of glyphosate (Roundup) herbicide and other chemical pesticides around your home. Chemical herbicides and GMO farming practices work together to make bacteria more resistant to antibiotic drugs.

How Nature Kills Bacteria

Antibiotics are relatively simple chemicals. The mode of action of many antibiotics (i.e. interfering with bacterial reproduction and metabolic processes) is relatively subtle and is not a blatant attack on the bacteria. In contrast, your immune system intelligently seeks out bacteria and actively kills them in multiple and deliberate ways. Antibiotic drugs are also one-dimensional in their action. They work in one particular and narrow way, making it easy for bacteria to counteract.

Unlike man-made antibiotics, natural remedies tend to be chemically complex and work in more than one dimension. Natural substances are composed of multiple interrelated components that can work together in complex, synergistic ways to battle infections. Natural substances that control bacteria can have chemical complexity, multi-dimensional modes of action and powerful mechanisms to destroy bacteria or halt their growth. As a result of this complexity, bacteria have a much harder time adapting to natural substances than to simple man-made antibiotics.

Nature provides bacteria with the ability to evolve and easily become resistant to drugs, allowing them to survive. Fortunately, nature also provides many natural substances that kill bacteria and are very difficult for bacteria to resist. These natural substances evolved to keep bacteria in check and in balance with other life forms on the planet. It's no coincidence that these effective natural substances are readily available from plants and food sources that humans can use.

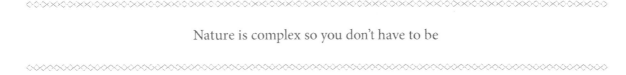

Nature is complex so you don't have to be

Humans were created and evolved along with bacteria as a part of nature, and nature provides mankind with all that it needs to survive and be in healthy balance with nature. The key is to tap into the power of nature and to relearn what man has known for thousands of years but has recently forgotten… that *food is medicine.*

8 What is Alternative Medicine?

Alternative medicine, which is similar to holistic, natural, complementary or integrative medicine, has been practiced for thousands of years around the world. It was in existence well before the recent advent of mainstream medicine, where surgery and pharmaceutical synthetic pills are used to treat a disease. Over the years, total reliance on chemical and surgical technologies by the mainstream medical system has led to the dismissal of alternative health options as either outdated or ineffective.

However, most people in the world do not use mainstream medicine. In fact, the World Health Organization (WHO) estimates that 80% of the world's population (about 3 billion people) relies upon alternative medicine as their primary form of healthcare[15]. The New England Journal of Medicine notes that one-third of all doctor's visits in the United States are to holistic doctors, not medical doctors. There are five homeopathic hospitals in Great Britain run by the British National Service. And, in Germany, one out of three prescriptions is an herb and in France, many medical doctors routinely prescribe essential oils[16].

In France, natural remedies and treatments are considered normal and routine. French doctors incorporate both herbal medicine and the full extent of modern medical knowledge and skill in their approach to medical care. Treatment using herbs and essential oils is even covered by health insurance plans. People in France can go to pharmacies where they can choose from formulas consisting of essential oils and herbal tinctures (made under a doctor's prescription) or they can choose more mainstream pharmaceutical products. Natural medicine is taught in colleges, universities, and medical schools.

Treating the Person, Not the Disease

So why are people increasingly moving towards alternative and holistic medicine? The reasons are pretty simple: it is safe and it works! Holistic medicine treats each person as a whole, with their own individual challenges and needs. In contrast, mainstream medicine tends to focus on the disease rather than the person, viewing the disease as an isolated issue to be fixed. There are pros and cons to both types of medicine, depending on what you need at the time.

For example, mainstream medicine works well for trauma and emergency situations. You do not call your herbalist if you have just broken your leg. You need an emergency room doctor. Alternative and holistic medicine are much more effective in treating chronic disease, prevention, and in dealing with the needs of an individual. These areas are all interdependent and are precisely where alternative medicine excels. True health is about supporting the body and creating health within the body, not simply fighting disease.

Alternative medicine is not taught in mainstream medical schools, therefore, most doctors have little to no training, experience or knowledge using alternatives. As a result, mainstream medicine is short changing the health of millions of people by not addressing prevention and the root cause of disease.

A key principle of alternative medicine is that the body is able to rid itself of a disease process if supported properly and brought into balance. The focus of natural health is both therapeutic and preventative. As your body strengthens and heals from the inside, disease is no longer able to thrive and health is regained.

Mainstream medicine emphasizes the treatment of SYMPTOMS.
Alternative medicine includes addressing the ROOT CAUSE of a disease.

The Biggest Mistake People Make

Most infection sufferers who begin using alternative medicine only focus on finding a silver bullet remedy, or a more natural replacement for their antibiotics. Unfortunately, this is the same mistake that mainstream medicine makes: focusing on the disease, not the person.

It's a very easy mistake to make. Almost everyone has been programmed by drug companies, the media and their doctors with the ideal that taking pill X will cure illness Y. Using this same idea with alternative medicine can handicap some of its most important benefits.

The full power of alternative medicine is not just in the remedies themselves. Remedies are just one piece of the puzzle. The full potential of alternative medicine comes from seeing the body as a whole and

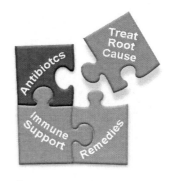

Alternative medicine is not a replacement for mainstream medicine; it is a broader approach to health and healing.

supporting the body's inherent healing ability. Strengthening the immune system, using remedies and detoxification may all be parts of the puzzle. Antibiotic drugs, if and when needed, may also play a part. Unlocking the full potential of alternatives is the purpose of the 3 Action Steps in chapter 1.

To fully understand alternative medicine, a fundamental shift is needed in the way most people view health and wellness. But it's a shift worth making because alternative medicine has many unique and powerful benefits when addressing stubborn diseases like Staph and MRSA.

Natural Approaches: Pros and Cons

The table below compares the key pros and cons of alternative and mainstream medicine. Both approaches are valid and can serve an important role with MRSA or Staph infections. Be aware that the two approaches are not mutually exclusive. In fact, you can get the most options by using a combination of both alternative and mainstream medicine.

	Mainstream Medicine	Alternative Medicine
Pros	• Best option for surgical emergencies, trauma care and acute life threatening illness • Best option for replacement of hips, knees and other damaged body parts • Best for re-constructive surgery • Effective at quickly masking symptoms to provide immediate relief • Prevention of some diseases by immunization (with side effects) • Widely available and covered extensively by health insurance • The default option, requiring minimal self-direction, training or specialized knowledge on the part of the patient	• Focus on proactive measures • Treats the cause of illness and disease in addition to the symptoms • No antibiotic resistance problems • More cost effective and economical • Targets whole body as an interrelated system • Boosts the immune system • Most effective options for chronic and degenerative conditions, such as cancer • More successful with viral, autoimmune and many kinds of mental illness • Generally safe with minimal side effects when used according to directions • Excellent success record for chronic diseases and long-term prevention • Open, inclusive view of medicine

	Mainstream Medicine	Alternative Medicine
Cons	• Does not treat the underlying cause • Poor track record on healing chronic diseases and disease prevention • Treatments are often invasive and have undesirable side effects • Can be very expensive, especially longterm • Treats the body in parts, not as a whole, interrelated system • Medical schools are structured into organ-specific departments, with little relationship with each other • Often discourages and dismisses other medical approaches and alternatives	• Requires more personal education and self-direction for optimal success • Not taught to most doctors and most patients never hear about alternative options or methods • Can take longer to see results because addressing the root cause of an illness is more involved than simply masking the symptoms • Healthcare insurance coverage is usually less comprehensive and challenging • Some alternative methods have not been scientifically studied, but many have

Approaches to Alternative Medicine

The terms alternative, holistic, natural, complementary and integrative are often used synonymously, however, there are some important differences between each approach. All these approaches share some things in common, such as a focus on prevention and a focus on finding the root cause of a health challenge. While they are all alternative to some extent, each approach has a slightly different emphasis on how alternatives are used.

Alternative medicine in it's most basic form is the use of healing techniques that are beyond the scope of mainstream or allopathic medicine. Holistic medicine focuses on treating the patient as a whole rather than focusing only on the disease or the affected part of the body. Complimentary medicine considers alternatives as an add-on or supplement to mainstream medical treatment, not as a standalone substitute for mainstream medicine. Integrative medicine strives to combine both mainstream and alternative approaches together as needed.

Alternative Medicine Modalities

There are many different alternative modalities that can be used for infections. A few of the most important ones will be briefly outlined in this section. There are other modes of practicing alternative medicine not listed below, such as Ayurvedic medicine, biofeedback, homeopathy, massage therapy, reflexology, bodywork, hydrotherapy, aromatherapy, and various other forms of energy medicine.

While licensed naturopathic doctors are probably your best choice for addressing your infection naturally, you may also choose to find another type of practitioner to help you regain overall health and balance your body.

Naturopathic Medicine

Naturopathic medicine focuses on the body's inherent ability to heal itself. Naturopathy seeks to treat the cause of a disease rather than simply suppressing its symptoms. Licensed doctors of Naturopathic medicine receive a degree from a four year accredited medical college. Naturopaths may use herbal medicines, homeopathy, dietary modifications, hydrotherapy, and lifestyle counseling to achieve healing. The chapter "Naturopathic Medicine: Safe & Effective Healthcare" on page 61 has details on naturopathic medicine.

Traditional Chinese Medicine (TCM)

Traditional Chinese Medicine has been practiced for over 3000 years and over one quarter of the world's population now uses one or more of its component therapies. TCM, with its unique diagnostic methods, systematic approach, abundant historical literature and materials, has attracted much attention from the international community. TCM combines the use of medicinal herbs, acupuncture, and the use of therapeutic exercises such as Qi Gong. It has proven to be effective in addressing many chronic diseases, including cancer, allergies, heart disease and AIDS. TCM also focuses on the individual and looks for and corrects the underlying causes of imbalance and patterns of disharmony.

Chiropractic

Chiropractic work primarily involves the adjustment of the spine to alleviate pain and improve general health. It was practiced by the early Egyptians and in 1895 was developed in America by Daniel David Palmer. It is now the most common form of alternative medicine in the United States. Chiropractors not only manipulate the spine and joints, but also advise their patients on lifestyle and diet matters. They believe that humans possess an innate healing potential and that all disease can be overcome by properly activating this potential.

Handling Infections Naturally

There are many natural ways to address Staph and MRSA and the troublesome symptoms that accompany these infections. Be sure to see the Action Steps in chapter 1 for a step-by-step guide of the most important things to focus on. Remember to be patient. Natural solutions can often take longer than fast-acting antibiotics, but the benefits can far outweigh a little extra time.

In subsequent chapters, you'll learn about specific alternative remedies people have had success with for infections. These remedies are based upon the author's personal experience, research, and the positive experiences of others with infections. The selected remedies are not a complete list, but they do represent good options to start with for the majority of people.

Natural remedies are not drug products and most have not been approved by the FDA for treating diseases. Overall, natural remedies have a much safer track record than drug products, but some remedies are not appropriate for everyone. If you are unsure or have questions about natural remedies and approaches, be sure to contact your physician or a qualified health care provider.

Why Natural is Often Better

Plants have complex components and contain many different substances that affect the human body in very controlled and balanced ways. For example, one component of a plant may act as a stimulant while another component causes you to calm down. The net result is a balanced and self-correcting natural system with built-in feedback loops. If one action is too strong, the counteracting substance is immediately available for the body to use. The synergy and multi-dimensional effects of natural substances help explain why many natural infection remedies work so well and have such a good safety record.

Nature tends to follow patterns and use the same substances over and over again in seemingly unrelated ways. A specific class of genes has been discovered that predetermines a limited range of variation available to evolution. Because of this, the range of compounds that a plant can produce is not unlimited but will follow a clear pattern and remain within specific boundaries. For example, the bark beetle secretes a substance to attract other beetles. This same substance is secreted by hornets as an alarm signal. This compound is also found in citrus fruits and hops and has narcotic effects on mice.

In short, nature provides balanced, self-correcting systems where plants, animals and humans have evolved together over millennia to benefit safely and symbiotically from each another. Therefore, the burden of proof for safety falls much more heavily upon synthetic and unnatural drugs than on those natural plant-derived substances that have a long track record of safety.

MRSA and Staph Remedy Requirements

There are many alternative remedies for infections, but there are some special considerations when choosing such a remedy for support with Staph and especially MRSA. Below are some special requirements a remedy should meet for optimal support with these infections.

Active Against Staph Bacteria

There are many different kinds of bacteria and the remedy should have a track record of activity against *Staph aureus* bacteria. Fortunately, many of the most well recognized natural remedies for infection have broad activity against many kinds of bacteria as well as viral and fungal or yeast infections.

Potency

There are hundreds of different natural substances with at least some amount of activity against bacteria and many others with secondary infection support properties. Some of these remedies can play an important role in MRSA Staph recovery, especially in a supportive role, such as immune support or biofilm support.

However, few remedies have sufficient potency or strength to make a real difference against stubborn infections when used medicinally. Staph and especially MRSA can cause tenacious and resilient infections that often require particularly strong medicinal-strength remedies to make a dent in the infection. While less potent supportive and preventative remedies can play a vital role in recovery, it's equally important to have strong medicinal-strength options, especially for more severe infections.

Gentle on Beneficial Flora

One of the best ways to support your immune system is to maintain a healthy balance of probiotic organisms and beneficial flora inside your gut and on your skin. Some natural remedies may be disruptive to your beneficial flora when taken in high amounts. Of course, the same is also true of many drugs and antibiotics. One of the biggest benefits of natural remedies is the ability to target the infection-causing bacteria while leaving the beneficial bacteria alone. Remedies that are balanced and gentle on the gut are especially important for children and the elderly who have weaker or less developed immune systems and more delicate systems.

Activity Against Biofilms

Biofilms are likely a big reason why some people struggle with recurring infections. Unfortunately, most antibiotic drugs have a hard time penetrating biofilms and are not very effective against them. Luckily, some alternative remedies have natural activity against biofilms. Such remedies can provide an added measure of support for people with a history of recurring infections.

Alternative Remedy Safety and Precautions

Most natural remedies have a long history (often thousands of years) of safe use by humans. In contrast, pharmaceutical drugs are only decades old and are often untried and unproven in the long-term. Pharmaceuticals can also have a lengthy list of side effects. In contrast, most of the alternative remedies in this book have side effects like boosting the immune system, removing harmful toxins from the body and energizing and oxygenating the body.

However, just because something is natural does not necessarily mean it's safe. Natural remedies must be used appropriately while taking any needed precautions. It's also best to stick with tried-and-true remedies whenever possible that have well established safety records, well known precautions and well understood effects on the body.

Don't let precautions scare you. Precautions simply mean to use a remedy with care, awareness and respect in order to have the best possible experience. Unfortunately, this level of awareness is often lacking in the use of mainstream medications, which often have many potential and dangerous side effects and unknown interactions with other drugs.

Necessary Precautions

Subsequent chapters detail alternative remedies that have worked for recurring infections, including MRSA. However, there are no guarantees that a specific remedy will work for you or be safe for you. Also, the precautions listed for each alternative remedy are not all-inclusive. Be sure to refer to the product label and consult with your doctor, especially if you are pregnant or nursing.

While the author is comfortable using any of the methods in this book, it is prudent that you discuss any remedies, supplements or dietary changes you're considering with a qualified healthcare professional before use, especially if you are pregnant, nursing or have any preexisting health conditions. You should always have a health care provider monitor your progress no matter what remedies or treatment methods you choose to use.

9

Alternative Remedies

This chapter outlines several natural and alternative remedies that meet the important Staph and MRSA requirements for potency, effectiveness and safety that were detailed in the previous chapter. These requirements include strong infection-fighting qualities, being gentle on intestinal flora and providing support for the immune system.

The remedies in this chapter can be used alone, in combinations or in blends. While single remedies can be very helpful, blends combine the benefits of multiple natural products into a single remedy. Because most common remedies lack the strength to fight stubborn infections, you'll find details below on what to look for when selecting the most potent products.

Keep in mind that you don't need to use every remedy listed in this chapter. For a step-by-step guide on which remedies to use, see "Action Step 1: Bacteria Control" on page 9 in chapter 1. This chapter provides the details needed to use several specific remedies safely and effectively. However, use chapter 1 to guide you regarding how to choose the best remedy for your particular needs.

Use chapter 1 to help you choose a remedy.
Use this chapter for details about your chosen remedy.

This chapter will show detailed protocols and usage amounts for specific natural products. Always follow the directions on the product label or the guidance of a healthcare professional if they differ from the protocols in this book.

Essential Oils

Essential oils include several of the strongest infection-fighting remedies available. Some essential oils are broad-spectrum, with antibacterial, antifungal and antiviral properties. Oils have wonderful side effects like boosting the immune system and energizing the body. They are very powerful, very concentrated and contain hundreds and even thousands of chemical components. The topics of essential oil remedies and how to use them are covered in detail in subsequent chapters.

Olive Leaf Extract

Olive leaf has a long history of being used against illnesses in which microorganisms play a major role. It's effective against bacteria, viruses, yeast and parasites. In ancient Egypt, olive leaf oils were used in mummification to help preserve bodies from decay caused by bacteria and fungi. In the 1800's olive leaves were used in commercial European pharmaceuticals for malaria. By the middle of the 1900's, scientists researching this medicinal plant isolated the compounds responsible for its infection-fighting effects, including oleuropein.

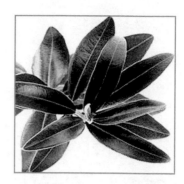

Olive leaf has antibacterial and immune supportive properties.

Oleuropein is a phenolic compound that makes olive trees vigorous and resistant to insect and bacterial infections. Research shows that oleuropein can play a similar role in humans with little risk of side effects. In fact, Upjohn Pharmaceutical Company conducted a safety study on a calcium derivative of oleuropein and found that even amounts many times higher than recommended had no toxic effects[17].

Olive leaf extract appears to be particularly potent against Staph and MRSA bacteria. In a 2010 laboratory study, 122 different species of bacteria were subjected to olive leaf extract. The results showed especially high activity against Staph and MRSA bacteria[18].

Olive leaf also has immune stimulating effects. The infection and immune-supporting qualities of this potent herbal product are especially beneficial given its safety record and lack of side effects. When blended with other botanical substances, olive leaf can support the body in multiple ways when battling infections.

Using Olive Leaf Extract

- Select a high potency product with at least 18% oleuropein content inside the extract. A good usage amount to start with for adults is approximately 1400 mg of extract twice per day, taken with meals. If the product is well tolerated, the usage amount may be increased to 2800 mg of extract twice per day for moderate infections. For severe infections, 2800 mg of extract three times per day may be used, if well tolerated.

- Drink lots of water to help prevent bacterial breakdown products from collecting in the kidneys.

- **Precautions:** Follow the manufacturer's guidance for complete precautions. Olive leaf extract can lower blood pressure. Consult with your physician if you are using blood pressure lowering medications. Olive leaf extract can lower blood sugar levels, so if you are hypoglycemic or taking insulin or on diabetic medications, consult with your physician. Olive leaf extract can reduce blood clotting. If you are taking anticoagulants, consult with your physician. Olive leaf extract may conflict with some antibiotics, consult with your physician if taking antibiotics.

Garlic

Garlic has both antibacterial and antiviral properties and is one of the strongest infection-fighting herbs. Garlic also stimulates the immune system, promotes balanced intestinal health and can improve cardiovascular health. Garlic has also been used safely and effectively for thousands of years in treating disease. Now modern science is studying garlic and its benefits for a number of major health problems, including many different kinds of infectious diseases.

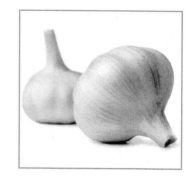

Garlic is one of the strongest infection-fighting herbs.

Garlic was used by the ancient Egyptians, Greeks, Romans and the Chinese to treat all types of infections, its use dating back over 5,000 years. As recently as World War II, garlic saved thousands of lives by protecting open wounds from getting infected. Even Louis Pasteur studied the strong antibacterial properties of garlic in 1858. As of today, there are over 2,000 studies on the infection-fighting qualities of garlic.

According to recent trails at the University of East London, patients who suffered for years with draining, chronic MRSA wounds were cleared of infection after a taking a course of a special extract of garlic. Most infections were resolved within eight to 12 weeks. Larger wounds took 18 weeks to heal, according to an article in the UK publication *The Sun* on June 12, 2008. A garlic product that contains the specially stabilized active ingredient allicin was used. See the following section "Stabilized Allicin" on page 95 for details on stabilized allicin remedies.

Garlic's Antimicrobial Ingredients

Garlic contains 27 known active ingredients and at least 35 other ingredients. Many of these ingredients are chemically complex and work together synergistically in the body to fight disease.

When garlic is crushed, bruised or cut, a reaction occurs that forms a compound called allicin, garlic's best known antimicrobial ingredient. Allicin is also responsible for garlic's distinctive odor. Allicin and several other compounds in garlic have strong antibiotic activity. In fact, garlic juice diluted as low at one part in 125,000 has been shown to inhibit the growth of bacteria[19]. Also, one milligram of allicin was found to equal the potency of 15 units of penicillin[20].

Unfortunately, allicin is rapidly oxidized after it is created and its antimicrobial potency does not last very long. However, garlic produces more than 100 active sulfur-containing compounds, proteins, and saponins when allicin oxidation takes place. While the allicin content is a common measure of garlic's potency, research is showing that S-allylcysteine and other active compounds in garlic are the most powerful ingredients.

There are many different kinds of garlic supplements, remedies and products. But not all garlic products contain the same amount of allicin. The amount of active components in fresh garlic and commercial supplements can vary widely, depending on where the garlic is grown and how the product is processed and prepared. Garlic oil, aged garlic and most powders contain limited or no active allicin. Garlic must be used fresh or specially processed to retain the allicin in a stable form.

Using Garlic

Herbalists generally recommend consuming three garlic cloves or equivalent garlic products daily, starting when symptoms of infection first appear. Garlic can be eaten raw or juiced, taken internally as supplements and used externally for skin infections. Cooked garlic is not nearly as effective as raw garlic. Garlic has been used successfully as a douche for troublesome vaginal yeast infections, a common secondary infection after taking antibiotics. Garlic can often be used along with other herbs or essential oils to create a broader range of therapy.

Below are general use guidelines for garlic and garlic products. These can be helpful for mild infections and for general immune support. The stabilized allicin product is covered in the following section.

- Whole garlic clove: Freshly mince 3 or 4 cloves of garlic per day and enjoy. Raw garlic can be added to a salad with an oily dressing to reduce possible irritation to the mouth

- Aged garlic extract: 600 - 1,200 mg throughout the day

- Freeze-dried garlic: 400 mg three times per day (for 1.3% alliin or 0.6% allicin standard concentrations)

- Liquid garlic extract: 4 mL per day, for a 1:1 w/v (weight/volume) standard

- Garlic tincture: 20 mL per day, for a 1:5 w/v standard

- Garlic oil: 0.03 – 0.12 mL three times per day

- Minced garlic for skin infections: Garlic can also be minced and blended with water before applying to an infected area. Be sure to use within an hour or two as its effectiveness diminishes rapidly. Be aware that garlic's phytochemical compounds are strong enough to burn the skin, so use with caution. Do not use on young children.

Garlic Precautions

Garlic is a very safe herb with a long and successful track record as a food and natural medicinal herb. However, just like any other herb or food, the possibility exists for side effects, allergies or interactions with other herbs, foods or drugs.

Excess garlic can hinder blood clotting and thin the blood and must be used carefully if you are taking anticoagulants, scheduled for surgery, delivering a baby or if you are taking certain anti-HIV drugs. Those with chronic digestive problems should be cautious using raw garlic because high amounts may irritate the intestinal tract. Pregnant women should exercise moderation with garlic, especially with high amounts, because garlic products may stimulate uterine contractions. Consult with a healthcare professional if you have questions about garlic use, safety and possible contraindications.

Children will require less garlic than adults. The amounts listed above are for adults. For proper guidance, consult with a healthcare professional experienced in using garlic with children.

Stabilized Allicin

Stabilized allicin is a specially formulated product derived from garlic which contains a potent, concentrated and stable form of allicin. Because the allicin in garlic is very unstable, specially formulated products are required to maintain the potency of allicin for any length of time. Most garlic products on the market are not in the stabilized form. The process of creating stabilized allicin concentrates the allicin from dozens of garlic cloves into a single drop of product, providing a formulation many times more potent than other garlic products.

Stabilized allicin has been proven to be effective against difficult infections that are resistant to antibiotics. In a 2004 study, a stabilized allicin extract killed all 30 strains of highly resistant MRSA as measured using 3 different laboratory tests[21].

In 2008, Dr. Ron Cutler and the University of East London (UEL) released the results from a human clinical study performed on 52 patients with hospital acquired MRSA. All 52 patients were treated with a form of stabilized allicin and all recovered fully from their MRSA infections. Many of the wounds healed in just 4 to 12 weeks and many of the patients had previously been treated with multiple antibiotics with no improvement[22]. The patient usage amount for the study was 1080mg of stabilized allicin internally, which is over 1000 times the potency of common freeze-dried garlic products. Liquid and cream forms of stabilized allicin were also applied daily on the infection site. As of 2010, 250 people have been successfully treated with stabilized allicin in the UEL study.

Using Stabilized Allicin

Below is a protocol table of general guidelines for using the liquid stabilized allicin formulation that was part of the UEL study. There are three levels of use, depending on the severity of the infection. The maintenance level is commonly used for long-term support with no current or recent infection challenges. The moderate and urgent levels apply to people with active infections. The moderate and urgent levels extend for several months to mirror the duration of use in the UEL study and to provide better support for biofilms and recurring infections.

The guidelines are for adults and children 12 years and older. The usage amounts may be divided or taken all at once each day; both methods provided the same results. For best results, the guidelines in the table below should be customized to best fit your own unique needs, including changing the amount and duration of use as needed.

Liquid Stabilized Allicin: General Use Protocol

Level	Usage Amount	Duration of Use
Maintenance	6 drops of liquid per day for generally healthy people. If you have a health challenge, 12 drops per day may be used for extra support.	For long-term use as a general preventative.
Moderate	**First 3 days:** Start with 1/2 tsp for the first 3 days to test for tolerance. **After 3 days:** Increase to 1 tsp daily with juice during meals.	A minimum of 5 months is generally used. After symptoms subside, continue using until you are clear of any signs of previous discomfort for 2-3 months depending on the level of desired result.
Urgent	**First 3 days:** Start with 1/2 tsp for the first 3 days to test for tolerance. **After 3 days:** Increase to 1 to 3 tsp daily with juice during meals.	A minimum of 5 to 12 months is generally used. After symptoms subside, continue using until you are clear of any signs of previous discomfort for 2-3 months depending on the level of desired result.

Different manufacturers provide products with varying amounts of stabilized allicin. Products with higher concentrations of allicin are a better value. There are also different formulations available, including cream, gel, liquid and capsule formulations. The liquid formulation typically has the most concentrated allicin content. The cream and gel formulations are better suited for topical applications for support with skin challenges. The cream and gel formulations are often used along with the liquid to provide both internal (systemic) and external (skin) support.

NOTE: See "Michelle's Recommended Products" on page 303 for product resources

Stabilized Allicin Precautions

Follow the manufacturer's guidance for complete precautions. Research shows that allicin can be taken with most medications with no adverse effects. However, if you are diabetic or taking blood thinners or blood pressure medication or if you have any questions about using stabilized allicin with your medications, then check with your doctor.

Symptoms of detoxification may occur when using stabilized allicin, which may temporarily increase symptoms. If this occurs, reduce the usage amount and build up slowly to the desired level according to your tolerance. See the chapter "Healing Crisis and Detoxification Support" on page 217 for more details about detoxification and how to address its symptoms.

The potency of stabilized allicin may cause a temporary stinging sensation when used on the skin. If irritation occurs and persists, rinse with cold water until discomfort has stopped and discontinue use.

Manuka Honey

Very different from regular supermarket honey, Manuka honey is a unique medicinal product with many infection-fighting and health-enhancing properties. People have found Manuka honey to be more potent than antibiotics for healing infected wounds. Manuka honey is safe, inexpensive, easy to find and simple to use and has activity against Staph and MRSA biofilms[23].

Researchers at the University of Waikato in New Zealand have found that Manuka honey's antibacterial activity stops the growth of MRSA bacteria. They've also found that Manuka honey has no adverse effects on healthy tissue and can be safely inserted into wound cavities and the sinuses to clear an infection. Such medicinal uses should never be attempted with ordinary supermarket honey.

Manuka honey is available in different strengths, depending on the quantity of the naturally occurring antibacterial agent in the honey. The higher the level of antibacterial agents, the more potent the honey. Dr. Thomas Henle of the University of Dresden, Germany discovered that Methylglyoxal (often designated with the initials MGO) is a key antibacterial compound in the honey that can kill bacteria like *Staph aureus*.

Manuka Honey Labeling Fraud

Because of manuka honey's popularity, adulteration with regular honey and labeling fraud have become a big problem in the last few years. There is little to stop a dishonest company from putting the words "UMF" and "active honey" on their product label to mislead people into buying an inferior quality product. One estimate is that approximately 80% of manuka honey products on the market are fraudulent[24]. Therefore, you have to be very wary about which brand of manuka honey you buy and where you get it.

One of the best ways to ensure genuine manuka honey is to look for products labeled with a license number from the UMF Honey Association. These licensed companies must follow strict testing, labeling and quality control guidelines and submit to audits by the association to maintain their license. Such rigorous controls ensure that manuka honey from a company that is licensed by the association is genuine manuka honey and is accurately labeled with a certified methylgloxal content. The following website has a list of UMF Honey Association licenses:

www.umf.org.nz/licensees

Finding Manuka Honey

High quality Manuka honey from New Zealand and Australia is readily available in sufficient potency for infection support. Use the following guidelines to find the best Manuka honey for your particular needs:

- Look for a UMF Honey Association license number on the label. Such a license ensures that the product is ligitimate UMF manuka honey.

- Look for a certified Manuka honey. This means that the level of the antibacterial agent has been tested and verified. Ideally, each lot of honey should be certified. If you don't purchase a certified honey, you may be getting regular table honey.

- Look for the designation UMF or MGO. UMF stands for Unique Manuka Factor and MGO is short for the antibacterial agent Methylglyoxal.

- Select a high UMF or MGO rating. UMF10 is the minimum to be of therapeutic value and corresponds to MGO 100.

  » UMF 10-15 (MGO 100 -250) is commonly used for external skin infections.

  » UMF 25+ (MGO 550) is a more potent choice for internal systemic support.

- The therapeutic properties of Manuka Honey increase with higher UMF or MGO ratings.

- Raw honey is preferable. Filtered and/or sterilized Manuka honey is also available if needed.

Using Manuka Honey

Manuka honey can be used on open wounds, skin infections and for sinus infections, but it can also be used internally for systemic support.

Wound Dressings

Below is a good method for using honey on wounds with dressings. The idea is to maximize contact between the wound and the honey by reducing the air-space in the gauze:

1. Clean the wound with hydrogen peroxide or as directed by your doctor.

2. Pre-soak a sterile gauze pad with manuka honey. Use approximately 20 mL (one ounce) for a 4 x 4 inch (10 x 10 cm) gauze pad.

3. Drizzle honey into the wound, including any cavities or depressions, and gently work the honey into the wound.

4. Cover wound with the pre-soaked gauze pad.

5. Cover the pre-soaked gauze pad with a waterproof dressing to reduce oozing of the honey onto clothing.

6. Secure the dressing to the skin using non-irritating adhesive or tape.

When using the method above, take care to avoid irritating the skin if you have frequent dressing changes. If bandages stick to the wound, replace the bandage more frequently, up to 3 times per day or as directed by your doctor. The section "Wound Dressing" on page 190 has more details about how to dress wounds.

Because every wound and infection is different, be sure to talk with your doctor for the best type and size of bandage or dressing to use and how often to replace it. If you have concerns, ask your doctor about any special precautions or steps to take before using the method above.

Internal Use

Manuka honey can be taken internally for systemic infection support and immune support. It is used just as you would any other kind of honey. Try on toast or in tea. Diabetics: take caution as you would with regular honey. Not for infants.

Sinus Rinses

Add approximately 1/2 teaspoon (or 2.5 mL) of honey to warmed sterile water with a teaspoon of salt. Add both to a neti pot or other sinus irrigation device and rinse nose and sinuses two times per day. Use a UMF 10-15+ for nasal irrigation. See the section "Sinus Rinsing" on page 191 for details about how to rinse the sinuses, including important safety precautions.

Manuka Honey Precautions

- Follow the manufacturer's guidance for complete precautions.

- Some people can have a rare allergic reaction to honey. Dr. Molan, director of the Honey Research Unit at the University of Waikato, has stated that "an allergic reaction may occur rarely, as happens with many foods, and diabetics should take into account the sugar content of honey, which is about 30% glucose." People suffering from eczema and bronchial asthma may be more sensitive to bee products. If you have ever had an allergic or hypersensitivity reaction to bee stings or bee products, you could have a reaction to Manuka honey too.

- Honey is a high-sugar food, so you want to moderate how much you consume. Sugar feeds infections and weakens the immune system, the last things you want if you have an infection. Using honey only for skin and sinus support is a safer option if blood sugar is a concern.

- Some people report a slight stinging or burning sensation when applying Manuka honey to wounds. If stinging occurs, it will usually subside within a few minutes. If it gets worse, remove the honey and rinse with warm water and try a lower UMF or MGO rated honey.

- Babies one year old or less should not ingest honey because of the risk of botulism (a type of bacteria commonly found in honey). Use only sterilized honey for babies.

Jarrah Honey

Manuka honey is not available in all parts of the world, especially in western Australia. Research has confirmed that honey from the Australian Jarrah forest has naturally high antibacterial properties. The Jarrah tree is actually a type of eucalyptus (*Eucalyptus marginata*), and as detailed in the section "Eucalyptus Oil" on page 142, eucalyptus has potent antibacterial properties.

Research performed by the Department of Agriculture and the Western Australia Beekeepers Association has found that Jarrah honey has been particularly effective in treating bacterial infections. Jarrah honey was found effective in treating wounds, burns and skin infections caused by Staph, MRSA, *E. coli* and Candida fungal infections. Jarrah honey can be used the same way as Manuka honey and has similar precautions as well.

Bee Propolis

Bees make a substance known as propolis, also known as *Russian penicillin*, which they use as construction glue for their hive. This substance also reduces the amount of bacteria in bee hives, serving as a natural defense for the hive. Propolis is a combination of beeswax and tree resins that have antibacterial qualities. Small amounts of propolis are found in honey. People have used propolis for over 2000 years on wounds and as a remedy for other ailments. Propolis was also used in traditional medicine practices in the 1600's in Europe.

Propolis has antibiotic and antiseptic properties and may also have antiviral and anti-inflammatory effects. It has also demonstrated activity against multiple strains of drug-resistant Staph bacteria in laboratory tests[25]. In addition to antibacterial properties, propolis also stimulates the immune system. You can find propolis in various forms in health food stores or better yet, get the raw form from beekeepers. Propolis is also available in capsule and tincture form to be taken internally. It can be used as a topical applicant for wounds. 500mg capsules, taken from 1 to 4 times daily, is a common practice for general infection support.

If you have had an allergic or hypersensitivity reaction to bee stings or bee products (including honey), you could react to propolis in the same way. People suffering from eczema and bronchial asthma may be more sensitive to bee products. In some individuals, frequent use of propolis can lead to reactions, such as swelling, fluid collection, redness, burning, eczema and fever.

Grapefruit Seed Extract (GSE)

Grapefruit seed extract was originally developed as an antiparasitic, but studies quickly showed it can inhibit the growth of fungi, viruses, and bacteria. The active ingredients of GSE are non-toxic and are extracted from the seed and pulp of grapefruit. The process converts the grapefruit bioflavonoids into an extremely potent compound that has been found to kill Streptococcus, Staph, Salmonella, *E. coli*, Candida, herpes, influenza, parasites, fungi, and more.

Using GSE

- GSE can be used internally as a natural broad-spectrum antibacterial.

- GSE has been added to cleaning sprays to make household disinfectants. GSE can also be added to laundry and to shampoo and body soaps for added antibacterial support.

- **GSE Precautions:** Follow the manufacturer's guidance for complete precautions. When taken daily, GSE seldom produces a significant allergic reaction, however, people who are allergic to citrus fruits should exercise caution in the use of GSE. Large amounts could lead to diarrhea.

Intravenous Vitamin C Therapy

The benefits of long-term vitamin C consumption in excess of the U.S. government recommended daily allowance (RDA) are widely acknowledged and include reduced risks of cancer, cardiovascular disease, and cataracts. Helpfulness has been reported for severe attacks of advanced human cancers and ulcerative colitis. Reports include intravenous (IV) usage amounts ranging from 50 to 150 grams per day, with no adverse effects reported.

Dr. Thomas E. Levy, a practicing physician for 25 years, is a board-certified internist and a fellow of the American College of Cardiology as well as an attorney. Dr. Levy's book *Vitamin C, Infectious Diseases, and Toxins: Curing the Incurable* outlines the work of Dr. Frederick Klenner who studied vitamin C and treating extremely ill patients with a variety of diseases. Dr. Klenner used mega-doses of vitamin C, intravenously (through an IV) on many patients who were extremely ill and often close to death. After injecting vitamin C, he found that most patients returned to health. Dr. Levy's book presents clear evidence that vitamin C affects disease and his book holds a lofty 1,200 scientific references. The website www.VitaminCFoundation.org is a good resource on vitamin C.

Using IV Vitamin C Therapy

High dose IV vitamin C is a valid MRSA treatment option, especially if you are admitted to a hospital and antibiotics have been unsuccessful. While most natural and alternative remedies can be challenging or impossible to administer in hospitals, IV vitamin C therapy may be administered with a little advanced preparation and planning. For tips and support on how to get IV vitamin C administered in a hospital, see the webpage www.doctoryourself.com/strategies.html.

Outside the hospital, it's easier to find a naturopath or other alternative healthcare professional who will administer high dose vitamin C intravenously. It is not possible to take enough by mouth to achieve the high levels of vitamin C required.

Colloidal Silver

Silver ions are naturally antibacterial and antifungal. Colloidal silver refers to microscopic particles of silver that are held in a liquid suspension. Prior to the 1930's when antibiotics arrived, colloidal silver was used widely by physicians as a mainstream antibiotic. Colloidal silver was used for everything from colds to infections. Silver creams have been used in burn clinics for over 100 years. Silver coins were placed in drinking vessels to reduce the spoilage rate of milk. While alternative medicine praises its use as an antibiotic, mainstream medicine considers silver somewhat of a poison. Colloidal silver has a safe and proven track record when used as a topical antibiotic, and many people use it internally with success.

Colloidal silver is antibacterial at concentrations of 5 parts per million or higher. One study showed a high level of activity of colloidal silver against highly resistant MRSA, however, the activity was dependent on the particle size of the silver[26]. Colloidal silver has even been approved by the EPA as an effective MRSA killing disinfectant for hospitals and medical centers.

Even with its long history as a remedy and present day approved uses, the FDA has issued warnings to colloidal silver manufacturers that they cannot claim it has any use as an antibiotic or for medicinal uses. In the 1940s, the FDA began its decades-long oppression of medicinal silver under the premise that it was unsafe. Of interest is that Curaid bandages use colloidal silver and were recently approved by the FDA for such use.

There are many colloidal silver products on the market today. However you should be careful and do your research before using colloidal silver, especially internally.

Using Colloidal Silver

Products with 20% ionic silver and the rest silver particles (silver particle size of 2 nanometers or smaller) are preferred for quality medicinal uses. Home machines that make colloidal silver do not make this quality of silver.

Colloidal silver has been used successfully for external infections. It can be found in sprays and creams for skin application. Colloidal silver has also been taken internally. According to Dr. James F. and Phyllis A. Balch, colloidal silver has been shown to be effective against more than 650 different disease-causing microorganisms[27]. Be sure to follow product indications and directions if you choose to use colloidal silver medicinally.

Colloidal Silver Precautions

Follow the manufacturer's guidance for complete precautions. Many sources indicate that high quality colloidal silver products are safe for external or internal use. However, a very rare medical condition called Argyria which causes an irreversible gray skin coloration can occur if large quantities of improperly prepared silver accumulate in the body. Despite the fact that silver is a heavy metal, there have been very few reports of toxicity, especially if the product is used as indicated.

Because silver is a heavy metal, and because it serves no natural need in the human body, some people feel that it should only be used externally for skin applications. While silver has well established antibacterial activity, it does nothing to support the body to fight infections in other ways, such as immune support. Unless other steps are also taken, such as immune support and addressing the root cause of the infection, silver may provide little protection against recurring outbreaks.

Viral Phage Therapy

A bacteriophage or phage is a live virus that targets and invades bacterial cells and can cause them to self-destruct. Unlike viruses that cause a cold or flu by infecting cells of the human body, these viruses only attack bacterial cells, not human cells. Phage therapy is the therapeutic use of these bacteriophages to treat infections like MRSA. The side effects are typically less than those associated with using antibiotics and phages don't appear to create any resistance issues in bacteria.

Phage therapy is not widely known in the United States, but research centers can be found in Poland and the Republic of Georgia. This technology has been in use in the Republic of Georgia for many years and is starting to enter the U.S. and Canada. The phages have been modified to target MRSA or other strains of pathogenic bacteria. This is a relatively new technological for infection control and may require additional long-term safety studies before it is accepted in the U.S.

Phage Therapy Pros and Cons

Phage therapy operates using valid microbiological principles and thus far has been relatively free from side effects. The therapy can be quite successful and the author has heard first hand accounts of how well the therapy has worked. However, any time a genetically engineered organism is used, especially a virus, there is always the potential for unanticipated consequences.

While phage therapy appears to be quite successful in the short term, the therapy alone does nothing to change the conditions inside the body that allowed an infection in the first place. Therefore, the therapy may not help against long-term recurring infections. Stopping an active infection is certainly important, and phage therapy may be an effective way to do it. However, unless other steps are also taken, such as immune support and addressing L-forms and biofilms, the infection may come back again later.

Other Herbs and Botanicals

The herbal remedies described in this section can provide benefits during an infection, especially when combined with more potent antibacterial remedies.

Ginger

Ginger has been used to relieve colds and flu. Ginger may also stimulate the immune system and aid its ability to fight infections. Ginger can also help with stomach upset and has aided many people with nausea from antibiotic use. As a precaution, be sure to consult with your doctor if you take blood anticoagulants and want to use ginger.

Turmeric

Some people have experienced good results with MRSA using the herb turmeric. Turmeric has antimicrobial, anti-allergic, anti-inflammatory, antioxidant, anti-ulcer, antiviral, anti-cancer, and immune-stimulant actions. One of the main active ingredients is curcumin, which has demonstrated strong activity against MRSA bacteria[28].

Turmeric is available bottled in prepared capsules for internal use. Look for brands that contain 95% or more curcumin. For powdered turmeric, a common usage amount is 1 teaspoon of turmeric powder in half a glass of warm water taken internally 3 times per day. This amount can be continued for several days or more. You can find turmeric powder in bulk at health food stores or Indian food stores.

Follow the manufacturer's guidance for complete precautions. Turmeric can cause constipation for some people. Magnesium may alleviate constipation. Turmeric may cause dehydration, especially at night, so be sure to drink several glasses of plain water after taking turmeric. Turmeric is a natural blood thinner so do not take it with anticoagulants. Turmeric stimulates the secretion of bile and should be avoided if you have a blocked bile duct.

Goldenseal

In addition to being an immune system stimulant, goldenseal is well established as an antibacterial and antiviral agent. A key immune-like compound called berberine has been found in goldenseal (and gentian) and is supportive of the immune system. Goldenseal has been shown to be antibacterial and has multiple mechanisms of activity against MRSA[29,30]. One study showed that berberine can boost the anti-MRSA effectiveness of some antibiotics when the drugs and berberine are used together[31].

For support of the intestinal flora, goldenseal's ability to restore mucus membrane integrity inside the stomach and intestines can be beneficial. Goldenseal also stimulates the release of bile because of its bitter alkaloid content. Bile is important in the detoxification process as it helps remove toxins from the body through the intestines.

Because of the potential negative GI effects from using too much goldenseal, this herb is best blended along with other beneficial plants rather than using it by itself in high amounts. Adding goldenseal to an herbal blend is the best way to provide the right amount of bile stimulation and detox without side effects.

Milk Thistle

Milk thistle is a widely respected detoxification aid that also helps protect liver cells. Supporting the optimal functioning of the liver further enhances detoxification effects. The liver takes the brunt of detoxifying the body. Many antibiotic and pharmaceutical drugs and some herbal preparations when used over time can stress the liver, making liver support and detoxification even more important. Because of milk thistle's cleansing effects, it can be a helpful addition to herbal blends for dealing with infections.

Cordyceps

Cordyceps has a long history of being used in ancient China, Nepal and Tibet as a medicinal fungi or mushroom. Pharmaceutical companies use cordyceps as the source of the drug Cyclosporine, an important transplant anti-rejection drug. However, cordyceps is also useful as an herbal remedy for immune support and to boost energy during the recovery stage after an infection.

Laboratory studies show that cordyceps promotes T-cell growth and helps lymphocytes to survive longer. This multi-dimensional action on the immune system can be a great benefit when the body is fighting an infection.

Echinacea

Echinacea offers support for your body's immune system and is also antibacterial. Studies have demonstrated echinacea's effectiveness against bacterial, fungal and viral infections. Echinacea also reduces inflammation and can be effective in treating various skin problems, including wounds, eczema, acne, boils and psoriasis. This herb can also decrease the recovery time from an infection.

Echinacea is generally not taken for prolonged periods of time as a regular preventative. Taking it longer than 3 to 4 weeks will make it lose its effectiveness. Echinacea is best avoided if you have an allergy to ragweed or have an autoimmune disorder.

Botanical Herbal Blends

Blending multiple botanical herbs together into a single product can provide unique benefits beyond those available from any single herb by itself. Synergistic blends of botanicals can provide excellent broad-spectrum support and maximum therapeutic potency.

For example, herbs that provide broad-spectrum antibacterial action can be blended with herbs that assist with detoxification of bacterial waste products. Botanical substances that modulate or support the immune system can also be added to provide multiple dimensions of benefit.

Active botanical substances can have a complex array of major, minor and trace ingredients. A single herb can also have multiple modes of action and create different effects in the body. Therefore, skill, experience and expertise are required to formulate herbal blends that are both safe and effective for their intended use. When combining more than one herb, the complex web of interactions between all the individual components must be considered.

Quality, potency and proper balance of the formulation all matter when choosing a botanical blend for infection support. Below are important qualities to look for in a botanical blend:

- Is the product tested for purity, along with certificates of analysis?

- Is the product potency stated on the label? Is it a professional grade formulation?

- Does the product have a history of safe clinical usage? Is the product used by naturopathic or medical doctors for infection support?

- Is the product made in a facility that follows Good Manufacturing Practices (GMP) to control the product quality and consistency?

- Are there artificial ingredients, preservatives, fillers, colorings, additives or common allergens in the formulation?

Olive Leaf Blend

One particular botanical blend is formulated for controlling bacteria with several herbs chosen for their synergistic antibacterial, immune support, restorative and detoxification properties. This herbal blend includes Olive Leaf Extract (at least 18% Oleuropein, 1375 mg per capsule), Garlic, Goldenseal, Milk Thistle, Cordyceps and other complementary herbs. It is gentle, easy to use, safe for all ages and broadly active against many types of infections.

Biocide Blend

Another botanical blend is formulated for broad-spectrum antibacterial and immune system support that targets the intestines and supports digestion. This concentrated liquid herbal blend contains Bilberry Extract, Black Walnut, Noni, Echinacea, Goldenseal, Gentian, Oregano Oil, Shiitake, Grapeseed Extract and other complementary botanicals.

Botanical Blend Protocol

The Olive Leaf Blend and the Biocide Blend can be combined with a specially formulated Probiotic Blend to produce a 3-part protocol for broad-spectrum infection control. The probiotic in the 3-part protocol is detailed in the section "Probiotic Flora Blend" on page 214.

The Botanical Blend Protocol in the following table consists of three remedies and five different usage amounts, depending on the severity of the challenge and the age group. For adults who are new to the protocol, starting with the beginning usage amount for the first few days will help ensure that the blends are well tolerated before taking higher amounts.

The moderate usage amount is ideal for active infection challenges in adults. However, if extra support is needed, then slowly increasing to the maximum usage amount over a few days can be helpful. Make sure the blends are well tolerated before moving up to the maximum amount. The moderate or maximum usage amounts may be used until symptoms resolve. After the infection has cleared, the maintenance amount may be used by adults as a long-term preventative and for ongoing immune support.

Children's usage varies depending on the child's age. The amounts for children are smaller than for adults and are based on the child's body weight. Note that the Olive Leaf Blend and Probiotic Blend should not be taken by very young children.

Follow the manufacturer's guidance for complete precautions. The Botanical Blend Protocol and it's components have not been tested or approved for use by those who are pregnant and is not recommended during pregnancy. Nursing mothers should use 1/2 the adult amount for both the herbal and biocide blends. Consult a healthcare practitioner qualified to recommend herbal medicine in any case that is severe or unresponsive. Do not use the herbal or biocide blends before surgery as some herbs may have a blood thinning effect.

Usage Amount	Biocide Blend	Olive Leaf Blend	Probiotic Blend
Beginning	1 - 2 drops three times per day. Take half an hour before meals.	1 capsule twice per day. May be taken at the same time as the Biocide Blend	5 pumps in a quarter cup of water, twice per day. Take at least 1 hour apart from the Biocide or Olive Leaf blends as the herbs can reduce the probiotic potency if taken at the same time. If using other probiotic products, take this at the same time.
Moderate	3 - 5 drops three times per day. Take half an hour before meals.	2 capsules twice per day. May be taken at the same time as the Biocide Blend	
Maximum	6 - 10 drops three times per day. Take half an hour before meals.	2 capsules three times per day. May be taken at the same time as the Biocide Blend	
Maintenance	5 drops once per day. Take half an hour before meals.	1 capsule once per day. May be taken at the same time as the Biocide Blend	5 pumps in a quarter cup of water, once per day. Take at least 1 hour apart from the Biocide and Olive Leaf blends.

Usage Amount	Biocide Blend	Olive Leaf Blend	Probiotic Blend
Children	**Children under 12:** 1 drop for every 10 pounds of body weight per day, in divided amounts*. Take half an hour before meals. **Severe cases:** up to 2 drops per 10 pounds of body weight per day may be used if well tolerated. **Maintenance:** half a drop per 10 pounds of body weight per day may be used for long-term immune support. *** Divided amounts:** Divide the usage amount to twice a day. Example: a 40 lb child could take 2 drops AM and 2 drops PM, for a total of 4 drops a day.	**Children under age 12 use.** Use the Biocide Blend only. **Ages 7 - 12:** children who can swallow a capsule may use half a capsule twice per day. **Teens:** 1 capsule twice per day. Gradually work up to the usage amount listed for children less than age 12.	**Do not use the Probiotic Blend with children under age 2.** Consider a probiotic product made especially for infants or babies instead. **Age 2 - 12:** 2 pumps in a quarter cup of water. Gradually work up to the usage amount listed for children less than age 12.

◇◇

NOTE: See "Michelle's Recommended Products" on page 303 for product resources

◇◇

Energetic Medicine

Energetic medicine is a complement to the other therapies listed in this book. Energetic medicine comes in two different forms, one that can be physically or scientifically measured (like sound or vibrational therapy), and one that has yet to be measured (such as prayer). Any type of energy medicine technique is usually considered *alternative* by conventional medical standards, however, such techniques are gaining popularity in the United States. Many people repeatedly experience that prayer and spirituality help maintain a sense of purpose, meaning, and hope in the face of pain, suffering, and uncertainty.

Energy medicine practitioners believe that illness is caused in part by disturbances of the bodies subtle energies. For example, more than 2,000 years ago, Asian practitioners postulated that the flow and balance of life energies called *Qi* are necessary for maintaining health and they developed tools to restore them. Herbal medicine and acupuncture originated from such practitioners. Acupuncture is the stimulation of specific points on the body by a variety of techniques, including inserting thin metal needles though the skin. It is intended to remove blockages in the flow of Qi and restore and maintain health.

Energy medicine can help balance and restore the body which will be helpful for any disease process as well as your mental, spiritual and emotional state. For a good starting place to discover the many options available, go to the National Center for Complementary and Alternative Medicine (CAM) & NIH website at: https://nccih.nih.gov/health/integrative-health. Some of the most common energy medicine techniques include the following:

- **Reiki** therapists claim that Reiki enhances immunity and the body's ability to heal itself.

- **Prayer,** either performed by you or someone praying for you. See the section "Prayer and Meditation" on page 235 for more on this topic.

- **Qi gong**, a Chinese practice of energizing the body is gaining popularity in North America.

- **Healing touch**. The therapist is purported to identify imbalances and correct a client's energy by passing his or her hands over the patient.

- **Acupuncture** stimulates and restores the energy flow in the body.

- **Acupressure** is similar to acupuncture, but uses no needles, only pressure on the skin. For more information on a simple acupressure technique you can perform yourself, see "Emotional Freedom Technique (EFT)" on page 311.

10 Essential Oil ABCs

Essential oils are the aromatic and volatile liquids extracted from the flowers, leaves, seeds, stems, bark and roots of herbs, shrubs and trees through a process called distillation. These oils are highly concentrated and one of the most potent forms of botanical medicine. Essential oils are in essence the plant's immune system which protects it against other plants, insects and bacterial or fungal infections.

Because plants are constantly changing their chemical composition to help them adapt to the ever-changing environment, the resulting essential oils also change in composition over time. This evolving nature combined with inherent chemical complexity has created a superior natural antibiotic with little room for bacteria to develop resistance.

In this chapter, you'll discover the basics of how essential oils work and the different ways they can be used for infection support. You'll also learn how to detect worthless and potentially dangerous oils, and most importantly, how to find genuine essential oils that are safe and effective.

What are Essential Oils?

Essential oils are extremely concentrated which makes them very powerful[32]. For instance, it takes 60,000 roses to make just one ounce of rose oil[33]. In fact, essential oils are 70 times more concentrated than what is found in the plants they are extracted from[34]. Essential oils are so potent that just one drop can have powerful health effects on the body. Amazingly, once applied topically, essential oils are absorbed through the skin and travel systemically throughout the body within seconds[35]. For example, some users note that oils applied on their feet can be tasted in their mouth in less than a minute. Essential oils also have very pleasing and therapeutic aromas which led to the term *aromatherapist* to describe people who specialize in the application of oils for health and wellness purposes.

Essential oils are not to be confused with perfume or fragrance oils. Essential oils are distilled from plants, while perfume oils are artificially created in a laboratory. Perfume oils offer no therapeutic or healing properties.

The main components of most essential oils belong to a class of natural chemical compounds called terpenes and phenylpropanoids. Terpenes are also the basic unit of structure for a number of important compounds in the human body, including steroids and vitamin A. The close chemical similarity between essential oils and crucial biological molecules provides a hint as to why essential oils are often so medicinally potent[36]. The table below shows the relationship between terpene structure, essential oils and other compounds required for bodily functions.

Class of terpene	Found in
Monoterpenes	Essential oils
Sesquiterpenes	Essential oils
Diterpenes	Essential oils and resins, Vitamin A, phytol
Triterpenes	Steroids, heart glycosides
Tetraterpenes	Carotenoids, xanthophylls
Phenylpropanoids	Essential oils, amino acids

While terpenes and phenylpropanoids make up the bulk of essential oil ingredients, hundreds of minor and trace components, some of which are extremely potent, are responsible for many of the medicinal and antibacterial properties of essential oils[37]. In particular, the smell of essential oils is commonly due to minute trace components in the oil. Some of these components have a noticeable odor at concentrations as low at 0.0002 parts per billion.

Modern Medicinal Uses of Essential Oils

Essential oils have been used for thousands of years, dating back to the ancient Egyptians and possibly beyond[38]. According to ancient Chinese manuscripts and Egyptian hieroglyphics, essential oils were used to heal the sick, making oils one of the oldest forms of medicine known to man. Two thousand years ago, frankincense and myrrh essential oils were gifts brought to baby Jesus and other essential oils were referenced many times throughout the Bible. In some ancient cultures, essential oils were literally more valuable than gold.

Today, essential oils such as eucalyptus and tea tree have been proven effective at stopping MRSA in hospital patients, both alone and in combination with antibiotic drugs[39]. Tea tree has also proven to be an effective alternative to mupirocin nasal ointment and triclosan body wash for MRSA decolonization[40].

Much of the research done on essential oils has been performed in France. Julie Lawless is an aromatherapy expert and she notes that French medical doctors and French hospitals routinely prescribe essential oils as an alternative to using antibiotics. They use essential oils primarily for respiratory infections, but they've also been found useful against skin infections, digestive system infections, and infections of the urinary tract and reproductive organs.

Of all of the illnesses and health problems that exist today, essential oils are widely regarded by oil experts to be particularly effective for use against infectious diseases, including MRSA and Staph[41]. Several oils in particular have broad and potent antibacterial and infection-fighting properties[42] and a large percentage of all known essential oils have at least moderate antimicrobial effects. This level of antimicrobial activity is no surprise, given that the key role of essential oils in nature is to protect plants from infectious and invasive organisms. This makes essential oils one of the most powerful and beneficial allies available today for infection support.

Antibiotic Resistance and Essential Oils

Plants have evolved and adapted to life on Earth over great expanses of time. Essential oils derived from these plants have hundreds and sometimes thousands of active chemical compounds in specific ratios and amounts that work together in complex, multi-dimensional and self-balancing ways. On the other hand, antibiotic drugs have been around for less than a century and typically have only one synthetic active ingredient and a simple one-dimensional mode of action. Mainstream medicine and the industrial farming industry have overused, abused and misused antibiotics for decades, giving bacteria more opportunities to become resistant[43]. Bacteria are very crafty and intelligent and can arm themselves easily against such a simple and often improperly used weapon as antibiotic drugs.

Fortunately, bacteria have not shown the ability to overcome hundreds of chemical components as found in essential oils. According to internationally recognized essential oil experts, there have been no superbugs created by therapeutic, high quality essential oils. The same cannot be said of antibiotics, as bacteria have learned to become resistant to many of these so called *miracle drugs*[44]. As more superbugs learn to resist more antibiotics each year, the importance of antibiotic alternatives such as essential oils becomes more clear.

Activity Against Biofilms

Two ways that MRSA and Staph bacteria can resist treatment and cause recurring infections are biofilms and L-form *stealth* bacteria. The U.S. National Institute of Health (NIH) states that biofilms are linked to 80% of recurring infections[45]. L-forms of cell wall deficient bacteria, are another way that MRSA and Staph evade treatment and cause recurring infections[46].

Fortunately, essential oils have activity against biofilms and stealth bacteria. As bacteria developed the ability to create biofilms in nature, so too plants evolved the ability to counteract this threat. In particular,

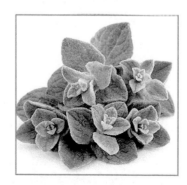

Oregano oil provides potent infection support and contains compounds that attack biofilms.

tea tree oil and the key active ingredient in oregano oil have shown activity against biofilms of Staph bacteria[47, 48].

While there are dozens of essential oils that can be beneficial for infection support, this book highlights only the most potent, effective and safe oils and methods. Keep in mind that the mainstream medical community has not yet recognized the importance or benefits of essential oils or most other alternative therapies, despite the growing scientific research on their effectiveness against infections. Therefore, as is true of most alternative remedies, your doctor is unlikely to be familiar with essential oils.

Essential Oils Uses

The great variety of essential oils, along with their potent, liquid form, lend these concentrated plant extracts to a variety of uses. Because of the nature of essential oils, their medicinal components are readily absorbed through the skin and into the bloodstream. For example, significant amounts of an essential oil can enter the bloodstream though skin application and air diffusion.

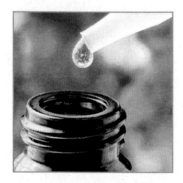

The liquid form and highly concentrated nature of essential oils lends them to many different uses.

Below are some of the most common ways that essential oils are used for medicinal, therapeutic purposes or to support overall health and wellbeing. Detailed protocols for use of specific oils will be covered in the chapter "Essential Oil Protocols for Use" on page 137.

- **External or topical skin application** is the most common way to use essential oils. Because a few popular oils are hot or spicy (capable of burning the skin), they are diluted in a carrier oil before applying to the skin. For details, refer to "Applying Essential Oils Topically" on page 129.

- **Bathing** with essential oils can provide many benefits, including skin decolonization of bacteria. The general bathing procedure will be covered in "Bathing With Essential Oils" on page 134.

- **Inhalation of oils** via a diffuser is another popular method of use that is detailed in the section "How to Air Diffuse Essential Oils" on page 132.

- Essential oils are often **added to personal care products** such as soaps, lotions and shampoo. Oils can also be added to **laundry** wash water and to homemade **cleaning** and sanitizing products to aid in bacterial control around the home. Personal care product uses are detailed in the chapter "Essential Oil Protocols for Use" on page 137.

- **Oral or internal use** of essential oils can be performed safely when using the proper oil quality and taking the proper precautions. For an overview of the pros, cons and alternatives to internal use, see the section "Taking Essential Oils Internally" on page 130.

What You Must Know to Find Safe and Effective Oils

When using essential oils for demanding infection or health related purposes, quality, purity and potency are all critically important to ensure safety and effectiveness[49]. Unfortunately, essential oils are one of the most adulterated, confusing and misleading products in the wellness industry.

The majority of essential oils produced around the world are laboratory-made for the perfume and cosmetic industry and are wholly inappropriate, ineffective, and downright dangerous for medicinal and therapeutic uses, especially for internal uses[50]. The essential oils generally used in North America, as found in health food stores, bath, culinary, and beauty shops, are also not suitable for most medicinal uses.

A Note About Store-Bought Oils

People who are new to essential oils are usually tempted to drive to the nearest health food store and buy the first oils they find. It's also tempting to try an inferior quality essential oil in an attempt to save time or money. Unfortunately, your safety and your health could be at risk from using the wrong grade of oil.

The majority of store-bought essential oils are not made for or intended for medicinal, therapeutic or internal uses. Moreover, reading the product label or the manufacturer's website or brochure probably won't tell you how safe, effective or appropriate the oil is for controlling infections. If you want to get the right kind of oils for infection support that are both safe and effective, then there are some key things you need to know, as outlined in the sections below.

Essential Oils to AVOID

95% of all essential oils on the market are not appropriate for medicinal uses. To make matters worse, essential oil labeling can be very confusing and misleading. The following tips will help you to understand what essential oil labels and claims really mean and will help you avoid inferior oils:

Be Wary of 100% Pure or Therapeutic Oil

The terms *100% pure* and *natural* sound like good things, right? Unfortunately, oils that are labeled as *pure* or *100% pure* are allowed to have as little as 51% essential oil by law. Therefore, the word *pure* on the label doesn't really mean anything. It's a common practice by many companies to use an extender oil like almond or safflower oil as a base to dilute the essential oil in order to cut costs or to restrict the range of potential uses. This creates a slower acting oil that is much less effective for some types of uses. Extender oils can also become rancid quickly, reducing how long the essential oil will last.

There are also no laws regulating how the term *therapeutic* is used on labels or advertising materials. You must know what additional factors to look for to help ensure a true therapeutic oil.

Be Wary of Certified Aromatherapy Grade or Perfume Oils

Some oils are certified as being *aromatherapy grade* oils, but this does not necessarily mean they are therapeutic grade oils. The criteria that define aromatherapy grade do not guarantee sufficient quality for therapeutic and medicinal uses.

Avoid Synthetic Oils

Synthetic oils are chemically created in a laboratory. The terms *pure* and *100% pure* can also be used for synthetic essential oils. Most essential oils also contain some artificial synthetic ingredients. Such ingredients are not made from actual plants and should be avoided. At best, they will not be effective. At worst, such oils will be toxic and harmful to your health if used medicinally.

Be Wary of AFNOR and ISO Certified Oils

Standards for essential oils have been developed by the Association French Normalization Organization Regulation (AFNOR). Some oils indicate International Standards Organization (ISO) certification on their label. AFNOR certified oils pertain to perfume and fragrance grade oils but are irrelevant to medicinal oils. Therefore, AFNOR certification on the label is a good sign of a perfume or fragrance oil, and should thus not be used for therapeutic or medicinal purposes.

ISO certification has to do with the internal controls, customer support and business management systems of a business organization or company. However, ISO certification has nothing to do with the actual quality of the essential oil or other products the company makes. Therefore, ISO certification is helpful, but doesn't mean much on its own with respect to therapeutic quality.

Avoid Absolutes and Chemically Extracted Oils

Perfume oils are generally extracted using heat and chemical solvents to speed extraction times and boost product yields. Absolute essential oils are extracted with a solvent, usually alcohol or a not-so-nice chemical called hexane. Absolutes are not suitable for therapeutic use.

Unfortunately, chemicals such as hexane and other chemical residuals from extraction remain in the essential oil and will enter your body when used therapeutically. Therapeutic quality essential oils should be steam distilled only, never chemically extracted.

Avoid the Incorrect Plant Species

Inferior oils are sometimes made by blending oils extracted from different parts of the plant that can be hazardous to your health if used medicinally. Some oil products are made from cheaper or less therapeutic plant species and then misleadingly labeled as a therapeutic grade oil.

Lavender oil is a prime example, where hybrid *lavandin* species are often used instead of the genuine and authentic *Lavandula augustifolia vera* species. To help avoid a possibly toxic or ineffective product, only use oils from the plant species mentioned in the chapter "Essential Oil Protocols for Use" on page 137 or those recommended by an essential oil expert or health professional.

What to Look For in Essential Oils

As you can tell, not all essential oils are created equal. When using essential oils for health related purposes, you want to use a genuine therapeutic essential oil, preferably organic or wild-crafted. And for the most potent healing oils, you also need the right growing and harvesting conditions. The soil, irrigation, location, elevation, weather and time of harvest can all increase or decrease the chemical healing properties within the plant, and should be included and recognized by the manufacturer as a factor of oil quality.

The best way to ensure the quality of an essential oil is to investigate the source of an essential oil, starting with the grower and progressing through the distiller, broker, seller/bottler and finally to the retail source. You can also recognize genuine therapeutic grade oils by the product's aromatic body, the price, by those who endorse it and by its organic certification (if available). Endorsement by a doctor, pharmacist or research facility trained in reading gas chromatograms of essential oils is ideal. The following tips will help you to identify genuine therapeutic grade essential oils.

Only Use Steam Distilled Oils

Therapeutic quality essential oils should be steam distilled using water, low heat and low pressure to retain as much of the living essence of the plant as possible. Steam distillation is a slow, inefficient and a much more expensive process than other extraction methods, but the extra quality, effectiveness and therapeutic safety are well worth the added cost.

Some oils are being extracted using a new method called supercritical fluid extraction, which uses carbon dioxide as an extraction agent. Such oils are quite expensive and their therapeutic qualities have not yet been well established.

Look For GC and GC/MS Testing

Some oils come with a certification of *premium therapeutic grade*. Absence of this certification may mean adulteration of an authentic essential oil. Therapeutic essential oils should be tested by a third party professional using gas chromatography (GC) and/or mass spectrometry (GC/MS) analysis.

GC and GC/MS tests determine which chemical components are in the oils. Such tests seek to indicate the purity of the oil, the presence of any adulteration and the percentage of the individual naturally occurring chemical constituents of the plant. These tests can also detect impurities such as pesticides and if synthetic oils have been added.

Ideally a third-party professional should conduct GC and GC/MS testing, not the manufacturer of the oil. Manufacturers who certify the oils themselves have been known to manipulate the testing data. Third-party testing is always best and lends more credibility to the testing results.

It is very important to recognize that GC testing by itself is of little value unless a controlled standard is used to compare the GC test results with. A database of reference GC standard chromatograms must be used to get the most benefit out of GC test results. Likewise, the people looking at the results and comparing them to the reference standards must be very knowledgeable and experienced to discern the oil's quality. Each oil is different and has its own unique GC *fingerprint* of quality. The often subtle clues of adulteration and impurities are unique to each type of oil, requiring extensive experience and expertise on the part of the oil's tester.

Get Organic and Wild Crafted Oils When Available

Whenever possible, choose an organic and/or wild crafted essential oil. Organic essential oils are produced from plants that are grown in accordance with organic agricultural standards. Such plants should be free of pesticides, which can be concentrated during the distillation process. Wild-crafted plants, which means the plants were grown wild in nature, should also be free of pesticides.

Some oils are not available as organic or wild-crafted. And some high-quality growers and distillers may be small, family run farms that have not yet received organic certification. If available, both organic and wild-crafted oils are preferable to non-organic and farmed plants. Amazingly, some therapeutic oils are labeled as organic, but use chemicals to extract the oils from the plant, which leaves unhealthy chemical byproducts in the *organic* oil. Therefore, organic designation by itself is not the sole indicator of an oil's quality or medicinal safety or effectiveness.

Advantages of EOBBD Tested Oils

EOBBD is an indicator of high standards for premium, therapeutic grade essential oils and helps ensure an oil's medicinal value[51]. EOBBD stands for *Essential Oil Botanically and Biochemically Defined* and indicates a rigorous series of tests and quality control measures. This testing was historically carried out by a single laboratory in France to ensure essential oils of sufficient quality to be used for medical purposes by physicians. The original EOBBD laboratory has ceased its certification. However, testing to the same standards of EOBBD purity is possible if the correct reference GC chromatograms are used in addition to following the strict parameters and quality requirements below:

- **Botanical definition** – verification that the correct plant species was used.

- **Confirmation of producing organ** – the essence formed in the plant varies depending on the producing organ, such as flowers, leaves, fruits, stems or roots.

- **Extraction method** – water vapor extraction should be used, employing the correct volume, pressure, distillation time, harvest freshness and other parameters.

- **Growing and cultivation** – the growing location and conditions, cultivation methods and harvesting and soil microbiological analysis are all defined and certified.

- **Biochemical analysis** – the exact molecular fingerprint of the oil is measured using gas chromatography-mass spectrometry (GC-MS) and compared against a reference library for identification, purity and correct levels and ratios of major and minor molecular components.

Formulator Expertise and Experience

In the realm of essential oils, there's no substitute for experience and expertise on the part of the person who formulates the oils. Although EOBBD testing and other signs of a therapeutic quality are helpful and important, such quality indicators fail to paint the full picture of an oil's quality. Several additional factors can have a noticeable impact on an oil's potency. Such factors must be combined with proper sourcing and formulating to provide the highest quality oils.

For example, an essential oil's quality can be affected by several environmental factors such as the geographical region, humidity, altitude, climate, soil health, growing conditions and harvest method and season. Even the time of day the plant is harvested can affect the oil's therapeutic value. Such factors are not part of standard testing and quality practices. Therefore, it's up to the formulator to know how these factors affect each individual oil and source products accordingly.

A good example of the importance of the growing environment is lavender essential oil. Unless lavender is grown in acidic and fungal soil at a high altitude, the therapeutic quality of the oil will be reduced. Growing lavender in normally fertilized bacterial soils at lower altitudes changes the ratios of its chemical components, making it less therapeutically active, or not therapeutically active at all. Some manufacturers get around this problem by adding synthetic components to the oil to bring the ratios back within normal range: an adulteration short-cut that compromises the pure nature and the medicinal effects of the oil.

The Cost of Quality

Cost is usually a reliable indicator of a genuine therapeutic essential oil. These oils are simply more expensive because of the higher cost involved to grow, produce and test a higher quality oil. Synthetic oils and the use of cheap extenders dilutes the true oil in a product, thus lowering production costs. The use of chemical solvents and heat speeds up the extraction process and yields more oil product, both of which lower production costs. Growing species of plants that are hardier (though less therapeutic) and growing those plants in large farms using pesticides and industrial farming practices further reduces products costs. The end result is cheap, synthetic perfume-grade oils, which make up the bulk of the oils being sold today around the world.

As a pricing example, a 10 ml bottle of tea tree essential oil, priced at $5 indicates a perfume grade or adulterated oil that should not be used for therapeutic purposes. A premium grade, therapeutic tea tree oil will cost somewhere near $15 to 25.

See the section "Michelle's Recommended Products" on page 303 for product resources.

11 Essential Oil Safety, Techniques and FAQs

This chapter is a must read before you start using essential oils. You'll discover hands-on details and techniques about how to use, apply, dilute, ingest and diffuse essential oils. Also covered are important safety considerations for topical and internal use, as well as using oils with children, pets and the elderly. You'll also find answers to the most frequently asked questions about using oils.

Armed with these techniques, knowledge and proper precautions, you'll be ready to start using essential oils with confidence. Be sure you read the chapter "Essential Oil ABCs" on page 111 for how to find genuine therapeutic oils, the only oils that should be used for any health-related purpose. Detailed protocols for how to use specific essential oils, including oil usage amounts and administration protocols, can be found in the next chapter "Essential Oil Protocols for Use" on page 137.

Essential Oil Safety

Essential oils are very safe when used properly and according to well-established methods. However, essential oils are potent medicinals, and they should be treated with respect. The subsections that follow will outline several key principles, practices and precautions that will help you get the most benefit when using essential oils. This section isn't meant to scare you. Essential oils have a wide margin of safety when used in an educated manner. So be mindful of the precautions but also be confident in your use of essential oils.

Less is More

The principle of *less is more* is especially true of essential oils. There are many protocols where the most medicinal benefit is actually achieved by diluting an essential oil rather than using it full-strength. While essential oils are generally well tolerated for the majority of people, taking too much of an oil for too long a period of time can increase the risk of skin sensitivity, stomach upset (when taken orally), detoxification symptoms and other potential side effects.

Some essential oils can also cause stress to the liver, gall bladder or other organs of the body if used orally in large amounts and/or for long periods of time. Therefore, if using orally, using the least amount of an essential oil to achieve the desired effect is prudent. For this reason, it's best to limit the usage amount and duration of use to established protocols and levels as shown in the chapter "Essential Oil Protocols for Use" on page 137, or as specified by the oil manufacturer or a healthcare professional.

First: Test It

It's a good idea to test an essential oil first to make sure you react well to it. Testing a small amount of the oil on your skin before using the full sized usage amount is especially important if any of the following applies to you:

- You are new to using essential oils.

- You have sensitive skin or are using the oil around an infection.

- You are elderly.

- You are using the oil during pregnancy or on a baby or small child.

- You are about to use an unfamiliar oil.

You can test an oil by putting a small dab onto the tip of a tooth pick, then wiping a little bit of the oil onto your arm or leg. If you notice no ill effects after a few hours, test again with a single drop of ¼ diluted oil. You can make the ¼ diluted oil by adding one drop of essential oil to 3 drops of a carrier oil (such as grapeseed oil) and then using just one drop of the mixture. If there is still no reaction after a few hours, then consider proceeding by working up to the desired usage amount per the section below.

Second: Scale Up the Usage Amount

If you test OK for a new or unfamiliar oil, consider working up to the recommended amount slowly over a few days. Gradually scaling up to the recommended target usage amount will give you a better chance to deal with any negative side effects if they occur.

Start with the lowest usage amount of the protocol you are using, or even a fraction of the usage amount to be more conservative. For example, if you want to take an essential oil internally at a usage amount of 4 drops per day, start with just one drop the first day, move up to 2 drops the second day and finally take the full 4 drops on the third day. As an example for skin application, if the desired usage amount is 100% tea tree oil on a wound, start with ¼ tea tree diluted in a carrier oil the first day, followed by ½ diluted tea tree the second day and finally full strength tea tree oil on the third day.

Keep in mind that the duration of scale up and the usage amount dilutions you use are not set in stone but are flexible. If you are experienced with using essential oils, then the scale up process may be shortened or not used at all to best fit your needs. On the other hand, if you have a history of being very sensitive to essential oils, then extending the scale up time may be a good idea.

Avoid Unsafe Oils

You can avoid many potential safety concerns by only using the highest quality essential oils of the proper medicinal grade. Quality is of the utmost importance for therapeutic uses, especially internal ingestion. All of the oil protocols in this book are based on the use of high quality therapeutic grade EOBBD essential oils. Oils of lesser quality can be toxic, dangerous and may cause serious side effects. Only use the highest quality therapeutic grade essential oils internally or on your body.

If you choose to use essential oils that do not meet the criteria in the section "What You Must Know to Find Safe and Effective Oils" on page 115, then contact the manufacturer of the oil for the proper protocols for use. Each oil company can have different protocols, usage amounts and methods of use that vary from the information in this book.

Hotness Ratings

Because of the chemical composition of essential oils, they may sting or feel as if they are burning when applied topically to the skin. Even mild oils may cause skin irritation if used undiluted, or if applied to the same area of skin for too long. The so-called *hot* or *spicy* oils require a few extra steps and precautions before using them, especially on the skin.

The three hotness ratings listed below refer to how sensitizing, irritating or *hot* an oil may feel on the skin of an average person. Be aware that each person is different and your reactions to an oil may vary. Unfamiliar essential oils should always be tested for skin sensitivity prior to use by diluting it in a carrier oil (such as olive oil) and then applying to a small area of skin.

If an essential oil burns or is too hot on the skin, the burning can be relieved by rinsing the area with a carrier oil, as detailed in the section "What If an Essential Oil Burns?" on page 135.

- **Mild.** Mild oils are generally gentle and safe on the skin. Mild oils are ideal for babies, small children and the elderly or for use on sensitive skin areas. Dilution of the oil may still be required for very sensitive areas, such as the face or nose, armpits or groin areas.

- **Medium.** Oils of medium hotness can cause irritation on sensitive skin areas unless diluted properly. Medium hotness oils should be used cautiously on babies or elderly skin.

- **Hot.** Hot oils require extra care and are best to avoid for most skin uses. Hot oils are generally unsuitable for children and the elderly. Hot oils are generally placed into a capsule and diluted for internal uses.

Potential Side Effects

Even though essential oils are quite safe when used properly, some mild side effects may occur under certain conditions. These side effects are largely avoidable if you follow established protocols, start slowly and use proper quality oils. The list below covers more common potential side effects.

Be under the care of a qualified health practitioner to monitor your progress when using any natural remedies, especially if you have any medical condition.

Detoxification

Botanical products, including essential oils, can stimulate the body to release long-held toxins or infection by-products that have stored up in various tissues. This process is called detoxification, and while it is generally beneficial, it can cause undesirable symptoms if it progresses too quickly. Taking large amounts of essential oils can cause uncomfortable detox symptoms. Detox symptoms may include fatigue, headache, diarrhea, gas, rashes, mild lethargy and flu-like symptoms. If you experience a detox reaction, reduce the amount of oil you are taking until symptoms subside. Afterward, you can increase the amount you are using again. Detox is more likely for internal use of oils than for topical use. For details about the symptoms, causes and controlling of detox, see the chapter "Healing Crisis and Detoxification Support" on page 217

Seizures

If you have a history of seizures, avoid or take special care when using basil, fennel or lavender or any other essential oils. Lavender aroma can potentially trigger an epileptic event in some people. If you choose to use one of these oils and have a history of seizures, only use them when another person is present to watch your response. Start with a low usage amount and scale up slowly and cautiously.

Sun Sensitivity

All citrus oils, including lemon and orange, and most oil blends containing citrus oils are photo-sensitizing, meaning they can cause a sunburn. Keep the area of the skin where citrus oils have been applied out of direct sunlight for 48 hours after application to avoid sunburn.

Eyes, Nose, Ears and Sensitive Areas

Some oils can feel hot when applied to the skin, especially on sensitive areas. Some oils are irritants and should not be used in these areas. Essential oils are concentrated and potent and must be used cautiously on any area of sensitive skin. Keep oils away from your eyes, and only use mild and diluted oils near sensitive areas like your nose, ears, lips, arm pits and genital areas.

Rashes, Hot Oils, Burning and Stinging

Some oils are hot and are irritants to the skin like oregano, cinnamon, clove and thyme oils. Never apply these oils undiluted to the skin. If you get direct skin contact with a hot essential oil or an oil that is irritating you, do not wash it off with water as water will drive the oil deeper into the skin and increase the burning. Instead, apply a carrier oil like a vegetable oil to the affected area immediately. Carrier oils can reduce oil related burning or stinging sensations.

Occasionally, people can develop a localized skin sensitivity to a particular essential oil. Sensitivity is most common when an oil is used daily for a long period of time on the same area of skin.

If you develop a rash or dermal sensitivity to an essential oil with any use or with repeated use, discontinue using the oil, switch to a different essential oil or try another type of remedy. Note that some rashes could also be the result of detoxification through the skin due to the cleansing properties of the oil.

Liver Stress or Toxicity

Some oils when used orally can stress the liver if taken in large amounts or for long periods of time. Other oils should never be taken internally as they are toxic. Liver stress (or congestion) is most common with oils such as oregano and thyme but can happen with any oil when overused. Liver stress is unlikely through topical application of essential oils.

If you choose to use oils orally, remember that *less is more*. Your doctor or Naturopath may deviate from the standard protocols if she is familiar with essential oils and your condition. If you experience adverse symptoms or show signs of liver stress, then discontinue use. Refer to section "Taking Essential Oils Internally" on page 130 for more details. You can also refer to "Liver Support" on page 176 for ways to support a healthy liver.

Stomach Upset

Some people find that stronger oils, such as oregano, can cause stomach upset when taken internally. The risk of upsetting your stomach can be reduced by using a capsule with a carrier oil to dilute the oil or ingesting the capsule along with food.

Reactions with Medications

If you are taking antibiotic drugs or other prescription medications, avoid using essential oils within two hours before or after taking your medication. Some oils can interfere with your body's ability to absorb certain medications. Always consult with your healthcare provider when taking any supplement or natural products along with medications.

High Blood Pressure

Be mindful that peppermint may increase blood pressure, so avoid prolonged use of this oil if this is of concern. You can help offset peppermint's effect by immediately layering lavender oil on top after the topical application of peppermint. Oil blends containing peppermint should have minimal effect on blood pressure due to the low concentration, but caution is still prudent.

Pregnancy Precautions

Extra care should be exercised when using any natural products during pregnancy, including essential oils. Some experts believe oils should be avoided the first 3 months of pregnancy. Others say that it's wise to avoid internal or undiluted topical use of oils throughout pregnancy. Yet other oil experts believe that most oils are generally safe to use in moderation during pregnancy.

It's best that you speak with your doctor about the use of any essential oils when pregnant. See more information in the safety section at the National Association for Holistic Aromatherapy: https://www.naha.org/

Pet Precautions

Dogs, cats and horses can get MRSA and Staph infections from people. As with people, essential oils can be very therapeutic for companion animals with the proper protocols and adjustments. However, not all oils are safe for use on animals. Dogs and horses generally tolerate oils quite well. However, essential oils should not be used on cats as they have a poor tolerance for oils.

Of note, there are reports of cats reacting poorly to essential oils, but a few vets have been using high quality oils with cats and have had great results. It's possible the poor reactions in cats may have been due to using inferior oils (those with toxic extraction solvents) or that too much oil was used on the cats. It's important to remember that animals are small and much more sensitive to most remedies than people are.

If you plan to use essential oils on your pet, talk to an aromatherapist or holistic veterinarian who understands the safe use of essential oils. Below are general guidelines for using essential oils with pets.

- **Tea tree and thyme oil may be toxic** to some animals. Use caution when cleaning with these oils around animals, especially floors or surfaces the animal touches.

- **Do not use hot oils like** clove leaf/bud, garlic or thyme, or wintergreen.

- **Less is more, especially with animals.** Dilution of essential oils is required for dogs. Their weight must be used to calculate the amount of oil to use. Follow the protocols in the section "Essential Oil Protocols for Pets" on page 164.

- **Do not use essential oils on cats, birds, fish, reptiles and pet rodents (rats, gerbils, etc).**

- **Cats do not tolerate oils** because they do not metabolize oils in the same way that humans, dogs, or other animals do. Excess accumulation of essential oils can occur in cats. This can happen quickly through internal or external application, or from continuous inhalation, including nearby air diffusion of oils. The result can be liver or kidney damage or even death.

- **Tea tree** may be toxic to cats.

- **When diffusing oils** remove any animal of concern out of the room where essential oils are being air diffused. If you have a cat in the home, consider diffusing lavender, eucalyptus or the spice blend in place of tea tree for control of airborne bacteria.

- **Do not use oils around sensitive areas** like the eyes, ears or genitals of pets.

Precautions for Children

Essential oil protocols must be modified for children as they are more sensitive to oils. When used correctly, topical use and inhalation of oils are generally very safe. However, some oils are not appropriate for children, especially hot, spicy oils which can more easily burn their skin and accidentally get near their eyes or nose.

Some oil experts advocate using oils internally on children for infections when appropriately diluted from adult usage amount. Other doctors and experts do not advise any oral use of essential oils in children. If you wish to use oils internally on your child, be sure you first discuss it with your doctor or holistic physician.

CAUTION: Children with asthma or respiratory illnesses may be more susceptible to diffused oils which could irritate airways and possibly lead to an asthma attack. If you have concerns, start with a low amount in the diffuser and slowly work your way up, stopping if any adverse symptoms appear.

Regarding the cautionary statement above, children have also found relief from asthma using oils. Like adults, not every child reacts the same way to essential oils. Essential oils have a wide margin of safety when used in moderation and with proper precautions. For details about using essential oils with children, see the section "Children, Babies and Elderly Protocols" on page 160.

Other Precautions

- **Elderly.** As a general rule, dilute oils twice as much as the normal adult usage amount. If this extra dilution is well tolerated, a gradual increase to the normal adult usage amount may be attempted. Use organic or natural grape seed carrier oil to dilute. For details, see the section "Children, Babies and Elderly Protocols" on page 160.

- **Labels.** Be sure to follow any specific cautions that appear on the label of an essential oil. Keep essential oils away from fire, flame, heat or sparks and keep bottles caped tightly and stored in a cool, dark, dry place. Keep essential oils away from children and pets.

Techniques for Using Essential Oils

Essential oils are a powerhouse when it comes to dealing with infections. This is due to their complex chemical composition and their high penetration into the skin when used topically, and the lungs when inhaled. The following section covers different ways to use and apply essential oils.

Pouring a Single Drop of Oil

Some oils are thin and pour very quickly while others are thicker and pour slowly. To pour one or two drops, quickly rotate the essential oil bottle upside down and immediately rotate it back right side up again in one fluid motion without spending time in the upside down position. This is a quick motion, typically 0.5 to 1 second to rotate upside down and right side up again. The slower you rotate the bottle, the more drops will come out.

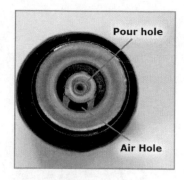

The pour hole and air hole of an essential oil bottle.

For better pouring control, keep the air hole of the bottle toward the sky when pouring, which will keep extra oil from pouring out of the air hole. If the bottle is close to empty, keep the air hole facing down instead of up, allowing oil at the bottom of the bottle to exit through the air hole. To make pouring easier, firmly tap the upright bottle a few times to get rid of air bubbles in the air hole or the pour hole just prior to pouring. When the bottle is nearly empty, the plastic liner can by pried up around the edges and removed to get the last drops out.

Diluting Essential Oils in a Carrier Oil

The most effective way to use some essential oils is to dilute them first. Essential oils can be diluted by mixing them with a *carrier oil*. Dilution reduces the essential oil's concentration or potency to the level which is most safe and effective for a given method of use. Carrier oils which are often used include grape seed oil, jojoba oil, sunflower oil, coconut oil, olive oil or combinations of such oils. Organic cold-pressed grape seed oil is one of the most versatile, inexpensive and readily available carrier oils. The following techniques can be used to dilute an essential oil. The choice of dilution technique depends on personal preference and how you intend to use the essential oil.

- **In the hand.** One of the quickest ways to dilute an essential oil for general topical uses is to pour the desired number of drops of essential oil and carrier oil into the palm of your hand and mix briefly with your fingers.

- **In a vessel.** The required drops of essential and carrier oils can be poured into a small cup, vial or any other conveniently sized or shaped container and then mixed briefly. Make sure the container is compatible with essentials oils (glass is best).

- **In a capsule.** For internal uses, it's easiest to dilute the essential oil directly inside a veggie capsule, as detailed in the section "Capsule Filling Technique" on page 132.

- **Dilution rates.** As an example, a 50% dilution is the same as a 1:1 dilution of essential oil to carrier oil. This is the same as 1 drop of essential oil plus 1 drop of carrier oil. A 25% or ¼ dilution of essential oil is 1 drop of essential oil plus 3 drops of carrier oil.

Applying Essential Oils Topically

Oils are applied to the skin either undiluted (neat) or diluted, depending on the protocol being used. If applying undiluted essential oil, the oil can be poured directly from the bottle to the affected skin area. Alternatively, the oil can be placed in the palm of one hand then applied with either a finger from the other hand, a cotton swab, or a small gauze pad. After applying the oil, it can be rubbed into the affected area briefly and gently. If tolerated, mild essential oils like tea tree may be applied to the skin neat multiple times per day, or when changing wound dressings.

If applying a diluted essential oil, the same method described above for neat oils can be used after the oil is diluted in a carrier oil.

CAUTION: If an essential oil stings or is too *hot* on the skin, rinse it away with grapeseed oil or another carrier oil. Never rinse with water! Water will make the burning worse.

How to Increase Skin Absorption

When dealing with skin infections such as cellulitis, deep boils or abscesses, there are a couple ways you can help push the oils deeper into the affected areas of the body. First is cabreuva essential oil. When applied on top of another essential oil, cabreuva oil can help push the first oil deeper into the skin, enhancing its effects. A second way to increase skin absorption of essential oils is to apply a warm, wet compress to your skin after applying the essential oil. Because oil and water do not mix or dissolve into each other, the water in the compress will repel the essential oil away, forcing it deeper into your skin.

CAUTION: Infected, inflamed or wet skin may be more sensitive when applying essential oils. Be sure to dilute any essential oil 1:1 (50/50) or more with a carrier oil, and see how your skin reacts.

Topical Foot Application

Some people apply oils topically to their feet as an alternate to internal ingestion. Some oil experts say that the bottom of your feet have an abundance of large skin pores which allow the essential oil to enter into your bloodstream. Other experts believe it's not the pores, but inhaling the oils while applying them that provide the most internal benefit. Either way, topical application does get some oil internally in the body. And because the sole of the foot is less sensitive, you can also use hotter oils without discomfort. This technique is also useful for children or the elderly.

1. Gently rub the essential oil onto the bottom of the feet until absorbed. Breathe in the aroma.

Use the oils diluted or undiluted as appropriate.

2. If following an internal use protocol, instead of taking the oil internally, apply the oil to the bottom of the feet. Use the same amount, time of day and duration of use specified in the internal protocol, unless topical application is not advised.

3. Cover your feet with socks or slippers to keep the oils on your feet rubbing onto the floor.

Taking Essential Oils Internally

With proper care and precautions, essential oils are powerhouses when it comes to supporting the body systemically with broad-spectrum antibacterial support against Staph, MRSA, fungal and viral infections.

There are varying opinions on the internal use of essential oils. Some doctors and essential oil experts are advocates of internal use. Some doctors only use oils internally for infections that do not respond to herbal remedies. Yet other doctors and oil experts are more conservative and do not recommend that oils be taken orally. From the FDA's point of view, essential oils that are *generally regarded as safe* (GRAS) are safe for human consumption as a food additive.

The author and her family have used essential oils internally off and on, in moderation with great success for many years. They are the preferred *go-to* remedy for many ailments. As mentioned previously, the vast majority of essential oils are not true therapeutic grade oils and should never be taken internally. Inferior oils contain unsafe impurities, adulterants, synthetic ingredients or residual solvents that are toxic or carcinogenic. See "What You Must Know to Find Safe and Effective Oils" on page 115 for full details.

Because oils are very potent, be under the care of a natural healthcare professional when using any essential oil internally or if considering internal use with children.

Unsafe Oils for Internal Uses

Not every essential oil is safe for human consumption. Just because an oil is pure or of the highest therapeutic quality does not mean that it is appropriate for oral use.

Two common examples of oils that should never be taken internally include birch and wintergreen. While therapeutic-grade birch and wintergreen oils can be used safely on the skin, they should never be taken internally. Also, some oils, such as eucalyptus and tea tree, can cause problems if ingested and therefore are best to avoid for internal use. But eucalyptus and tea tree oils are very safe for skin, air diffusing and other non-internal applications.

GRAS Oils

The Food and Drug Administration (FDA) considers a group of 50 essential oils to be *Generally Regarded As Safe* (GRAS) for food and cooking uses, which includes incidental ingestion. GRAS means the FDA considers the oils safe for ingesting for non-drug purposes. Only GRAS oils should be taken internally, unless directed to do otherwise by a medical professional.

GRAS Essential Oils				
Angelica	Dill	Laurus nobilis	Orange	Sage
Basil	Eucalyptus globulus	Lavender	Oregano	Sandalwood
Bergamot	Frankincense	Lemon	Patchouli	Spearmint
Chamomile, Roman	Galbanum	Lemongrass	Pepper	Spruce
Chamomile, German	Geranium	Lime	Peppermint	Tarragon
Cinnamon Bark	Ginger	Melissa	Petitgrain	Tangerine
Citrus rind (all)	Grapefruit	Marjoram	Pine	Thyme
Clary Sage	Hyssop	Myrrh	Rosemary	Valerian
Clove	Juniper	Myrtle	Rose	Vetiver
Coriander	Jasmine	Nutmeg	Savory	Ylang Ylang

Internal Use Techniques

The most common way to take essential oils internally is using the capsule method as detailed in the next section. Below are two other methods to use essential oil internally

- **Honey and spoon method.** This method is best for oils that are relatively mild, not too hot, and when only taking a drop or two of essential oil. Place some honey on a spoon and add a drop or two of the essential oil. Mix briefly with a fork and then ingest. Manuka honey is ideal.

- **The lick trick method.** An easy way to take oils orally is called the *lick trick*. Simply place 1 or 2 drops of essential oil onto the back of your hand and use your tongue to lick the oil into your mouth. This method is best for relatively mild oils that are not too hot.

Internal Use Alternatives

There are pros and cons to using essential oils internally, including the potential for liver or organ stress with some oils. And depending on the oil and the health challenge, there can be more effective ways to use an oil besides internal ingestion. If you prefer to not ingest essential oils, two safe and effective alternative techniques are detailed in the section "Is There an Alternate to Taking

Essential Oils Internally?" on page 136. For long-term internal use, remedies that have fewer risks may be a prudent option, including several of the herbal remedies described in the chapter "Alternative Remedies" on page 91. You can also refer to "Liver Support" on page 176 for ways to support a healthy liver.

Capsule Filling Technique

Only use veggie capsules (*veggie caps*) with essential oils, not gel capsules. Gel capsules will melt when exposed to essential oils. Capsule sizes 0 or 00 are best for ease of filling and swallowing. Note that some oils are thin and pour very quickly while others are thick and pour slowly. The steps to fill a capsule with essential oils are below.

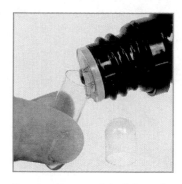

Pouring an essential oil from the bottle into an empty vegetable capsule (or *veggie cap* for short).

1. Hold the longer half of an empty veggie capsule directly underneath the pour spout of the essential oil bottle.

2. Rotate the oil bottle upside down to pour the desired number of drops into the capsule.

3. Fill the remaining capsule volume with a carrier oil and then press the other half of the capsule (the lid or shorter half) on top to close the capsule. The exact amount of carrier oil used is not important.

4. Shake the capsule a couple times to mix.

5. Swallow the capsule with food. Avoid crushing or biting into the capsule while swallowing.

6. Filled capsules may be stored in a refrigerator for up to one day with the capsule lid facing up.

How to Air Diffuse Essential Oils

Air diffusing is one of the most powerful ways to benefit from the medicinal and therapeutic effects of essential oils. Air diffusing is most commonly done using a simple device called a cold air diffuser. The diffuser turns the liquid oils into a vapor that is gently blown into the air, spreading the vapor throughout the room. When you breathe the air, the oil droplets pass into your lungs, quickly absorbing into your bloodstream. Not only is it supportive to your body, it's also helpful for the reduction of airborne bacteria.

Cold air diffusers can be found at some health food stores or online. **Only use a cold air diffuser.** Diffusers that heat the oil will decrease or eliminate the effectiveness of the oil. Some diffusers can be programmed to shut off after a period of time or to diffuse in intervals. Other diffusers allow oil bottles to be directly connected for ease of operation.

Below are steps for air diffusing an essential oil. Refer to the chapter "Essential Oil Protocols for Use" on page 137 for details about diffusing each type of essential oil. Also refer to the air diffuser's operation manual for additional instructions.

- Pour several drops of the essential oil into the diffuser oil chamber.

- Turn the diffuser on and set to the desired vapor level.

- Most air diffusion protocols involve diffusing the oil for intervals of 10-15 minutes several times throughout the day.

- Periodic cleaning and unclogging of a cold air diffuser may be needed. Some essential oils have thick components that can eventually clog a diffuser. To clean or unclog a simple diffuser, the glass atomizer or nozzle can be soaked in rubbing alcohol or washed with soap and water. Dry all parts completely before reassembly. If the instruction manual has cleaning instructions, then follow the manual rather than the method described here.

- If you have cats, birds or small mammals, remove them from the room before diffusing.

- Be aware that using diffusers for long periods of time may cause a detoxification reaction.

CAUTION: Children with asthma or respiratory illnesses may be more susceptible to diffused oils which could irritate airways and possibly lead to an asthma attack. If you have concerns, start with a low amount in the diffuser and slowly work your way up, stopping if any adverse symptoms appear.

Systemic Support with Air Diffusion

Air diffusion is an alternative to the internal use of essential oils. The absorption process in the lungs is highly efficient, allowing relatively large amounts of oxygen (and some essential oil) to pass into the blood, where they can circulate throughout the body.

There are a few limitations to air diffusing essential oils instead of taking oils internally. Only mild or moderately spicy oils should be air diffused. Spicy or *hot* oils such as oregano and thyme should not be air diffused because they can burn the eyes and nose and can be sensitizing. While these and other hot oils may be highly potent at controlling bacteria, air diffusing is not the safest way to use them.

Sinus Rinsing Technique

Essential oils can be used along with sinus rinsing methods to help control Staph and MRSA sinus infections and to assist with nasal decolonization. Because the nose and especially the sinuses are very sensitive, only mild essential oils in small amounts should be used. One or two drops of either tea tree or eucalyptus oil is commonly added to the sinus rinse solution to provide extra bacterial control. For sinus rinsing details and instructions, including important safety precautions, see the section "Sinus Rinsing" on page 191.

Bathing With Essential Oils

Adding essential oils to your bath is a great way to benefit from oils in multiple ways. Oils such as tea tree can add extra bacterial control to your bath, support infected skin areas, and help in your skin decolonization efforts. Oils can also be very calming and relaxing when added to your bath, especially lavender oil.

A typical way to use essential oils for a full sized bath tub is to add 5 drops directly to a scoop of dry bath salts, then stir the dry salts to mix before adding the salts to the bath water. Avoid adding essential oils directly to the bath water because the oil is more likely to float on top and disperse poorly. The amount of oil you use is not set in stone and can be adjusted to fit your needs, so long as the bath water is well tolerated without burning or stinging your skin.

TIP: Add oils to your bath water after you are in the bathtub. This will prevent the oils from getting on any sensitive areas as you enter the water.

To protect sensitive skin areas, mild essential oils are typically best for bathing, such as tea tree, eucalyptus or lavender. Oils that are very hot or spicy like oregano, thyme or cinnamon are best avoided for bathing. Eucalyptus oil, while being mild, should be kept away from facial areas to prevent burning or stinging, especially around the nose or eyes.

Sometime spot bathing with a cloth is better than using a bath tub, especially for babies or children. For spot bathing, 1 or 2 drops of an essential oil may be added to a tablespoon of dry bath salts and stirred into a small wash basin. For larger basins, a few more drops of oil can be used, according to your needs and how well the oil is tolerated on the skin.

Frequently Asked Questions

What is a Carrier Oil?

A carrier oil is an inert, vegetable oil used to dilute the concentration of an essential oil. Common carrier oils include grape seed, jojoba or coconut oil. Olive oil can be used, but has a thick viscosity when placed on the skin. Diluting an essential oil with a carrier oil will reduce potential burning on sensitive skin areas, but it does not dilute the effect of the essential oil. Diluting can also aid absorption of the essential oil when taken internally. Dilution is also required for some oils and protocols to increase the effect of the oil. See the section "Diluting Essential Oils in a Carrier Oil" on page 128 for more details.

What If an Essential Oil Burns?

If an essential oil burns when rubbed on the skin, you can dilute the burning effect with a carrier oil such as olive oil, grape seed oil or vegetable oil. Many oils should not be used undiluted to begin with. **Never rinse with water**. Rinsing with water will make the burning worse. For internal uses, if an essential oil burns the mouth, rinse the mouth with a teaspoon of carrier oil. Rinsing with or drinking water will make the burning worse.

What are Blends?

Essential oils, like herbal remedies, come in many different types with many different properties. Just as herbal botanical blends can provide powerful products for infection support, essential oils can also be formulated into blends for enhanced, broad-spectrum support. Blends have multiple kinds of essential oils that are mixed together by a formulator. Some blends are particularly useful for support with fungal, viral or bacterial support. Specific blends of oils will be detailed in the chapter "Essential Oil Protocols for Use" on page 137.

In most cases, blends should only be made by a professional formulator who is knowledgeable of essential oil constituents and the nuances of blending. One essential oil may have constituents that compete with or counteract the constituents of another oil. Blends must therefore be make with great care and expertise to avoid dangerous or ineffective blends and combinations.

How Exact are Oil Usage Amounts?

Most of the usage amounts for each essential oil specified in this book are approximate. The amount of oil you use for each protocol can be adjusted somewhat without compromising safety or effectiveness. Staying close to the specified usage amounts is recommended, but not critical for most people. For example, if a protocol specifies a usage amount of 3 drops of essential oil, any amount between 2 and 4 drops should be fine for most people. The protocols in this book are a rule of thumb only and not set in stone.

Who Can Use Essential Oils?

- **Anyone with an active infection** can use essential oils to support their body to fight infections on multiple levels. Adults, children and the elderly require different usage amounts and protocols for use.

- **Anyone sharing a home with an infected person** can use the oils for prevention support. Specifically, taking the lowest usage amount of some oils may help with prevention and immune support until the infected person has recovered.

- **Caregivers for someone who's infected** can also benefit from using essential oils.

- **Anyone wanting to prevent infections** can use oils to support the body in fending off many types of bacterial, viral and other infectious challenges.

Can Essential Oils be Used With Antibiotics?

If you are using essential oils internally at the same time you are using antibiotic drugs, it's good practice to take the essential oil 2 hours before or after your antibiotics. Taking oils or other natural products at the same time as the antibiotics may diminish the effects of the drug. This precaution is a general rule of thumb.

Of interest, several laboratory studies show that some essential oils can have a synergistic effect when used along with antibiotic drugs, with the combined effectiveness being greater than the sum of the oil and antibiotic alone[52]. Certain essential oils have also been found to reduce the resistance of Staph and MRSA bacteria to antibiotic drugs. One study showed that essential oils can weaken the cell wall of resistant bacteria, allowing antibiotic drugs to better penetrate the bacteria[53].

While the majority of oil-antibiotic combination studies show that essential oils can help antibiotics work better, in a few cases, essential oils may reduce the effect of specific antibiotics. In one laboratory study, rosemary oil reduced the effectiveness of the antibiotic ciprofloxacin (Cipro) against *Staph aureus* bacteria[54]. Because there may be potential for some oils to interfere with some antibiotics, it's best to work closely with your doctor when taking antibiotics along with essential oils.

Is There an Alternate to Taking Essential Oils Internally?

Air diffusing and foot application are two excellent ways to get systemic support from essential oils without having to ingest oils. Topical and diffusion methods go internally to some extent because of the high penetration of oils through skin and the high permeability of the lungs.

For details on the foot application technique, see "Topical Foot Application" on page 129. For more information about diffusion essential oils, see the section "How to Air Diffuse Essential Oils" on page 132. For protocols on specific essential oils, see the chapter "Essential Oil Protocols for Use" on page 137.

See the section "Michelle's Recommended Products" on page 303 for product resources.

12 Essential Oil Protocols for Use

This chapter will give you detailed protocols for using essential oils to support your body to heal from infection challenges. You'll also learn important modifications and special uses for children, the elderly, expecting mothers and for pets.

As discussed previously, not all essential oils are created equal. Some oils and brands of oils can cause harm if used according to the methods in this book, especially for internal uses. Read the section "What You Must Know to Find Safe and Effective Oils" on page 115 before buying any essential oils or using any of the protocols below. Likewise, be sure to read the safety and important oil use techniques in the chapter "Essential Oil Safety, Techniques and FAQs" on page 121 before using any essential oils or following any of the protocols below.

Which Oils to Use

There are several essential oils with notable activity against Staph and MRSA. There are many other oils that can provide support for the challenges that often accompany these infections. However, it's often easier to get started by focusing on just a few key oils rather than trying to do everything all at once. If you are unfamiliar with essential oils, then consider starting with just one or two of the essential oils listed below to keep things simple.

- **Tea tree oil** used topically is an ideal place to start if you are new to essential oils. Tea tree oil is ideal for sensitive skin areas like the nose, face, armpits and groin. Tea tree is also great for bathing to control skin bacteria and air diffusing for airborne bacteria reduction. This oil is mild and generally safe for children and the elderly, especially when diluted.

- **The Antibacterial Blend** is a specific combination of several essential oils for broad-spectrum bacterial support. It can be used topically, diffused or taken internally. This blend is stronger than tea tree in antibacterial activity, but it is also a little hotter and may sting on sensitive skin areas unless diluted. If you can only use one essential oil, the Antibacterial Blend is a good choice. This blend may be used undiluted on less sensitive skin areas, however, it is usually diluted for skin application. This blend is also ideal for internal support and was formulated to be potent yet balanced and well tolerated.

- **The Broad-Spectrum Internal Protocol** uses the Antibacterial Blend in combination with two other oil blends for very broad internal infection support. The three blends are the Antibacterial Blend, the Antifungal Blend and the Spice Blend, all of which are detailed later in this chapter on pages page 145, page 147, and page 148, respectively.

- **Oregano oil** is very powerful for internal support, but it can be potentially taxing on the liver with prolonged use. Unless you are familiar with using essential oils, it may be best to consider other oils or blends before using oregano oil.

- **The Stealth Bacteria Blend** was formulated for special support with L-forms and biofilms that can play a role in recurring infections. This blend should be considered as an add-on or an addition to the use of other more potent infection-fighting oils. For added infection support plus L-from support, consider following the "Stealth Bacteria Protocol for Adults" on page 158.

In, On and Around for Essential Oils

The *In, On and Around* principle was introduced in chapter 1, in the section "Action Step 1: Bacteria Control" on page 9 . The same principle can also be applied when using essential oils. Below is a list of essential oils that can work well with the *In, On and Around* principle:

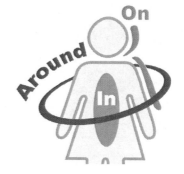

The *In, On and Around* principle can be effectively applied to the use of essential oils.

- **In.** The Antibacterial Blend, Broad-Spectrum Internal Protocol, or Oregano may be used for internal support. The Stealth Bacteria Blend is a helpful add-on for support with biofilms and L-forms.

- **On.** Tea tree, eucalyptus or diluted Antibacterial Blend oils may be used for topical skin support. The cabreuva oil can help enhance the effect of oils applied to the skin.

- **Around.** Tea tree, oregano, lemon and lavender are helpful for cleaning and sanitizing for home bacterial control. Tea tree and eucalyptus are ideal for air diffusing for airborne bacterial support.

How Much Oil To Use

The essential oil usage amounts in the protocols later in this chapter are rules of thumb only. As with many other natural remedies, essential oil usage amounts are flexible rather than precise. The best usage amount for you may differ from other people and may vary from the standard protocols. While the usage amounts in this chapter are well-established guidelines, always adjust the usage amounts based on how you feel, your natural doctor's advice, and what works best for you.

TIP: Often the best way to set a specific oil usage amount is to listen to your body. You can modify a usage amount or stop a protocol as needed based on how you feel and the results you experience.

How Long, How Often and When

- **How often.** Most of the skin application methods in this chapter can be used multiple times per day, every day, until the infection clears. Tea tree oil and the Antibacterial Blend (diluted if needed) are two examples of oils that can be used topically multiple times per day. The Broad-Spectrum Internal Protocol is used three times per day, taking a different oil blend at specific times as detailed in the section "Broad-Spectrum Internal Protocol for Adults" on page 156.

- **How long.** For oils taken internally in moderate or high usage amounts, limiting the duration of use to a set number of days is best, as specified in the protocols later in this chapter. For long-term daily prevention support, the lowest level of the Broad-Spectrum Internal Protocol (1 drop of each blend per day) can be used indefinitely if well tolerated, either taken using an internal method or applied to the bottom of the feet.

- **When.** For some essential oils, the time of day to use the oil is important, as detailed in the Protocols later in this chapter. If you are taking antibiotic drugs, it's generally best to take essential oils 2 hours before or after your antibiotics. Taking the oils at the same time as the antibiotics may diminish the effects of some antibiotic drugs. If you are taking probiotics, it's generally best to take essential oils 2 hours before or after your probiotics. For internal ingestion, taking oils with food can help aid absorption and reduce the risk of stomach upset.

Before You Get Started

As powerful, versatile and beneficial as essential oils may be, they are often not enough by themselves to stop a stubborn bout of Staph or MRSA. The same is true of all remedies and treatments, including antibiotic drugs. While treating the infection is obviously important, other steps are usually needed beyond treatments for best results. Relying solely on essential oils or any other treatment or remedy increases the risk of the infection coming back again later. To get the best results with your infection, be sure to follow the Action Steps in chapter 1.

Speak with your doctor about the use of any essential oils when pregnant, since it has not been guaranteed that they are safe during pregnancy.

Essential oils are powerful allies to have in your medicine chest, and countless people rely on them for all kinds of health issues beyond infections. Be aware that the protocols in this book are a rule of thumb only and your tolerance to an essential oil may differ from the average person. While some oils may be safe when pregnant or nursing, be sure to first consult with a physician. Also consult a physician before using oils on children. Be sure to read "Essential Oil Safety, Techniques and FAQs" on page 121 before you start using any oil.

For maximum safety, the internal use of essential oils should be limited in duration and should be done under the care of a healthcare professional, especially if you have any medical conditions. Only the highest quality therapeutic grade essential oils should be considered for internal uses.

Essential Oil Protocols for Adults

This section provides detailed usage amounts, methods for use and important precautions for individual essential oils and essential oil blends that are suitable for adults. If you prefer not to ingest essential oils, refer to "Is There an Alternate to Taking Essential Oils Internally?" on page 136.

The adult usage amounts in this section are not suitable for babies, children, the elderly or for pets. See the "Children, Babies and Elderly Protocols" on page 160 and "Essential Oil Protocols for Pets" on page 164 as applicable.

NOTE: It is not necessary or recommended to use every essential oil in this section, nor is it necessary to follow every protocol listed for each essential oil. Only use the oils and protocols that meet your particular needs based on the preceding sections and the Action Steps in chapter 1. Always follow the directions on the product label or the guidance of a healthcare professional if they differ from the protocols below.

Tea Tree Oil

- **Hotness rating:** mild. Non-irritating and ideal for sensitive skin areas.

- **Antibacterial, antiviral and antiseptic** properties. Active against MRSA[55].

- **Ideal for skin** applications (cuts, infections and skin decolonization).

- **Ideal for children, the elderly** and for air diffusing.

- **Best oil to start with** if you are unfamiliar with essential oils.

- **Not for internal use.**

Tea tree oil (*Melaleuca alternifolia*), which is sometimes called melaleuca oil, has been used for centuries by the Aborigines of Australia and later by the British settlers. As early as 1923, human clinical trials in Australia began to provide scientific evidence of tea tree's antibacterial and antiseptic properties. Tea tree oil was even made a standard issue for all soldiers in the Australian army during World War II. A 2004 study showed that tea tree was superior to common topical treatments for eradicating MRSA carriage on the skin[56].

There are over 300 different species of tea tree native to Australia. *Melaleuca alternifolia* is regarded as one of the highest quality species for therapeutic use. Manuka oil is sometimes confused with tea tree but it is not the same oil. Manuka oil is distilled from the Manuka New Zealand tree.

Other uses for tea tree oil include support for colds, flu and common bacterial and viral infections. Tea tree has also been used for cuts and scrapes, athlete's foot, fungal infections, acne control and even warts.

Precautions

Keep out of reach of children. Avoid contact with eyes. Keep the oil away from cats. Some people may have an allergic reaction, including rashes and itching, when applying tea tree oil. If a reaction develops, stop the use of tea tree oil. Not for internal use.

Children and the elderly: Follow dilutions and use directions in the "Children, Babies and Elderly Protocols" on page 160.

Type of Support	Tea Tree Usage Amounts and Protocols for Use
Skin or topical	1-2 drops of tea tree oil can be applied directly onto any skin infection area, 3 or 4 times per day while infection lasts. Tea tree can be diluted with a carrier oil, especially it if stings a bit. You can also add a few drops of tea tree oil into warm water and use as a wound wash. See "How to Increase Skin Absorption" on page 129 if desired for deep infections like abscesses and boils. **Prevention:** Use on cuts or scrapes to help prevent infection.
Nose infection	Add 2 drops of tea tree oil to 2 drops of carrier oil. Dilute with more carrier oil if it stings a bit. Apply to the inside of nostrils with a Q-tip. Can also add rosemary and lavender oil for extra support. See "Natural Remedy Protocol for the Nose" on page 201 for full details.
Bathing	Add 5 drops tea tree oil directly to a scoop of dry bath salts, stir the dry salts to mix, then add the salts to the bath water (full size tub). Do not add oils directly to the bath water. Can be used with every bath while infection lasts.
Air diffusing	For respiratory or airborne bacteria support, cold-air diffuse 15-20 drops of tea tree oil in 10-15 minute intervals several times throughout the day while infection lasts. May be diffused with equal amounts of eucalyptus oil for enhanced effect.

Type of Support	Tea Tree Usage Amounts and Protocols for Use
Sinus infection	Add 1 drop of tea tree oil to neti pot. Irrigate sinuses using neti pot, 1 or 2 times per day while infection lasts. 1 drop of eucalyptus oil can be added for enhanced effect. See "Sinus Rinsing" on page 191 for neti pot instructions:
Mouth infection	Add 1 drop of tea tree oil and ½ teaspoon sea salt to 1 cup of warm water and mix well. Rinse mouth and discard, several times per day while infection lasts.
Bone infection	Apply tea tree oil to the skin over the infected bone using the skin protocol above. Moisten a small towel with warm water. Apply the warm moist compress to the skin to help drive the oil into the body. Continue the compress until the cloth is cool. Cabreuva oil may also be applied after tea tree for added skin penetration effect.
Vaginal infection	Combine 5 drops of tea tree, 2 drops lavender oil and **1 ounce (30 mL) of carrier oil** together and mix. Douche or irrigate with the mixture daily while infection lasts. Mixture may also be applied to a tampon prior to insertion. Oil mixture may feel warm or sting slightly, but should only be temporary. **CAUTION: Rinse with more carrier oil if burning or stinging is experienced.**
Personal care products	Add at least 20 to 30 drops of tea tree oil to 8 - 12 ounces of personal care product in the bottle (hand and body washes, lotions and shampoos). Shake or mix well.

Eucalyptus Oil

- **Hotness rating:** medium

- **Antibacterial and antiviral** properties.

- **Ideal for adults,** air diffusing and lung support.

- **Not for internal use.**

Native to Australia, eucalyptus (*Eucalyptus radiata*) are among the tallest trees in the world. Eucalyptus oil is steam distilled from the leaves. This oil has long been used for respiratory infection support and for controlling airborne bacteria. Eucalyptus oil can support the body to open the lungs and help clear congestion. The oil has expectorant, mucolytic and decongestant properties which are supportive during colds, coughs, sore throat, sinus problems and respiratory disorders. Eucalyptus has also been used to loosen bronchial secretions. The oil's antiseptic and antiviral properties have been used for control of airborne bacteria and viruses. Eucalyptus has been shown to have strong antibacterial activity against MRSA in laboratory studies[57]. One study showed that tea tree and eucalyptus combined together to create a powerful synergy against MRSA (Dr. Eugene Sherry, University of Sydney). There are many species of Eucalyptus oil on the market but *Eucalyptus radiata* is one of the safest varieties.

Precautions

Keep out of reach of children. Eucalyptus oil should not be applied to the facial areas, especially the nose or eyes. Nor for use on the face of small children or infants (use tea tree oil around the nose and eyes instead). Some people may have allergic reactions, including rashes and itching, when applying eucalyptus oil topically. If a reaction develops, stop the use of the oil.

Children and the elderly: Follow dilutions and use directions in the "Children, Babies and Elderly Protocols" on page 160.

Type of Support	Eucalyptus Usage Amounts and Protocols for Use
Skin or topical	Dilute eucalyptus oil 1:1 in a carrier oil and apply 1-2 drops of the diluted oil directly onto the skin or a sore or wound, 3 or 4 times per day while infection lasts. If the oil stings, dilute even more with a carrier oil before applying. You can also add a few drops of the oil into warm water and use as a wound wash.
Bathing	Add 5 drops eucalyptus oil directly to a scoop of dry bath salts, stir the dry salts to mix, then add the salts to the bath water (full size tub). Do not add oils directly to the bath water. Can be used with every bath while infection lasts.
Air diffusing	For respiratory or airborne support, cold-air diffuse 15-20 drops of eucalyptus oil in 10-15 minute intervals several times throughout the day while infection lasts. May be diffused with equal amounts of tea tree oil for enhanced effect.
Sinus infection	Add 1 drop of eucalyptus oil to neti pot. Irrigate sinuses using neti pot, 1 or 2 times per day while infection lasts. 1 drop of tea tree oil can be added for enhanced effect. See "Sinus Rinsing" on page 191 for neti pot instructions:

Oregano Oil

- **Hotness rating:** very high

- **Potent antibacterial**, antifungal and antiviral properties.

- **Ideal for adults,** internal and sanitizing purposes.

- **Best for internal use only.**

- **Not for children or babies.**

Oregano is sometimes called the *big gun* of infection-fighting essential oils. This oil has broad and potent activity against a wide range of bacterial species that cause infections[55]. The species *Origanum vulgare* is high in the naturally occurring phenolic compound called carvracol. Carvacol has been found to be more effective than 18 pharmaceutical drugs and is very active against MRSA[60]. Georgetown University researchers have found that oil of oregano appears to reduce infection as

143

effectively as traditional antibiotics. Oil of oregano at relatively low usage amounts was found to be efficacious against Staph bacteria and was comparable in its germ killing properties to antibiotic drugs such as streptomycin, penicillin and vancomycin[61]. Oregano is also a strong surface sanitizer.

While oil of oregano has potent antibacterial and antifungal properties, in its pure or undiluted form this oil is very hot and irritating to the skin. Oregano must never be used on the skin without diluting it significantly in a carrier oil. This oil is also prone to sensitizing the skin with prolonged topical use. For these reasons, oregano oil is a poor choice for skin applications on young children and the elderly. Because oregano can be a skin irritant it is best suited for internal ingestion after diluting it in a carrier oil and placing it into a veggie capsule.

Oregano oil with a carvacrol content of 70% or more is strongly therapeutic. However, natural carvacrol content this high is very uncommon and hard to find in most commercial oregano oil products. Most commercial oregano oils are pre-diluted in a carrier oil, limiting the product's potency and the potential uses. Pure wild-harvested oregano from specific locales in Turkey is the most potent source of oregano oil.

Precautions

Keep out of reach of children. Oregano oil that is 100% pure and undiluted is very irritating to the skin. Keep away from eyes and mucous membranes. If skin irritation develops wash away using a carrier oil and discontinue use. Use sensibly and carefully. Do not air diffuse. Avoid use with children. Avoid use if pregnant.

When using oregano oil internally, foul smelling feces is common as the body may dump dead bacteria and associated toxins. Oregano is best suited for temporary use only during the acute phase of an infection. Short-term use is recommended to avoid sensitizing the skin and reduce the risk of undesirable changes in liver metabolism that can occur with prolonged use.

If you accidentally get undiluted oregano oil on your skin or in your mouth, wash with olive oil, vegetable oil or another carrier oil. Never use water to wash off essential oils because water will make the burning worse. Do not use in bath water. Never touch your face after handling oregano oil before washing hands well.

Type of Support	Oregano Oil Usage Amounts and Protocols for Use
Internal support	**Mild infections:** 1 drop internally, 3 times per day. Should be added to a veggie capsule diluted with carrier oil. Avoid long-term use. **Moderate infections:** 3 or 4 drops internally, 3 times per day for **30 days only**. Add to a veggie capsule diluted with carrier oil. Avoid long-term use. **Severe (life-threatening) infections:** 10 drops internally, 3 times per day for **3 days only**. DO NOT EXCEED 3 DAYS. Add to a veggie capsule diluted with carrier oil. After the first 3 days, follow the *moderate infection* usage amount above for 30 days if needed.
Sanitizing	Add 10-20 drops of oregano oil, 2 cups water and a detergent or soap of your choice into a spray bottle. Mix well immediately before each use and spray onto surfaces to be sanitized. Wipe off excess and allow to air dry. Keep away from skin and face. For added sanitizing activity, some or all of the following oils may be added to the spray bottle along with the oregano oil: • 10 drops thyme • 10 drops clary sage • 20 drops lemon oil

The Antibacterial Blend

- **Hotness rating:** medium-high

- **Potent antibacterial** properties. Blended specifically for superbug support.

- **Ideal for both internal and external uses.**

- **Best oil choice** if only one essential oil is used.

A blend of several individual essential oils, the Antibacterial Blend is specifically formulated for broad-spectrum antibacterial support and for superbugs like Staph and MRSA. This blend is suited for internal use and can also be applied to the skin where support is needed, either neat (undiluted if tolerated) or diluted in a carrier oil for sensitive skin areas. The blend can also be air diffused to control airborne bacteria and added to bath salts for extra antibacterial action.

The constituents combined in the Antibacterial Blend have a powerful ballistic-type action that seeks out harmful pathogens throughout the body and renders them ineffective. This blend is composed of a synergistic combination of antibacterial and immune supportive oils including nutmeg (*Myristica fragrans*), thyme (*Thymus vulgaris*), rosalina (*Melaleuca ericifolia*) and rosemary (*Rosmarinus officinalis*). Thyme in particular has strong activity against actual clinical isolates of MRSA[57].

The Antibacterial Blend is also used as part of the "Broad-Spectrum Internal Protocol for Adults" on page 152 and the "Stealth Bacteria Protocol for Adults" on page 154.

Precautions

Keep out of the reach of children. This oil can be somewhat hot or spicy and may cause skin sensitivity in some people. Test this oil on a small area of skin first before using. Avoid using this oil near the eyes and dilute before using on sensitive skin areas. Do not allow near the face of children, spot bathing may be better.

Children and the elderly: Follow dilutions and use directions in the "Children, Babies and Elderly Protocols" on page 160.

Type of Support	Antibacterial Blend Usage Amounts and Protocols for Use
Skin or topical	Dilute the Antibacterial Blend 1:1 (50%) with carrier oil and apply topically on and around boils, sores or abscesses, 3 or 4 times per day while infection lasts. Dilute with additional carrier oil if too hot on the skin. Use caution on sensitive skin areas. See "How to Increase Skin Absorption" on page 129 if desired for deep infections like abscesses and boils **Prevention:** Use on cuts or scrapes to help prevent infection.
Bathing	Add 5 drops of the Antibacterial Blend directly to a scoop of dry bath salts, stir the salts to mix, then add the salts to the bath water. Do not add oils directly to the bath water. Use with every bath while infection lasts. Spot bathing may be preferred for sensitive skin areas.
Air diffusing	For respiratory support or airborne support, cold-air diffuse 15-20 drops of the Antibacterial Blend for 10-15 minute intervals several times throughout the day while infection lasts. Reduce or discontinue if burning or irritation occurs.
Internal support	**Mild infections and long term maintenance:** 1 drop internally, 3 times per day. Should be added to a veggie capsule diluted with carrier oil. Long term maintenance can be used if well tolerated. **Moderate infections:** 3 or 4 drops internally, 3 times per day for **30 days only**. Should be added to a veggie capsule diluted with carrier oil. After 30 days, if infection has resolved, consider using the maintenance usage amount above as a long-term preventative. **Severe (life-threatening) infections:** 10 drops internally, 3 times per day for **3 days only**. DO NOT EXCEED 3 DAYS. Should be added to a veggie capsule diluted with carrier oil. After the first 3 days, follow the *moderate infection* usage amount above for 30 days if needed. After 30 days, consider using the maintenance usage amount above as a long-term preventative if needed.
Bone infections	Apply to the skin over the infected bone using the skin protocol above. Moisten a small towel with warm water. Apply the warm moist compress to the skin to help drive the oil into the body. Continue compress until the cloth is cool. Cabreuva oil may be applied after the Antibacterial Blend for added skin penetration effect.

Type of Support	Antibacterial Blend Usage Amounts and Protocols for Use
Personal care products	Add 20 to 30 drops to each 8 - 12 ounce bottle of personal care product, such as hand and body washes, lotions and shampoos, and shake or mix well.

The Antifungal Blend

- **Hotness rating:** high

- **Potent antifungal** properties. Blended specifically for yeast and fungal infection support.

- **Ideal for internal use.**

The *Antifungal Blend* is for support with yeast and fungal infections and is ideal for internal use. Fungal infections are common after having Staph or MRSA or after taking antibiotic drugs. This blend supports immune function and convalescence. The constituents in the blend help flush pathogenic invaders from the entire body including the urinary and respiratory systems. This blend is best suited for internal use because it has a high hotness rating. However, the blend can be used on the skin if diluted adequately and used with care. This blend is composed of a combination of the antifungal and immune supportive oils cinnamon bark, black cumin, frankincense and ravensara.

The first two ingredients (cinnamon bark and black cumin) exhibited strong anti-MRSA properties in laboratory studies[58]. Cinnamon bark studies also show inhibition of oral Candida yeast, while black cumin showed antifungal effects against Candida yeast and Aspergillus mold species. The Antifungal Blend is also used as part of the "Broad-Spectrum Internal Protocol for Adults" on page 152 and the "Stealth Bacteria Protocol for Adults" on page 154.

Precautions

Keep out of the reach of children. This oil is hot or spicy and may cause skin sensitivity, dilute before using on the skin. Test this oil on a small area of skin first before using. Avoid using this oil near the eyes. Avoid use on the face of children, spot bathing may be better. Do not use during early pregnancy.

Children and the elderly: Follow dilutions and use directions in the "Children, Babies and Elderly Protocols" on page 160.

Type of Support	Antifungal Blend Usage Amounts and Protocols for Use
Skin or topical	For fungal skin infections, dilute the Antifungal Blend 1:1 (50%) with carrier oil and apply topically where needed, 3 or 4 times per day while infection lasts. Dilute with additional carrier oil if too hot on the skin. Use caution on sensitive skin areas.

Type of Support	Antifungal Blend Usage Amounts and Protocols for Use
Bathing	For fungal skin infections, add 5 drops of the Antifungal Blend directly to a scoop of dry bath salts, stir the salts to mix, then add the salts to the bath water. Do not add oils directly to the bath water. Use with every bath while infection lasts. Spot bathing may be preferred for sensitive skin areas.
Internal support	**Mild infections and long term maintenance:** 1 drop internally, 3 times per day. Should be added to a veggie capsule diluted with carrier oil. Long term maintenance can be used if well tolerated. **Moderate infections:** 3 or 4 drops internally, 3 times per day for **30 days only**. Should be added to a veggie capsule diluted with carrier oil. After 30 days, if infection has resolved, consider using the maintenance usage amount above as a long-term preventative. **Severe (life-threatening) infections:** 10 drops internally, 3 times per day for **3 days only**. DO NOT EXCEED 3 DAYS. Should be added to a veggie capsule diluted with carrier oil. After the first 3 days, follow the *moderate infection* usage amount above for 30 days if needed. After 30 days, consider using the maintenance usage amount above as a long-term preventative if needed.
Personal care products	Add 20 to 30 drops to each 8 - 12 ounce bottle of personal care product, such as hand and body washes, lotions and shampoos, and shake or mix well.

The Spice Blend

- **Hotness rating:** high

- **Potent antiviral** properties. Blended specifically for cold, flu and other viral infection support.

- **Ideal for internal use**.

The *Spice Blend* is ideally formulated for support for secondary viral infections and general infection support. Viruses cause infections such as the cold and flu that can be easier to catch if your immune system has been weakened by recent Staph or MRSA or from taking antibiotic drugs. This blend also provides broad general antibacterial infection support in addition to support for the immune system.

The Spice Blend is best suited for internal use because it has a high hotness rating. However, the blend can be applied to the skin where support is needed if diluted adequately in a carrier oil and used with care. This blend can also be air diffused with care. This blend is composed of a synergistic mix of the antiviral, antibacterial, anti-inflammatory and immune supportive oils cinnamon, lemon, lime, mandarin orange, oregano and ravensara essential oils. Cinnamon and oregano have strong anti-MRSA activity[58]. The Spice Blend is also used as part of the "Broad-Spectrum Internal Protocol for Adults" on page 152 and the "Stealth Bacteria Protocol for Adults" on page 154.

Precautions

Keep out of the reach of children. This oil is hot or spicy and may cause skin sensitivity, dilute before using on the skin. Test on a small area of skin first before using. Do not use if pregnant. Avoid diffusing or using near the eyes. Avoid use on or near the face or in the throat of children less than 30 months of age.

Children and the elderly: Follow dilutions and use directions in the "Children, Babies and Elderly Protocols" on page 160.

Type of Support	Spice Blend Usage Amounts and Protocols for Use
Skin or topical	For viral skin lesions, dilute the Spice Blend at least 1:1 (50%) with carrier oil and apply topically on the area of need, 3 or 4 times per day while infection lasts. Dilute with additional carrier oil if too hot on the skin. Use caution on sensitive skin areas.
Air diffusing	For respiratory support with viral infections, cold-air diffuse 15-20 drops of the Spice Blend for 10-15 minutes every 3 or 4 hours throughout the day while infection lasts. Reduce or discontinue if eye or nose burning or irritation occurs.
Internal support	**Mild infections and long term maintenance:** 1 drop internally, 3 times per day. Should be added to a veggie capsule diluted with carrier oil. Long term maintenance can be used if well tolerated. **Moderate infections:** 3 or 4 drops internally, 3 times per day for **30 days only**. Should be added to a veggie capsule diluted with carrier oil. After 30 days, if infection has resolved, consider using the maintenance usage amount above as a long-term preventative. **Severe (life-threatening) infections:** 10 drops internally, 3 times per day for **3 days only**. DO NOT EXCEED 3 DAYS. Should be added to a veggie capsule diluted with carrier oil. After the first 3 days, follow the *moderate infection* usage amount above for 30 days if needed. After 30 days, consider using the maintenance usage amount above as a long-term daily preventative if needed.
Personal care products	Add at least 20 to 30 drops to each 8 - 12 ounce bottle of personal care product, such as hand and body washes, lotions and shampoos, and shake or mix well. When using products containing this blend, take care to avoid the eyes and avoid use around the face of children less than 30 months of age.

Stealth Bacteria Oil Blend

- **Hotness rating:** mild

- **Ideal for L-form and Biofilm** support.

- **Ideal for external and internal use**.

Staph, MRSA and other types of bacteria can mutate into L-forms, allowing them to hide in the body for long periods of time, causing reinfections. L-forms are nearly immune to antibiotic drugs and difficult to treat. They may be a signification reason for recurring infections after antibiotic treatments.

Research is relating L-form bacteria to a host of chronic and degenerative diseases, including cancer. The Centers for Disease Control (CDC) have recognized the correlation between infections and chronic diseases. The Stealth Bacteria Blend contains 10 essential oils chosen to address L-form bacteria and rogue human cells. This formula is high in sesquiterpene constituents. These constituents are adept at seeking out rogue cells in the body, strengthening compromised cells to regenerate properly and aiding detoxification. This blend is composed of a synergistic combination of tissue healing and infection-supportive oils such as frankincense, helichrysum, copaiba and brazium oils.

This blend is best suited for internal use to seek out hidden L-form bacteria, but it can also be applied to the skin. The Stealth Bacteria Blend is also used as part of the "Stealth Bacteria Protocol for Adults" on page 154.

Precautions

Keep out of the reach of children. Avoid contact with the eyes.

Type of Support	Stealth Bacteria Blend Usage Amounts and Protocols for Use
Skin or topical	In addition to using either tea tree oil or the Antibacterial Blend, 1-2 drops of Stealth Bacteria Blend may be applied onto a sore or wound, 3 or 4 times per day. If the oil is too hot or strong, dilute with a carrier oil before applying.
Internal support	If not using the Broad-Spectrum Internal Protocol or the Stealth Bacteria Protocol, then the Stealth Bacteria Blend may be taken by itself, up to 4 drops internally, 2 times per day. Can be taken orally in a veggie capsule.

Cabreuva Oil

- **Hotness rating:** mild

- **Enhances skin penetration** of other oils.

- **Ideal for external use**.

150

This fragrant oil from the Brazilian cabreuva tree is relatively unknown to most essential oil users. To ensure maximum potency, cabreuva oil should be distilled from the wood chips of the tree rather than the less effective method of distilling from the watered-down substance of the tree. While antimicrobial itself, this oil helps amplify the properties of other essential oils when used together.

Cabreuva oil has antibacterial, antiseptic, antiulcer and skin penetration enhancing properties. It's unusually high concentration of nerolidol also helps it amplify the effects of other essential oils by helping them penetrate the skin or body tissues. Cabreuva oil has demonstrated an ability to help the body create bone marrow, repair tissue, heal ulcers, destroy pathogenic cells, eliminate mold or Candida overgrowth, and replicate red and white blood cells. This oil also provides a hormone like impact to assist the body in balancing the thyroid and protect the thyroid from bacterial attacks.

Cabreuva oil is best suited for skin support and for airborne bacteria. Layer it on the skin after other oils to enhance thee primary oil's effectiveness. Talk with your holistic doctor for internal use instructions.

Precautions

Keep out of the reach of children. Avoid contact with the eyes. **Children and the elderly:** Follow dilutions and use directions in the "Children, Babies and Elderly Protocols" on page 160.

Type of Support	Cabreuva Oil Usage Amounts and Protocols for Use
Skin or topical	Apply a primary oil of your choice for infection control, such as tea tree oil, to the affected area of skin. Next, apply 1 or 2 drops of cabreuva oil onto the same area. The cabreuva will help push the underlying oil through the skin. You can also use cabreuva alone on affected skin areas for mild and gentle infection support. Repeat the above protocol 3 or 4 times per day while infection lasts. If it is too strong or stings, dilute with a carrier oil before applying.
Bathing	Add 5 drops cabreuva oil directly to a scoop of dry bath salts along with 5 drops of a primary oil of your choice, such as tea tree oil or the Antibacterial Blend. Stir the salts to mix, then add to the bath water (full size tub). Do not add oils directly to the bath water. Can be used with every bath while infection lasts.
Air diffusing	For respiratory or airborne support, combine 15-20 drops of cabreuva oil with 15-20 drops of the primary oil of your choice, such as tea tree or eucalyptus oil. Diffuse the mixture in 10-15 minute intervals throughout the day while infection lasts.
Scars	First apply the primary oil of your choice for scar control, such as lavender or helichrysum oil, to the affected area of skin. Next, apply 1 or 2 drops of cabreuva oil directly onto the same area and message in. The cabreuva will help push the underlying primary oil through the skin. You can also use cabreuva alone for scar support. For old scars, repeat the above protocol 2 times per day for 3 to 6 months.

Helichrysum Oil

- **Hotness rating:** mild
- **Tissue healing and regeneration** properties.
- **For external use.**

The species *Helichrysum italicum* is excellent for trauma, helps regenerate nerves, increases lymphatic drainage, aids in wound regeneration, helps prevent and reduce scars, is antibacterial, anti-inflammatory, and is a very gentle oil.

Precautions

Keep out of reach of children. Keep away from eyes.

Type of Support	Helichrysum Oil Usage Amounts and Protocols for Use
Wound healing and tissue regeneration	Apply 1-2 drops directly onto the skin or a sore or wound, 3 or 4 times per day while condition lasts. Can be diluted in a carrier oil if desired.
Scar prevention	Apply 1-2 drops on afflicted area or use method below 2 times daily for 10 days.
Old scars	Combine 1 drop of helichrysum oil, 15 drops of flax seed oil and 1 teaspoon of hazelnut oil. Apply the mixture 2 times daily for 3 to 6 months.
Irritated skin	Apply 1-2 drops diluted in a few drops of carrier oil or hazelnut oil and apply on location.

Lavender Oil

- **Hotness rating:** mild
- **Tissue soothing and repair** properties.
- **Calming and emotional support** properties.
- **For external use.**

Lavender (*Lavandula angustifolia*) is one of the most widely known essential oils and can be used in many different ways. Lavender has respectable antibacterial properties and has been shown to be effective against MRSA and Staph bacteria[62]. Lavender is also well recognized for its calming and relaxing qualities and for its pleasing aroma. Lavender is especially useful for soothing damaged skin, sunburn and insect bites.

Lavender also supports tissue regeneration when used topically. Lavender provides excellent aromatherapy to reduce stress, which also helps support the immune system. Lavender is generally safe for long-term topical use.

Precautions

Keep out of reach of children. Keep away from eyes. Some medical professionals recommend limiting the use of lavender oil during the early stages of pregnancy.

Type of Support	Lavender Oil Usage Amounts and Protocols for Use
Skin or topical	Apply 1-2 drops of lavender oil directly onto minor cuts, scrapes or insect bites to control stinging and promote healing. Can be applied several times per day. Can be diluted in a carrier oil. **Prevention:** Use on cuts or scrapes to help prevent infection. **Children:** Dilute 1 drop oil to 3 drops carrier oil for children less than 24 months in age. Dilute 50/50 in carrier oil for children less than 36 months of age.
Bathing	For a relaxing bath, add 5 drops of lavender oil directly to a scoop of dry bath salts, stir the dry salts to mix, then add the salts to the bath water (full size tub). Do not add oils directly to the bath water. Can be used with every bath while infection lasts.
Air diffusing	For stress reduction and general immune support, cold-air diffuse 15-20 drops of lavender oil in 10-15 minute intervals throughout the day while infection lasts.
Personal care products	Add 20 to 30 drops to each 8 - 12 ounce bottle of personal care product, such as hand and body washes, lotions and shampoos, and shake or mix well.

German Chamomile Oil

- **Hotness rating**: mild

- **Anti-inflammatory** properties.

- **Immune stimulant** effects.

- **For external use.**

German chamomile (*Matricaria recutita or Matricaria chamomilla*) is one of the most anti-inflammatory of all the essential oils. It is also a very calming oil. German chamomile applied topically helps rid the body of toxic bacterial metabolic wastes and is supportive of the healing process. It has successfully been used for calming sensitive and inflamed skin and for helping difficult to heal wounds. It is a mild oil and generally safe for children. This oil should not be confused with Roman chamomile, which is a different species with different properties and effects on the body.

Precautions

Keep out of reach of children. Keep away from eyes. Do not use chamomile oil during pregnancy because it can stimulate uterine contractions. Because chamomile stimulates the immune system, using it on rashes and hives resulting from an autoimmune response can make the symptoms worse. Use with caution if you are allergic to grass and ragweed. Before using any natural approach for rashes, be sure to test it first by applying a small amount on a small area of skin. Chamomile is nontoxic and nonirritating, however, it can cause dermatitis in some people.

Type of Support	German Chamomile Usage Amounts and Protocols for Use
Skin or topical	**Difficult wounds:** Dilute German chamomile oil 1:1 in a carrier oil and apply 1-2 drops of the diluted oil directly onto the skin, 3 or 4 times per day while the condition lasts. **Irritated skin/rashes:** Can be used as above or combined with equal amounts of helichrysum oil for added effect.
Scars	Combine equal parts of German chamomile oil and helichrysum oil. Add 1-2 drops of the mixture into several drops of hazelnut oil. Apply a few drops of the final blend topically on location 2 or 3 times per day. May require several weeks or up to a few months of use to see results with old scars.
Stomach upset	Mix one drop of German chamomile oil into a cup of water and drink.

Bay Laurel Oil

- **Hotness rating**: mild

- **Detoxification** support.

- **For external use.**

Bay Laurel (*Laurus nobilis*) is a powerful immune system booster and has antimicrobial properties. Bay Laurel is excellent for moving sluggish lymph. Bacterial bodies and toxins accumulate in the lymph during an infection, which can cause pain and inflammation. Applied topically over areas of the lymph nodes, this oil can enhance lymphatic drainage and support toxin elimination. Bay Laurel is also good for respiratory congestion and can help relieve fever when used in combination with eucalyptus oil.

Precautions

Keep out of reach of children. Keep away from eyes. Start slowly and avoid using large amounts of bay laurel on the lymph nodes to reduce the risk of detox symptoms.

Type of Support	Bay Laurel Usage Amounts and Protocols for Use
Skin or topical	Apply 1 - 2 drops of bay laurel oil on the lymph node areas twice daily, for 2 to 3 weeks while infection lasts. Use diluted in carrier oil for larger skin areas. Try a body brush or light massage to enhance stimulation and movement of lymph fluids..
Lymph drainage stimulation	**Foot massage:** Place 1 - 2 drops of bay laurel oil on the palm of the left hand. Massage the ball of the right foot with the palm of the left hand in a figure-8 motion, 30 times, rubbing in the oil. Repeat for the left foot. This protocol can be done alone, but a partner is helpful. **Groin massage:** Place 1 - 2 drops of bay laurel oil on the palms and lightly push on the skin starting from the groin area, moving either up toward the chest or down toward the knees. **CAUTION:** do not apply bay laurel directly on sensitive skin areas on or near the genitals. Dilution in a carrier oil can be used for sensitive skin. **Chest massage:** Place 1 - 2 drops of bay laurel on the palms and lightly push on the skin starting near the nipple, pushing outward away in all directions. Perform this protocol on both sides of the chest. **Shoulder massage:** Place 1 - 2 drops of bay laurel on the palms and push on the skin starting near the top of the shoulders and pushing down toward the back. This protocol is much easier with a partner.
Air diffusing	For immune and detox support, cold-air diffuse 15 drops of bay laurel oil in 10-15 minute intervals throughout the day while infection lasts. May be combined with an equal amount of eucalyptus oil for support with respiratory congestion.

Other Essential Oils

The following essential oils are also worthy of mention for MRSA and Staph support:

- **Thyme.** *Thymus vulgaris* is a strongly antibacterial oil. It is high in thymol and carvacrol content and has broad anti-infectious qualities. Like oregano oil, thyme is a *hot* oil and is sensitizing to the skin, therefore, thyme is best for internal use for adults. Thyme is also great for cleaning and surface sanitizing. This oil is not suitable for young children or skin uses.

  » Precautions: Keep away from eyes and out of reach of children. Only use on the skin when diluted. Not for use on children under 6 years old. Like oregano oil, it can lead to liver stress with prolonged internal use. Use with caution for cleaning if you have pets in the house (see "Pet Precautions" on page 126 for more details).

- **Geranium.** Like lavender oil, geranium (*Pelargonium graveolens*) has respectable antibacterial qualities but is very mild and gentle enough for children. Geranium also has antifungal properties, is used for pain relief from burns and bruises and has calming and relaxing qualities. It can be used for skin infections, air diffused or added to personal care products. Refer to the

Lavender oil protocol for instructions and dilution ratios.

> » Precautions: Keep out of reach of children and away from the eyes.

- **Rosemary.** Rosemary (*Rosemarinus officinalis*) has many of the same chemical compounds that tea tree oil has and is great for skin support and as an addition to personal care products. For adults, dilute 25% to 50% for topical skin applications. For children less than 24 months, dilute 1 drop oil to 3 drops carrier oil. For children less than 36 months, dilute 50/50 in carrier oil.

  > » Precautions: Keep out of reach of children and away from the eyes. Not for use on newborns. Do not apply undiluted to the skin. Long term use not recommended due to ketone content.

- **Myrrh.** *Commiphora myrrha* is also antibacterial, and it enhances the bacterial killing effects of white blood cells. Myrrh can be very useful for skin infections, pain relief, and is very safe for topical use in adults and children. Apply to affected skin areas and dilute with carrier oil if necessary. For children less than 24 months, dilute 1 drop oil to 3 drops carrier oil. For children less than 36 months, dilute 50/50 in carrier oil.

  > » Precautions: Keep out of reach of children and away from the eyes.

Broad-Spectrum Internal Protocol for Adults

This protocol uses three separate essential oil blends. Details about each blend are in the three sections "The Antibacterial Blend" on page 145, "The Antifungal Blend" on page 147, and "The Spice Blend" on page 148. The usage amounts in this protocol are for adults only. For **children and the elderly,** follow dilutions and use directions in the "Children, Babies and Elderly Protocols" on page 160

Is This Protocol for You?

It is not necessary or recommended that you follow this protocol or use the essential oils in this section. Only use the oils and protocols that you need based on the steps you choose to follow from the section "Action Step 1: Bacteria Control" on page 9 , the first step in chapter 1. This protocol is not meant to be used by itself as a stand-alone resource - for best results, combine it with the other Action Steps in chapter 1.

Start Slowly

If you are unfamiliar with an essential oil, start slowly and work up to the desired usage amount. If you experience adverse symptoms, then decrease the usage amount, frequency of use and/or duration of use. As with any natural remedy, listen to your body and stop taking anything that is causing you problems. Always consult with your health care provider if you have any concerns about using essential oils along with medications.

Using the Protocol

The protocol includes three different essential oil blends, each taken once per day internally at a specific time of day. The timing for each blend was developed to coincide with the life cycle of different infection challenges. For example, viral challenges are less active in the morning, so this is the ideal time to use the Spice Blend, which is optimized for viral support. Likewise, the other two blends are taken at a time of day which coincides with the inactive phase of the blend's target challenge, including fungal challenges and bacterial challenges.

There are three levels or usage amounts in the protocol, depending on the degree of support needed. The mild level is suitable for long-term maintenance. The moderate and severe levels should only be used for a maximum of 30 days and 3 days, respectively, to avoid stressing the liver. If the severe level is used, the moderate level may be used afterward if needed, followed by the mild level (if needed).

Because internal use of essential oils can stress the liver, it should be done under the care of a health-care professional. For maximum safety, only the highest quality therapeutic grade essential oils should be considered for internal use.

The protocol is best followed using the veggie capsule technique for ingesting the oils. See the section "Capsule Filling Technique" on page 132 for details on this technique.

Alternatives to the Protocol

This protocol is ideal for internal support against infections. However, one simple alternative for people on a budget is to use the Antibacterial Blend only, omitting the other two blends in the protocol. For those wishing to avoid the internal use of oils, topical foot application or air diffusion are two alternatives. Follow details in "Is There an Alternate to Taking Essential Oils Internally?" on page 136.

Precautions

Follow precautions for individual oils.

Level	Morning	Afternoon	Evening
Mild (maintenance)	1 drop of the Spice Blend internally.	1 drop of the Antifungal Blend internally.	1 drop of the Antibacterial Blend internally.

Level	Morning	Afternoon	Evening
Moderate	3 or 4 drops of the Spice Blend internally. **Continue for 30 days maximum.** After 30 days, the mild level may be followed if needed.	3 or 4 drops of the Antifungal Blend internally. **Continue for 30 days maximum.** After 30 days, the mild level may be followed if needed.	3 or 4 drops of the Antibacterial Blend internally. **Continue for 30 days maximum.** After 30 days, the mild level may be followed if needed.
Severe	10 drops of the Spice Blend internally. **Continue for 3 days maximum.** After 3 days, the moderate level may be followed if needed.	10 drops of the Antifungal Blend internally. **Continue for 3 days maximum.** After 3 days, the moderate level may be followed if needed.	10 drops of the Antibacterial Blend internally. **Continue for 3 days maximum.** After 3 days, the moderate level may be followed if needed.

Stealth Bacteria Protocol for Adults

This protocol was developed for internal support for long-standing and recurring challenges in which biofilms and L-from bacteria are likely involved. This protocol uses four separate essential oil blends. Details about each blend are in the four sections "The Antibacterial Blend" on page 145, "The Antifungal Blend" on page 147, "The Spice Blend" on page 148 and "Stealth Bacteria Oil Blend" on page 149. The usage amounts below are for adults only. For children, see the changes and usage amount reductions in the section "Children, Babies and Elderly Protocols" on page 160.

Is This Protocol For You?

It is not necessary or recommended that you follow this protocol or use the essential oils in this section. Only use the oils and protocols that you need based on the steps you choose to follow from the section "Action Step 1: Bacteria Control" on page 9 , the first Action Step in chapter 1. This protocol is not meant to be used by itself as a stand-alone resource. Please use the Action Steps in chapter 1 to know what to do and which remedies to use for your own particular needs.

Start Slowly

If you are unfamiliar with an essential oil, start slowly and work up to the desired usage amount. If you experience adverse symptoms, then decrease the usage amount, frequency of use and/or duration of use. As with any natural remedy, listen to your body and stop taking anything that is causing you problems. Always consult with your health care provider if you have any concerns about using the essential oils along with medications.

Using the Protocol

This protocol is an addendum to the "Broad-Spectrum Internal Protocol for Adults" on page 156. This protocol is identical to the Broad-Spectrum Internal Protocol, but with the addition of a forth essential oil blend, which is taken before bed. To follow this protocol, refer to the section "Broad-Spectrum Internal Protocol for Adults" on page 156 for the morning, afternoon and evening usage amounts, then add one bedtime usage amount each day of the Stealth Bacteria Blend, as shown in the table below.

There are three levels or usage amounts in this protocol, depending on the degree of support needed. The mild level is suitable for long-term maintenance. The moderate and severe levels should only be used for a maximum of 30 days and 3 days, respectively, to avoid stressing the liver. If the severe level is used, the moderate level may be used afterward, followed by the mild level

Because internal use of essential oils can stress the liver, it should be done under the care of a health-care professional. For maximum safety, only the highest quality therapeutic grade essential oils should be considered for internal use.

The protocol is best followed using the veggie capsule technique for ingesting the oils. See the section "Capsule Filling Technique" on page 132 for details on this technique.

Alternatives to the Protocol

For those wishing to avoid the internal use of oils, topical foot application or air diffusion are two alternatives. Follow details in "Is There an Alternate to Taking Essential Oils Internally?" on page 136.

Precautions

Follow precautions for individual oils.

Level	Morning	Afternoon	Evening	Bedtime
Mild	Follow the Broad-Spectrum Internal Protocol with the Spice blend.	Follow the Broad-Spectrum Internal Protocol with the Anti-fungal blend.	Follow the Broad-Spectrum Internal Protocol with the Anti-bacterial blend.	1 drop of the Stealth Bacteria Blend internally.
Moderate				3 or 4 drops of the Stealth Bacteria Blend internally. **Continue for 30 days maximum.** After 30 days, the mild level may be followed if needed.
Severe				3 or 4 drops of the Stealth Bacteria Blend internally. **Continue for 3 days maximum.** After 3 days, the moderate level may be followed if needed. **Note:** This usage amount is identical to the moderate level usage amount.

Children, Babies and Elderly Protocols

Essential oils are wonderful allies to help fight stubborn and painful infections in children. However, it's important to remember that small children and the elderly have more sensitive skin and weaker immune systems than adults. Children also have smaller bodies than adults, making it easier to overuse a remedy. Therefore, adult usage amounts of essential oils should be reduced or modified to be safe. Also, some oils that are safe for adults may be inappropriate for children.

Consult with your doctor or holistic physician before using essential oils internally with your child. For maximum safety, only the highest quality therapeutic grade essential oils should be considered. Always follow the manufacturer directions or the guidance of a healthcare professional if they differ from the protocols below.

Start Slowly

The adjustments in this section are rules of thumb only. An individual's tolerance to essential oils may vary, especially with babies. Start slowly and work up to the desired usage amount over a few days. If adverse symptoms are experienced, dilute the oil more, decrease the usage amount, or reduce the frequency or the duration of use. You may also choose to stop using the oil or try a different oil or a different remedy if adverse symptoms arise.

Alternatives to the Protocol

Topical use on the skin is a very safe way to use essential oils, especially when diluted in a carrier oil. Oils can also be placed on the feet or diffused as an alternative to internal use. See "Is There an Alternate to Taking Essential Oils Internally?" on page 136 for more details.

Precautions

Oils must be diluted when used on babies or children. Be sure to read the "Precautions for Children" on page 127 before you start using or diffusing oils with babies or children. Follow precautions for individual oils.

Age Groups	Usage	Children and Elderly Usage Amounts and Protocols for Use
• 0 - 2 years • 85 or older	Skin	• **Tea tree oil** is ideal for any skin infections because it is mild and gentle. Avoid any *hot* or *spicy* oils on skin. • **Dilute 75%** by mixing 1 drop tea tree oil with 3 drops of a carrier oil. Can be applied to sore or wound when wound dressing or diaper is changed, or 3 or 4 times per day while infection lasts. • If prolonged stinging occurs, rinse the essential oil away with olive oil or another carrier oil. Do not rinse with water. Dilute the essential oil 90% or more before reapplication.
	* Internal	• **Broad-Spectrum Internal Protocol** may be used with the following usage amount changes. To take internally, add diluted mixture to a cotton swab and swab the inside of the mouth, or add 1 drop of mixture to formula or food. Except for the usage amount, all other details of the Broad-Spectrum Internal Protocol are followed. Do NOT use capsules with babies because they cannot swallow them. • For **mild/moderate** challenges: **dilute 80%** by mixing 1 drop of the oil with 4 drops of a carrier oil. Take 1 - 2 drops of mixture internally for 30 days max. • For **severe (life-threatening)** challenges: **dilute 75%** by mixing 1 drop of the oil with 3 drops of a carrier oil. Take 3 drops of mixture internally for **3 days maximum**. • As an alternative to internal use, apply 1 - 2 drops of each oil mixture to bottom of feet for general systemic support.
	Other uses	• **Only mild oils:** Only use tea tree, eucalyptus, lavender or cabreuva oils because they are gentle. Avoid using hot or spicy oils. Eucalyptus oil should not be applied to the facial areas (especially around the nose or eyes). Use diluted tea tree oil around such areas instead. • **Bathing:** Add 5 drops of either tea tree oil or eucalyptus oil directly to a scoop of dry bath salts, stir the dry salts to mix, then add the bath salts to the bath water (full size tub). Bathe baby with you for skin and/or respiratory support. Note: adding the oil directly to the bath water can cause it to simply float on the surface and may cause skin irritation. • **Spot bathing:** 1 or 2 drops of oil may be added to a tablespoon of dry bath salts and stirred into a wash basin for spot bathing with a cloth. • Note **air diffusion** precaution in "Precautions for Children" on page 127.

Age Groups	Usage	Children and Elderly Usage Amounts and Protocols for Use
• 2 - 3 years • 75 85	Skin	• **Tea tree oil** is ideal for any skin infections because it is mild and gentle. Avoid any *hot* or *spicy* oils on skin. • **Dilute 50%** by mixing 1 drop tea tree oil with 1 drop of a carrier oil. Can be applied to sore or wound when dressing is changed, or 3 or 4 times per day while infection lasts. • If prolonged stinging occurs, rinse the essential oil away with olive oil or another carrier oil. Do not rinse with water. Dilute the essential oil 75% or more before reapplication.
	* Internal	• **Broad-Spectrum Internal Protocol** may be used with the following usage amount changes: to take internally, add diluted mixture to a cotton swab and swab the inside of the mouth, or add 1 drop of mixture to food or formula. Except for the usage amount, all other details of the Broad-Spectrum Internal Protocol are followed. Do NOT use capsules with babies because they cannot swallow them. • For **mild/moderate** challenges: **dilute 50%** by mixing 1 drop of the oil with 1 drop of a carrier oil. Take 1 - 2 drops of mixture internally for 30 days max. • For **severe (life-threatening)** challenges: **dilute 50%** by mixing 1 drop of the oil with 1 drop of a carrier oil. Take 3 drops of mixture internally for 3 days maximum. • As an alternative to internal use, apply 1 – 2 drops of each oil mixture to bottom of feet for general systemic support.
	Other uses	• **Only mild oils:** Only use tea tree, eucalyptus, lavender or cabreuva oils because they are gentle. Avoid using hot or spicy oils. • **Bathing:** Add 5 drops of either tea tree oil or eucalyptus oil directly to a scoop of dry bath salts, stir the dry salts to mix, then add the bath salts to the bath water (full size tub). Note: adding the oil directly to the bath water can cause it to simply float on the surface and may cause skin irritation. • Note **air diffusion** precaution in "Precautions for Children" on page 127.

Age Groups	Usage	Children and Elderly Usage Amounts and Protocols for Use
• 3 or older • Less than 75 years	Skin	Tea tree is preferred because it is gentle. Avoid *hot* or *spicy* oils on the skin. Undiluted essential oil can generally be used if well tolerated, otherwise dilute as necessary. Can be applied directly to sore or wound, 3 or 4 times per day while infection lasts.
	Internal	The **Broad-Spectrum Internal Protocol** can generally be used at mild and moderate usage amounts if well tolerated. Dilute 50% if not well tolerated. Essential oils may be added to food for children too young to swallow capsules.
	Other uses	Adult uses and methods for tea tree oil, eucalyptus oil, lavender and cabreuva can generally be used if well tolerated. The Antibacterial Blend and other hot oils should be diluted 50% or more for younger children. Avoid face contact with any hot oils even if diluted. Note **air diffusion** precaution in "Precautions for Children" on page 127.

Essential Oil Protocols for Pets

Pets can catch MRSA or Staph from an infected owner, from a MRSA/Staph carrier or from a kennel or vet clinic experiencing an outbreak. However, MRSA and Staph in pets usually appears to originate from people, not the animal. An infected or carrier animal then acts like a reservoir and can pass the bacteria back to their owners. Just like people, pets can carry MRSA bacteria without becoming infected.

For additional resources on pets, antibiotics and MRSA, check out the Bella Moss Foundation which promotes prudent antimicrobial use and hygiene in human and veterinary medicine. This foundation was started by Jill Moss following the death of her dog, Bella, from a badly managed MRSA infection. They help link pet patients and veterinary clients with best practice resources and access to good advice. You can find out more here: www.thebellamossfoundation.com.

Fortunately, the majority of MRSA infections in pets are not severe and tend to be limited to the skin. Mild and moderate infections often respond well without antibiotics by using good wound management and diligent hygiene and prevention techniques. Thankfully, essential oils are a wonderful option and can help pets with MRSA or other infections, especially dogs, horses and other large animals. Some pets with MRSA have been helped with oils when no other treatment option worked.

Of note, there are reports of cats reacting poorly to essential oils, but a few vets have been using high quality oils with cats and have had great results. It's possible the poor reactions in cats may have been due to using inferior oils (those with toxic extraction solvents) or that too much oil was used on the cats.

Be sure to review the precautions before using essential oils on or around your furry friends per "Pet Precautions" on page 126. There is a lot of information (and misinformation) on the web about essential oils and pets. To learn more, find information from holistic veterinarians or animal professionals who use essential oils with animals.

⬦⬦

Do not use oils on cats, reptiles, birds or small mammals without consulting a holistic veterinarian. Remove these animals from rooms before diffusing oils. For maximum safety, consult with a holistic veterinary professional before using essential oils on pets.

⬦⬦

Antibacterial Oils for Pets

There are some pre-made oil blends on the market that have been developed just for pets. Mild oils (not hot) for topical skin applications that have exhibited activity against Staph or MRSA are:

- **Lavender** - *Lavandula angustifolia*

- **Eucalyptus** - *Eucalyptus radiata*

- **Geranium** - *Pelargonium graveolens*

- **Rosemary** - *Rosmarinus officinalis*

- **Myrrh** - *Commiphora myrrha*

Be sure to dilute the essential oil in a carrier oil before applying topically. Only use the highest quality oils per the guidelines in the section "What You Must Know to Find Safe and Effective Oils" on page 115.

Body Weight Adjustments

Less is more when using essential oils with pets. Because of their small size, the optimal amount of essential oil is much less than for humans. In the protocols below, the usage amounts of essential oils are reduced according to the pet's body weight.

The adjustments in this section are rules of thumb only. Just as with people, a pet's tolerance to the essential oils may vary. Start slowly and work up to the desired usage amount over a few days. If your pet experiences adverse symptoms (anxiety, excessive licking of the area, skin irritation, vomiting, etc) then dilute the oil more, reduce the frequency of use, decrease the duration of use, or stop the oil and try another oil or another remedy.

Pet	Topical Skin Uses
Dogs under 100 pounds	<ul><li>Use 1 drop of oil for every 100 lbs of body weight.</li><li>For example, for a 10-lb dog, add 1 drop of essential oil to 9 drops of a carrier oil then use 1 drop of the mixture on the skin.</li><li>If one drop of oil mixture is not enough to cover the affected area, add more carrier oil.</li></ul>
Dogs and animals over 100 pounds	The same amount of oil as for adult people is generally OK for large animals, including horses and pigs.

◇◇

See the section "Michelle's Recommended Products" on page 303 for product resources.

◇◇

13 Vitamins and Minerals

This chapter introduces the most important vitamins and minerals that help your immune system and provide infection support. While vitamins and minerals are inside the foods you eat, most foods don't have enough to support your optimal health. Therefore, supplementing your diet with a few key vitamins and minerals can be very helpful.

Vitamins and minerals are generally not a front-line *remedy* for fighting infections. However, they play many crucial roles in your body's systems. For example, vitamin C is a powerful antioxidant that supports heart health and tissue repair in addition to it's anti-infection properties. Vitamin D is crucial for proper cellular function, helps the body ward off invading pathogens and helps reduce the risk of dozens of chronic diseases, including cancer.

There are many other important vitamins, minerals and nutrients that your body needs beyond the ones covered in this chapter. But for the majority of people struggling with an infection, the nutrients detailed below are the most important ones to examine first.

Vitamin D, the *Antibiotic Vitamin*

One of the most crucial nutrients your body needs to fight and resist infections is vitamin D. Not only does vitamin D have antibacterial properties, it also mediates infection-fighting responses in your body's immune system.

It's estimated that up to 85% of Americans are vitamin D deficient and many don't realize it.

The elderly are at particular risk of deficiency. Vitamin D deficiency is more pronounced in those living in northern climates with less sun. Sun exposure on your skin is the best source of vitamin D. You may have noticed that there is a correlation between getting sick with colds and flu in the winter and getting less sun in the winter. There has also been an increase in Rickets disease due to insufficient vitamin D levels. These trends are likely due in part to vitamin D deficiency.

Deficiency Linked to MRSA Colonization

An article in the *Epidemiology and Infection* journal indicates that vitamin D deficiency may underlie a vulnerability to different kinds of infections. Researchers discovered an antimicrobial chemical in vitamin D called cathelicidin that appears to punch holes in the external membrane of bacteria, killing the bacteria. In another study, people with low vitamin D levels showed an increased risk of MRSA nasal colonization[63].

According to a study in *Science*, vitamin D controls a key antimicrobial response in humans against the bacteria *Mycobacterium tuberculosis* (TB)[64]. This study proposed that vitamin D deficiency may be the reason that African-Americans are much more susceptible to TB. This makes sense as African-Americans have higher pigment or melanin levels in the skin, which leads to less vitamin D production.

Vitamin D Testing

Vitamin D can be toxic if you get too much of it. Before you start any vitamin D supplementation, get your vitamin D levels tested and consult with a qualified healthcare professional.

It's very important to get the correct kind of test. There are two vitamin D tests: 1,25(OH)D and 25(OH)D. 25(OH)D, also called 25-hydroxyvitamin D, is the best indicator of overall D status. A few drops of blood is used to determine the level of 25(OH)D.

Professional opinions vary regarding a normal and healthy level of vitamin D in the human body. The general consensus is that anything below 32 ng/mL (nanograms per milliliter) is deficient. According to some medical authorities, people with deficient levels of vitamin D can be at an increased risk for various cancers, infections, MS, type II diabetes and other degenerative diseases. Study results by vitamin D authority Dr. Michael Hollick show that the optimal level is 50-64 ng/mL[65]. A good source of vitamin D information is the *Vitamin D Council* at the following website: www.VitaminDCouncil.org.

Best Source of Vitamin D

Sunlight on your skin naturally creates vitamin D in your body. 15 minutes of sunlight each day should be sufficient. Sunlight is the best form of vitamin D, however, many people don't have the time or a warm enough climate to get enough sun exposure. If you sun yourself, be sure to avoid sunburns, and remember that sun block lotions block the UVB rays needed to generate vitamin D.

There are two kinds of vitamin D supplements to choose from: natural and synthetic. Natural sources contain D3, which is the same chemical form that your body makes when exposed to sunshine. The synthetic variety is Vitamin D2. Nearly all the prescription-based supplements contain vitamin D2, which is not the same as D3. Milk also contains vitamin D2. Vitamin D3 is converted to a useful form inside your body much faster than D2, making it the optimal form to take in most cases.

Using Vitamin D

400 IU or more of vitamin D per day is frequently recommended by mainstream doctors if you are under 50 years of age. The Vitamin D Council and many holistic doctors believe that adults actually need 5,000 IU per day and children need 1,000 IU per day to avoid deficiency[66]. For reference, a salmon serving contains about 360 IU, an egg has 25 IU and one tablespoon of cod liver oil contain 1300+ IU.

Recent research shows that excessive amounts of vitamin A may interfere with vitamin D absorption. Cod liver oil is a common natural way to supplement vitamin D. However, most brands of cod liver oil contain more vitamin A than vitamin D. Therefore, it is best to look for products with a low ratio of vitamin A to vitamin D.

Some holistic physicians also believe if you supplement with vitamin D, you should also be taking vitamin K2 or eating vitamin K2 rich foods. When you take vitamin D, your body uses vitamin K2, which is produced by bacteria in your gut. If you don't have enough K2, then your body can't utilize the vitamin D you're taking, resulting in vitamin D toxicity. Symptoms of vitamin D toxicity include excessive calcification and hardening of the arteries[67].

Talk to a natural or nutritionally-minded doctor, test your
25(OH)D levels and come up with a plan that is right for you.

Vitamin D Precautions

Vitamin D can be toxic to your body if you get too much. Vitamin D toxicity has also been associated with a deficiency in vitamin K2. Before you start any vitamin D supplementation, be sure you test your levels and work with a qualified health professional. The Vitamin D Council upper limit of Vitamin D intake per day is 10,000 IU for adults and 2,000 IU for children. Again, testing is required to tell you how much vitamin D supplement is safe and appropriate for you.

Vitamin C

Vitamin C can help control bacteria, boost your immune system and neutralize damaging by-products of metabolism in your body. In the immune system, vitamin C works as an antioxidant, protecting the body's cells against oxidative stress caused by infections. It may also have roles in regulating some immune cells of the body.

The U.S. Recommended Daily Allowance (RDA) for vitamin C is 90 mg for adult men and 75 mg for women. Some natural health doctors recommend taking between 200 and 1000 mg of vitamin C per day for added immune support. Plant-based buffered vitamin C or vitamin C complex are the best types to take. Ascorbic acid (the acidic form of vitamin C) can actually lower your body's internal pH, potentially making infections worse.

The best source of vitamin C is from the foods you eat. Some foods are particularly rich in vitamin C. Black currents and sweet peppers contain up to 200 mg of the nutrient per cup. Oranges, strawberries, kiwi and papaya are relatively high in vitamin C, ranging from 60 to 90 mg per cup. Kale, broccoli, sweet potato and Brussels sprouts also have significant C content (20 to 40 mg per serving).

Eating five servings of assorted fruits and vegetables can provide roughly 200 mg of vitamin C per day, depending on the nutrient content of the food. Raw organic foods that are grown locally and eaten fresh have the highest nutrient contents. If you eat few raw veggies and fruits, or if you eat non-organic or low-nutrient produce, then supplementation can help fill in the gaps in your vitamin C needs.

Just like vitamins D and K2, every nutrient, including vitamin C, works in combination with other nutrients in complex ways. For example, taking one nutrient can raise or lower the levels of several other nutrients. In this way, foods provide a balanced source of vitamins and minerals that work together to support optimal health. In contrast, taking high levels of isolated vitamins or minerals can potentially throw off the balance of other nutrients. For example, large usage amounts of vitamin C can lower copper levels in your body, which can cause challenges if you happen to be deficient in copper.

IV Vitamin C for Severe Infections

The benefits of long-term vitamin C consumption in excess of the U.S. RDA values are widely acknowledged and include reduced risks of cancer, cardiovascular disease, and cataracts. Vitamin C has been reported to help with severe attacks of advanced human cancers and ulcerative colitis. Intravenous usage amounts ranging from 50 to 150 grams per day have been used with no adverse effects.

Vitamin C expert Thomas E. Levy, a practicing physician for 25 years, is a board-certified internist and a fellow of the American College of Cardiology as well as an attorney. Dr. Levy's new book, *Vitamin C, Infectious Diseases, and Toxins: Curing the Incurable*, outlines the work of Dr. Frederick Klenner, who studied vitamin C for treating a variety of diseases. Dr. Klenner used *mega-doses* of vitamin C intravenously (through an IV) on many patients who were extremely ill and often close to death. After injecting the vitamin C, he found that most patients returned to health. Dr. Levy's book presents clear evidence that vitamin C affects disease and has 1,200 scientific references.

High amount IV vitamin C therapy is an option if you are in a hospital and not responding to antibiotic treatments. Mainstream medicine usually rejects the validity of IV vitamin C therapy, despite the large body of evidence showing its benefits. Therefore, if you want to use this therapy, you'll need to educate yourself and have lots of determination to get your doctor to support you.

Using IV Vitamin C Therapy

Find a naturopathic doctor (ND) or other qualified healthcare professional who has experience administering vitamin C intravenously. It is not possible to take enough by mouth to achieve the high levels of vitamin C that are required. For those living outside the U.S., this therapy is much more common and easy to receive.

For a great resource on vitamin C information,
see the website: www.vitamincfoundation.org

Iodine

Iodine is crucial for immune system function, but most people don't get nearly enough in their diet. The World Health Organization states that 2.2 billion people in the world are at risk of iodine deficiency. Iodine levels in U.S. soil have fallen 50 percent over the past 50 years. Because the soil is deficient in iodine, so is the food that grows in the soil. Studies have also shown that the iodine from iodized salt is actually counteracted by the bromine found in many types of bread. This is another major reason why people are becoming iodine deficient. In fact, bromine (common in breads as bromated flour), chlorine (added to water supplies) and fluorine (added to water supplies) all compete in the body for the same cellular receptors that iodine uses. These three elements (commonly called halides) block iodine from working in the body and promote iodine-deficiency.

Officially, the U.S. RDA for iodine is 150 micrograms per day. You may want to consider taking more than the RDA to catch up if you are deficient. However, too much iodine is not good for you, so testing is important before beginning iodine supplementation. There is a simple test you can take for determining your iodine levels and many holistic health professionals can help you with it.

Iodine plays vital roles for both thyroid functioning and your immune system health. Foods like seafood, kelp and dulce (seaweed) are great dietary sources of iodine. Few people in the U.S. consume enough iodine-rich foods to get enough iodine. Talk to a qualified nutritional minded healthcare practitioner, get tested, and come up with a supplement plan that works for you.

Zinc

Zinc is a very important trace mineral with a firmly established role in protecting the immune system and fighting bacterial and viral infections. Foods rich in zinc include whole grains, legumes and meats. Zinc supplementation for infections is often recommended for a three-month period, taking 20 to 30 milligrams per day for adults and 10 to 15 milligrams per day for children. Excess fiber, iron and calcium in your diet can diminish your body's ability to absorb zinc. Zinc is very safe in low usage amount supplementation of less than 50 milligrams per day.

14 Secondary Conditions and Challenges

Many people who have been dealing with MRSA or Staph also have symptoms like localized pain, stomach upset or diarrhea caused by antibiotics. Secondary infections like yeast, Clostridium difficile-associated disease (CDAD), and recurring MRSA and Staph infections due to hidden stealth bacteria are also common. Addressing these secondary conditions and symptoms with *symptom-specific remedies* can help speed your recovery and reduce future infections.

This chapter will give you step-by step protocols and remedies for specific symptoms, conditions and challenges associated with Staph and MRSA. Also in this chapter are methods to address the primary side effects of antibiotic drugs, ways to support your liver, and measures to assist with common secondary infections and recurring MRSA and Staph caused by biofilms and L-form bacteria.

Check with your doctor before using unfamiliar supplements or wellness protocols in case of interactions with medications you may be taking. If there are any contradictions between the protocols in this chapter and the directions from your doctor, then either follow the directions from your doctor or enlist your doctor's support in using the protocols of your choice.

Reducing Antibiotic Side Effects

Antibiotic drugs often cause uncomfortable and unhealthy side effects. These side effects need to be addressed for best results with an infection.

- Contact your doctor immediately if you have a reaction to an antibiotic. Skin rashes and other reactions can be severe and may need immediate medical treatment.

- An allergic reaction can turn severe very quickly and lead to shock and even death without proper medical attention. If you experience any of the following symptoms, call your doctor or go to an emergency room:

  » Wheezing, difficulty breathing (not just nasal congestion), difficulty swallowing due to tight throat, excessive drooling with difficulty swallowing, swollen joints or any other signs that you suspect may be a severe allergic reaction.

Skin Reactions

One of the most common side effects of taking antibiotics is skin irritation such as itchiness, rashes and hives. Below are actions to take and activities to avoid that can help ease the symptoms of a skin reaction, followed by specific mainstream and alternative remedies.

- Do not scratch the skin as this will only aggravate the problem.

- Keep the skin slightly moisturized. Use a mild hypoallergenic moisturizer that is fragrance free. A natural skin moisturizer is preferable.

- Avoid hot showers and baths, as this can aggravate the rash and make it worse.

- Use only natural and mild soaps.

- Avoid abrasive, itchy or overly warm clothing. Wear light and cool fabrics like cotton.

- If you are following a detox or cleansing protocol, consider cutting back as detoxification through the skin can make antibiotic skin reactions worse.

Mainstream Medicine Remedies

For moderate skin irritation that is not severe, a couple common mainstream medical treatments that your doctor may prescribe include:

- A **steroidal treatment**, such as prednisone, or a hydrocortisone cream.

- Non-prescription **Benadryl**. This is an over-the-counter allergy medication that may temporarily decrease an allergic rash and itching.

Alternative Medicine Remedies

For moderate skin irritation, several natural methods have been used with great success without side effects, including the remedies below.

- **Aloe vera.** Fresh leaves from the plant are always best. Slice or break open the leaves and apply liberally to the skin until recovered. Aloe is very safe for external uses over long periods of time.

- **Calendula ointment** can be found at health food stores. Apply topically and use as directed.

- **Witch hazel.** Witch hazel acts as an astringent and it can relieve itchy skin rashes. You can find it at your local health food store. Apply with a clean cloth and leave it on for 30 minutes.

- **Essential oils** of German chamomile and helichrysum mixed in a carrier oil can help relieve allergic skin reactions.

Diarrhea

Diarrhea is a frequent side effect of antibiotics. Antibiotic drugs kill off your protective gut bacteria, creating a flora imbalance leading to diarrhea. *C. difficile* associated diarrhea is another unfortunate side effect of antibiotic use (see more about *C. difficile* later in this chapter). There are several natural remedies to help reduce the frequency and severity of diarrhea. Different people seem to have better results with different remedies for diarrhea, so you may need to experiment to see which one works best for you.

In addition to the remedies listed below, the unpleasantness of diarrhea can be reduced by simply knowing where the restroom is. When traveling or running errands away from home, always know where the nearest restroom is, just in case you need it quickly.

The essential oils below can be taken internally by different methods, depending on your needs. See the section "Taking Essential Oils Internally" on page 130 for use details. Many of the remedies in the section below on stomach upset and nausea will also work for diarrhea.

- **Probiotics**. The most important remedy for diarrhea caused by antibiotics is to take probiotics daily. Probiotics directly replace the beneficial bacteria in your gut. For details on probiotics and how to use them, see the chapter "Probiotics: The Good Bacteria" on page 209.

- **Basil and marjoram** essential oils. Marjoram can be rubbed on the stomach and basil taken internally on the tongue for diarrhea reduction. Both oils are mild enough to be used full strength for most people, but always dilute the oils if they are too hot on the skin. A 50/50 dilution in a carrier oil, such as olive oil or grapeseed oil, is a good place to start.

- **Fennel** essential oil. Fennel essential oil taken internally can help reduce gas, nausea, vomiting, abdominal cramping and indigestion.

- **Coriander and dill** oils. These two essential oils are useful for diarrhea relief. Typically a few drops of each is taken internally and/or applied topically to the abdominal area.

- **Basil, peppermint, geranium and lavender** oils can be used topically for inflamed bowels. Two or three drops of each of the four oils can be mixed with 1 tablespoon of carrier oil. The blend can be massaged onto the abdomen, rubbed on both sides of the lower back, and applied to the bottoms of the feet for symptom relief.

Stomach Upset and Nausea

Antibiotics can cause upset stomach, nausea and gastrointestinal pain and they can irritate the stomach and upset the natural balance of flora inside your intestines. Your intestines are filled with important beneficial bacteria that help you digest food, make vitamins and support your immune system. Most antibiotic drugs kill off the good bacteria in your body along with the bad bacteria, creating an imbalance. The following remedies can be quite helpful to relieve stomach upset:

- **Probiotics.** The most important remedy for the gastrointestinal side effects of antibiotics is to take probiotics daily. Probiotics directly replace the beneficial bacteria in your gut. For details on probiotics and how to use them, see the chapter "Probiotics: The Good Bacteria" on page 209.

- **Heating pad or hot water bottle.** This simple remedy held next to the abdomen can help ease stomach upset and soothe pain. Make sure it's not too hot to avoid burning the skin.

- **Ginger.** Ginger has been used in China for more than 2,000 years to treat upset stomach, diarrhea and nausea. Ginger also has a long history of use in other cultures for nausea. Ginger can be taken as 2 to 4 grams of freshly cut root daily. Alternatively, 0.25 - 1.0 g of powdered root, 1.5 - 3.0 milliliters (30 - 90 drops) of liquid extract, or ginger capsules can be taken daily.

  Precautions: Ginger should be avoided in children under age 2. Adjust serving sizes for older children according to their weight (the adult servings listed above are for a 150 pound person). Follow manufacturer directions if they differ from above.

- **Essential oils.** Oils of tarragon (*Artemisia dracunculus*), rosemary (verbenone type) and marjoram (*Origanum magorama*) can be blended together to calm an upset stomach. Mix one or two drops of each oil into some water and take orally. Peppermint oil (*Mentha piperit)* or German chamomile oil can also be used for upset stomach - simply mix one drop of the oil into a cup of water and drink.

  Precautions: Children under age 3 should not use peppermint oil. Do not use if you are pregnant.

- **Peppermint tea.** Peppermint tea can soothe stomach upset and aid digestion. Peppermint tea is made from the dried leaves of the plant, with 1 to 2 teaspoons per cup of tea being a typical serving size. Steep the dried peppermint leaf for 5 minutes in a cup of hot water and drink.

- **Roman chamomile tea.** Roman chamomile (*Chamaemelum nobile*) tea is another common remedy for upset stomach. Pour 1 cup of boiling water over 2 to 3 tablespoons of the dried herb and steep for 10 minutes and drink.

- **Pharmaceutical medications.** There are medications that can also help with stomach upset, including Imodium and Pepto Bismol.

Liver Support

Your liver plays a vital part in maintaining your health and in recovering from an infection, but it's an organ that few people ever think about. Aside from aiding digestion, the liver helps flush bacterial toxins from your body after an infection. It filters your blood and removes toxins you get from the environment, from foods you eat and waste products from cellular and organ activity. The liver is also responsible for breaking down and removing any medications, including antibiotic drugs. The nourishment you get from eating food enters your blood by way of the liver, making it a key link in feeding your body's immune system.

Taking antibiotics, prescription and over the counter medications, and some essential oils makes your liver work harder. That extra effort can overload your liver and may create a backup of toxins in your body, slowing down your recovery and causing symptoms of liver overload.

In the short term, an overtaxed liver can cause symptoms like tiredness and fatigue, rashes, jaundice, nausea, headaches, hormonal imbalances, drowsiness after eating and digestion problems. Long term, a neglected liver can potentially lead to serious health challenges, including cirrhosis, type II diabetes, liver disease, liver cancer and chronic infections.

You can help support the health of your liver by eating the right kinds of foods and avoiding foods and toxins that burden the liver. Below are some of the most common foods and actions to take that provide nutritional support to your liver and aid in detoxification:

- Eating plenty of **raw organic foods** and minimally processed foods.

- Kale and **cruciferous vegetables** such as broccoli, cauliflower and brussels sprouts.

- **Garlic and onion** can aid metabolism and detoxification.

- Drinking plenty of **purified water** to support waste and toxin removal.

- **Healthy fats** play a vital role in the detoxification pathways and function of your liver. Supportive fats include Omega-3 oils like those found in flaxseed oil and salmon.

Foods, toxins and habits that increase the burden on your liver and should be avoided or minimized include the following:

- **Processed foods** which contain simple carbohydrates and simple sugars.

- **Alcohol**

- **Unhealthy poor quality fats** like hydrogenated oils, canola, soybean and corn oil.

- **Environmental toxins.** Avoid harsh disinfectants, pesticides, cleaning agents and other household products that contain liver-stressing ingredients (such as phenol and cresol in cleaners).

- **Lack of exercise.** When you exercise, toxins pass through the skin as sweat and are exhaled out through your lungs. If you don't exercise, these toxins must be dealt with by your liver.

You can also take specific herbs and spices to support your liver and to aid your body's detoxification processes, as listed below:

- **Milk thistle** is a widely respected detoxification aid that also helps protect and support liver cells. Because of its detoxification and liver support effects, it can be a helpful addition to herbal blends for dealing with Staph and MRSA infections.

- **Dandelion root** is also respected for nutritional liver support. You can find supplement blends specific to the liver that contain a combination of herbs that may include: milk thistle, dandelion root, beet leaf, stinging nettle or other herbs.

- **Spices** such as turmeric and ginger root help support proper liver function.

Liver Precautions

Some prescription drugs and over the counter medications are associated with liver toxicity. Tylenol (acetaminophen) is a good example of one drug that when taken beyond suggested doses (usually unintentionally) can cause liver toxicity. If you have or suspect you have issues with your liver, certain antibiotics, medications or essential oils may not be appropriate for you. Be sure to consult with your physician.

- **Antibiotic precautions**. The following antibiotics have been implicated in causing liver injury[68]:

  » **Isoniazid** used to treat tuberculosis infections.

  » **Augmentin** (a combination of amoxicillin and clavulanic acid).

  » **Sulfonamides** - sulfadiazine, sulfadoxine, and sulfisoxazole, and the combination drugs sulfasalazine and trimethoprim/sulfamethazole (TMP-SMZ).

  » **Fluoroquinolones** - ciprofloxacin and levofloxacin.

  » **Macrolides** - erythromycin, clarithromycin, azithromycin and telithromycin.

- **Essential oil precautions**. Some infection-fighting essential oils, such as oregano, thyme and clove, can stress the liver when taken internally in large usage amounts or for too long a period of time. Essential oils are generally safe for internal use when used according to established protocols. However, for maximum safety, essential oils should only be used internally for short periods of time during the active stage of an infection. Only plants that are safe for internal use, and only the highest quality medicinal or therapeutic grade of essential oils should be used internally.

Liver Cleanse

A liver cleanse can help the body to detoxify and *clean house*. Both recipes below are simple, refreshing and easy to add to your daily routine.

- **Liver cleanse essential oil recipe.** Combine juice from one fresh squeezed organic lemon (at least 1 tbsp or more), 1 drop lemon essential oil, and 1 drop peppermint essential oil. Mix together and drink. Can be added to a cup of hot water (not too hot), or to a cup of cold water. Use once per day before breakfast. May be used two times per day for more aggressive short-term support, first thing in the morning and right before bed. This recipe is often followed for three weeks at a time, then a one week rest, then started over again if needed and well tolerated.

- **Liver cleanse tea.** Manuka honey can be added to the liver cleanse recipe above to make a warm soothing tea. Simply add 1 teaspoon of manuka honey in the recipe above, but use the hot water recipe. Take every day, first thing in the morning for three weeks, then take one week off. After four weeks, the liver cleanse oil recipe above may be followed if needed and well tolerated.

Pain, Discomfort and Fever

MRSA and Staph can cause pain and discomfort in different forms, including painful boils, skin discomfort and fever. Mainstream medical treatments for pain include drugs that block the feeling of pain. On the plus side, many of these drugs work quickly, especially strong prescription drugs. However, stomach upset and liver toxicity side effects must be considered when deciding whether or not to use pain medications.

Natural Pain Relief Remedies

Several natural ways to address general pain relief and discomfort are listed below:

- **White willow bark** can be found at your local health food store. It contains the natural compound salicin (or salicylic acid), which is the chemical forerunner of aspirin. White willow bark shouldn't be given to children who have a fever that may be due to viral illnesses including the flu. It should not be used during pregnancy or for children under age two.

- **Bromelain.** The enzyme bromelain comes from pineapples and it is an anti-inflammatory that can help with some kinds of pain. Bromelain is available in many different forms and can be found in health food stores. Do not take it if you are currently on antibiotics, if you are pregnant, or on blood-thinners.

- **Essential oils** can work on multiple levels to provide pain relief. On the chemical level, some oils block the receptors for pain in the body, similar to how opiate pain medications work. On a physical level, other oils reduce inflammation and cause a soothing effect to reduce pain. Essential oils can also stimulate the brain and calm the emotions.

  » **For pain:** Lavender, myrrh, helichrysum and yarrow (*Achillea millefolium*) oils used individually, can provide pain relief. Dilute in carrier oil and apply externally on location.

  » **Headaches:** Peppermint (*Mentha piperita*) and lavender essential oils can be used for headaches. Take a drop of each and apply to the back of the neck at the base of the skull to soothe headache pain. Don't use peppermint if pregnant.

- **Energetic medicine.** For long-term chronic pain management, energy medicine, including acupuncture, has an excellent track record of success. Consult with an acupuncturist or practitioner of energy medicine to get details on how these techniques can help with chronic pain. Emotional freedom technique (EFT) is also a simple and effective practice you can do yourself at home (see "Emotional Freedom Technique (EFT)" on page 311 for details).

Fever Relief Natural Remedies

Fever is usually a defense mechanism of the body in trying to kill off bacteria or viruses. The high temperature is good because it will help kill the infectious agents. However, if a fever goes too high for too long, it can be dangerous or even deadly. For adults, a consistent fever of 103 degrees F or higher can be dangerous and medical attention should be sought.

Essential Oils

- **Peppermint** (*Mentha piperita*): Add a couple drops of peppermint oil and some sea salt to a basin of water. Use a sponge or washcloth and wipe gently across the forehead and body. Do not use peppermint if you are pregnant.

- **Bay laurel and eucalyptus oils** together can help reduce fever. Add 5 or 6 drops to bath salts for a cooling bath. Or use a couple drops of each with some salt in a basin of water. Use a sponge or washcloth and wipe gently across the forehead and body.

Foot and Head Wraps

Wrapping your feet in cold, wet towels is a traditional fever remedy. Laying a cold wet towel or washcloth on your forehead can also help you feel better.

Scar Healing

Scars can be the longest lasting reminder of a Staph or MRSA infection. Scars are more common with skin and surgical site infections. Scars can have a big impact on social life and self esteem and can last long after an infection has ended. The body has the natural ability to regenerate skin and heal scars, but this process is usually very slow. Also, the body's ability to heal scars can be slowed by a weakened immune system and by poor diet and nutrition.

Mainstream medicine offers several treatments to remove or lessen scarring, including cosmetic surgery, skin grafting, laser treatments, dermabrasion and collagen injections. Some silicon products have also been used in treating scars along with vitamins, minerals and other more natural ingredients.

Scar Natural Remedies

- **Helichrysum oil:** The essential oil helichrysum has a long history of consistent, predictable and effective use in healing skin scars. Helichrysum oil must be 100% genuine and authentic in quality for it to work well. Please see the chapter "Essential Oil Protocols for Use" on page 137 for more details on the use of this oil.

- **Manuka honey:** Manuka honey has skin healing and antibacterial properties for lingering wounds. Apply topically to scar. See the section "Manuka Honey" on page 97 for details.

- **Aloe vera:** The fresh liquid juice of the aloe plant contains potent anti-inflammatory and anti-bacterial compounds that can be very effective in wound and scar healing. Aloe has a history of use in supporting the healing of burns and skin Staph infections and is also an excellent choice for scars. Aloe shares many of the same medicinal properties as honey and can be used in similar ways as honey for skin application.

- **Diet and pH:** The stronger your immune system and nutritional health, the more energy your body has to heal and repair itself. This holds true for scars as well as infections and other diseases. See the chapters "Boosting Your Immune System" on page 223 and "Foods and Your Immune System" on page 237 for more details.

- **Antioxidants and vitamins:** Vitamins C, D and E and Omega-3 oils all play an important role in maintaining healthy skin and in healing scars. See the chapter "Vitamins and Minerals" on page 167 for details.

Co-Infections and Secondary Infections

Yeast, fungus, viruses and many types of bacteria can cause secondary infections that can strike after having a Staph or MRSA infection. Sometimes another infection (co-infection) will occur at the same time as a Staph infection. Dealing with another infection on top of a Staph infection puts added stress on your immune system and makes it harder to heal and recover. Taking steps to deal with co-infections and secondary infections make it easier to overcome Staph and MRSA.

Regardless of the kinds of infections you may be struggling with, steps you take to support and boost your immune system will help. Proper diet, supplementation, probiotics and the other steps in the Action Steps in chapter 1 can be very supportive of the healing process. In addition to immune support, specific remedies are also helpful, depending on the type of infection.

Because each type of infection is unique, there may be special methods and remedies that will work best. One of the benefits of many natural remedies is their broad level of activity against not just Staph bacteria, but also viruses, yeast and molds and other kinds of bacteria. The sections below provide a brief summary of the co-infections and secondary infections most likely to occur with Staph and MRSA, along with a few basic remedy and support methods for each.

C. diff. (*Clostridium Difficile*) Infections

One of the most common types of secondary infections is *C. difficile*. C. diff. is also one of the most dangerous and stubborn kinds of secondary infections you can have. C. diff. can be a miserable illness with diarrhea and loss of bowel control, a burning raw backside, gut cramping and constant frantic trips to the bathroom. Relapses are common with C. diff. and it can be difficult to treat and even fatal.

What is C. difficile?

Clostridium difficile (*C. difficile*, or C. diff.) is a bacterial infection that causes mild diarrhea and inflamed intestines (colitis). The infection is often called Clostridium difficile-associated disease (CDAD) or Clostridium difficile infection (CDI). C. diff. bacteria produce a toxin that causes the diarrhea and inflammation in the digestive tract.

C. diff. bacteria can form spores to protect themselves. These spores are like a protective armor that shield the bacteria while dormant, allowing them to survive for years. These spores make *C. difficile* more difficult to control and easier to transfer to others. *C. difficile* cannot be treated with standard antibiotics. Most common antibiotics will make the infection grow worse.

C. diff Causes and Risk Factors

Many people who take antibiotics for Staph or MRSA develop another type of bacterial infection caused by the antibiotics themselves. *C. difficile* affects 250,000 people annually in the U.S. and is a significant risk for many people who take antibiotics. Even if an antibiotic stops your Staph or MRSA infection, you could catch a *C. difficile* infection afterward.

There are many different kinds of antibiotics and some are more likely to cause C. diff. than others. Below is a list of the antibiotics most likely to cause *C. difficile*:

- **Fluoroquinolones.** This commonly-prescribed class of antibiotics includes ciprofloxacin (Cipro), levofloxacin (Levaquin), moxifloxacin (Avelox) and gatifloxacin (Tequin) to name a few. Fluoroquinolones are known for their numerous negative side effects.

- **Clindamycin.** This commonly prescribed drug often causes *C. difficile* infections.

- **Cephalosporins.** This class of drugs includes the antibiotics cephalexin (Keflex), cefuroxime (Ceftin) and cefaclor (Keflor).

- **Amoxicillin.** Also called Agmentin and Clavamox, these drugs and other B-lactam antibiotics can cause C. diff. infections.

Not everyone who takes one of the antibiotics above will develop a *C. difficile* infection. And some C. diff. infections are not caused by antibiotics. The risk factors that increase your chances of developing a *C. difficile* infection include a prior history of *C. difficile*, recent hospitalization, recent abdominal surgery or low stomach acid. Living in a nursing home and being age 65 or older is another risk factor for *C. difficile* exposure and infections.

C. diff. Symptoms

Below are the most common symptoms of a C. diff. infection. Note that even if you have some of the symptoms, you may not actually have the infection. However, if you have any of the following symptoms **in combination with** any of the risk factors listed in the preceding section, then you may have a *C. difficile* infection. Laboratory testing in combination with a physical exam, examination of your medical history, and examination of your risk factors are usually taken into account when diagnosing a *C. difficile* infection.

- Diarrhea
- Stomach cramps
- Fever
- Loss of appetite

- Blood or pus in stool
- Weight loss
- Nausea

- Characteristic odor of stool
- Fatigue
- Acute pain

C. diff. Diagnosis and Treatment

C. diff. diagnostic tests come in many types, each with pros and cons. None of the tests are 100% accurate and some are prone to false results. Therefore, many doctors prefer laboratory testing in combination with a close review of your symptoms and/or risk factors to diagnose *C. difficile*. However, some doctors diagnose these infections based solely on symptoms and medical history without any testing.

Only a few antibiotics are prescribed to treat C. difficile. Metronidazole (Flagyl), oral vancomycin (Vancocin) and more recently fidaxomicin are the three most commonly prescribed drugs. Some infections do not respond well to treatment and recurrences are common.

Controlling *C. difficile*

An important way to help control C. diff. is good hygiene and cleaning. Proper hand washing after using the bathroom and before eating or preparing food is crucial. Because C. diff. spores are so tough, most disinfectants cannot kill them.

There are natural remedies and control methods that can have good results with *C. difficile*. Probiotics are especially important to help re-balance the intestinal flora. Medicinal herbal remedies and antibacterial essential oils are helpful, so long as they are gentle on the gut and intestinal flora. Diet changes, especially limiting carbohydrates, sugar and refined foods, can also help. Many of the same methods and techniques in the Action Steps in chapter 1 are also beneficial for C. diff.

Yeast, Candida, Thrush and Fungal Infections

Thrush, yeast, Candida and other fungal infections are the most common secondary infections and occur as a result of taking antibiotics. Yeast and Candida are also co-infections that can complicate the healing process from MRSA or Staph. Also, the MRSA infection itself can weaken the immune system and leave a person more prone to fungal infections.

Yeasts and Candida thrive on sugar. It is crucial to stop feeding the yeast with sugar or large amounts of simple carbohydrates, which are found in most processed American foods. Getting the right amount of water (not soda or other drinks) is also very important. See the section "Water, Water Everywhere" on page 247 for details.

Remedies with activity against yeast and fungal challenges include the Antifungal Blend essential oil blend or oregano oil, which is especially helpful with Candida. The moderate level internal protocol for these two essential oils is a good place to start, as detailed in the sections "The Antibacterial Blend" on page 145 and "Oregano Oil" on page 143. The liver cleanse protocol in the section "Liver Cleanse" on page 178 can also help with Candida.

In addition, botanical herbal blends containing olive leaf and probiotic support are also an effective option for yeast and Candida infections. The moderate level protocol is also a good place to start for internal support as detailed in "Botanical Blend Protocol" on page 106.

Urinary Tract Infections (UTI) or Bladder Infections

Urinary tract infections (UTI) or bladder infections can occur after a recent bout of MRSA or Staph as antibiotic use eliminates many protective bacteria within the urinary system. *E.coli* bacteria originate in the intestines, and are the most common cause of UTIs after antibiotic use. Many of the infection and immune support methods in this book will also help with UTIs. For MRSA and Staph bladder infections, see "MRSA Bladder and Urinary Tract Infections" on page 195.

E. coli Bladder Infections

- **D-mannose** can be very helpful against UTIs in general. D-mannose is a type of sugar that makes the bladder more slippery so that bacteria have a harder time sticking to the inside surface. A product that combines D-mannose with cranberry extract is a great option.

- **Essential oils.** The Spice Blend essential oil or oregano oil have been shown effective against *E. coli*. The moderate level internal method for either of these oils can be used as a starting point.

- **Topical use of essential oils.** Another method entails diluting oregano essential oil in a carrier oil (1 drop oregano oil to 1 ounce carrier oil) and applying 2-3 drops of the mixture on the skin over the bladder. Add a warm damp cloth over the area to help push the oil into the body. Do not get this oil mixture near the genitals as it will burn! Oregano oil must be used with great caution and care on the skin to reduce the risk of burning and sensitization. See "Oregano Oil" on page 143 for details about this oil.

- **Oregon grape.** *Berberis aquifolium* can also be helpful for UTI and bladder infections. This herb contains berberine, which can stop bacteria from adhering to the intestinal walls and urinary tract. The herb is available as a tea, in dried capsules or as a liquid tincture.

- **Uva Ursi.** *Arctostaphylos uva ursi* or bearberry is one of the most commonly used antibacterial remedies for UTIs. It has antibacterial qualities and has been used successfully against recurrent bladder infections. This is an herb and can be found as capsules and liquid tinctures.

- **Probiotics.** Beneficial bacteria are crucial for support with all kinds of infections. Lactobacilli are normal and beneficial residents in the urinary tract and help protect your system from invading bacteria. Probiotics are not a treatment, but should be considered more as a preventative. See the chapter "Probiotics: The Good Bacteria" on page 209 for more info.

Klebsiella UTI Infections

Klebsiella bacteria are *gram negative* bacteria and are also a common cause of urinary tract infections in older women. These infections can get started after antibiotic use, or using urinary catheters. Some remedies that have shown effectiveness against Klebsiella include berberine, oregano essential oil and olive leaf.

Pseudomonas Infections

Secondary skin infections caused by Pseudomonas bacteria are a somewhat common secondary infection. Rosemary and lavender essential oils have activity against Pseudomonas. One protocol uses 2 drops of rosemary, 2 drops of lavender and mixes them with 4 drops of carrier oil to make a 50% dilution. The diluted oils are applied to the wound area 2 or 3 times per day. For support with lung and respiratory infections, lavender and rosemary oils are mild enough to air diffuse with little risk of irritation. These two oils will also naturally calm and relax, which provides further benefit. See "Essential Oil Protocols for Use" on page 137 for details on using essential oils. Additional infection support beyond these essential oils may be needed.

Recurring Staph and MRSA

One of the main problems that plague so many Staph and MRSA sufferers is recurring infections. While antibiotics and other mainstream treatments often stop the first infection, these treatments do nothing to prevent the infection from coming back again later.

Support of the immune system and gut flora, along with controlling bacteria inside the home, are important methods to reduce the risk of the infection returning. These important methods are described in more detail in the chapters "Boosting Your Immune System" on page 223, "Probiotics: The Good Bacteria" on page 209 and "Hand Washing and Hygiene" on page 269. However, a lesser known but equally important cause of recurrent infections are biofilms hiding inside the body. The section below will provide specific support methods for biofilms.

Biofilm and L-Form Support

Biofilms can be present inside boils, abscesses, wounds or internal infections. Biofilms are created by the bacteria themselves, are highly resistant to treatments and are a key reason why MRSA and Staph become chronic, recurring infections. Antibiotic drugs are not able to treat biofilms and in fact can cause biofilms to form. Biofilms help the bacteria to hide in your body and they have been implicated in up to 80% of chronic infections. If you've struggled with stubborn recurring infections or medical device infections, there's a good chance you have a biofilm infection.

L-forms are another strategy that bacteria can use to hide inside the human body and promote recurring infections. While L-forms are a relatively new area of study, strong links have been made between these so-called *stealth bacteria* and recurring outbreaks for many kinds of infections, including Staph and MRSA.

As with L-forms, studies on biofilms and natural treatments are limited, but some natural botanicals, enzymes and essential oils have been shown effective against biofilms and/or chronic infections. Essential oils containing carvacrol (in oregano and thyme oils), manuka honey and tea tree oil have shown activity against biofilms. Stabilized allicin from garlic has also shown action against MRSA and Staph biofilms. There's also evidence that some botanical blends can help fight biofilms. Specially formulated enzyme blends and chelating compounds have also shown great promise and have been formulated to break down the protective biofilm structures.

Once the biofilm structure is removed, the bacteria from the biofilm have nowhere to hide and are more vulnerable to antibiotics and/or natural treatment approaches. Supporting your immune system for long-term eradication is also an important tactic. Immune support and addressing biofilms with effective treatments may take up to several months to see results. Many of the natural therapies outlined in this book have some level of effectiveness against biofilms and stealth bacteria.

Success Strategies For Biofilm and Stealth Bacteria

Below are ways you can help support your body in handling stubborn biofilm and stealth bacteria infections:

- **Essential oils.** Internal support with oregano, thyme or the Antibacterial Blend essential oil should be considered during any active infection. External support on wounds or skin infections with tea tree oil. Refer to the chapter "Essential Oil Protocols for Use" on page 137 for protocols for these oils.

- **Enzyme blends.** New formulations of enzymes and chelating agents are now available. These blends disrupt and break down the biofilm so that treatments can reach the bacteria that were inside the biofilm. Using these enzyme blends in combination with antibiotics or the Botanical

Blend protocol has been shown effective.

- **Botanical herbal blends.** Blends that contain medicinal grade herbs like olive leaf and essential oils have had success against chronic recurring infections and other known biofilm infections when used internally. Refer to the "Botanical Blend Protocol" on page 106 for details.

- **Stabilized allicin.** Products containing stabilized allicin can be used for internal support. Stabilized allicin has been found to permeate inside biofilm structures. The more potent forms of stabilized allicin have provided great results against severe and chronic, non-responsive infections. See the section "Stabilized Allicin" on page 95 for specifics.

- **Manuka honey.** Manuka honey has been shown to stall biofilm formation, stop bacterial growth and aid wound and tissue healing when used on skin infection sites. See "Manuka Honey" on page 97 for more details about this approach.

- **Minimize the use of antibiotic drugs.** Antibiotics can drive bacteria like Staph to convert into the L-form state. Antibiotics that attack bacterial cell walls can encourage L-form growth, including penicillin, cephalosporin, cycloserine, bacitracin (or neosporin), vancomycin and daptomycin. Work closely with your doctor to assess whether or not you really need antibiotics.

- **Multiple antibiotic therapies.** As mentioned above, antibiotics that attack bacterial cell walls can help create L-form bacteria. However, some level of success against L-forms has been achieved by taking multiple antibiotic drugs for long periods of time. One such approach is called the Marshall Protocol as outlined in the section "Diagnosis and Treatment of L-forms" on page 72. Keep in mind that taking antibiotics, especially for such a long period of time, can cause side effects as well as weaken your protective intestinal flora and your immune system.

- **Make lifestyle changes slowly.** Radical dietary changes or taking many new supplements all at once can change the internal environment of your body too quickly and can cause bacteria to cope by changing to L-forms. Make beneficial dietary and lifestyle changes at a moderate pace, allowing time for your body to adjust.

- **Long-term maintenance.** After an infection has cleared, continued long-term use of low usage amounts of antibacterial remedies can help support the body to eliminate biofilms and L-forms. See "Maintenance and Preventative Remedies" on page 207 for details.

- **Support your immune system.** The key to long-term prevention of recurring infections is to make your body resistant to stealth bacteria and biofilms. See the chapter "Boosting Your Immune System" on page 223 for details on immune support.

NOTE: See the section "Michelle's Recommended Products" on page 303 for product resources.

15 Infection Management Techniques

Knowing how to properly handle specific types of infections like boils or open wounds goes hand-in-hand with using remedies and treatments. Other infection control techniques, such as reducing airborne MRSA and decolonizing your skin or nose using non-toxic methods and also important. This chapter details the following infection management methods and techniques:

- Dressing wounds

- Caring for boils and abscesses

- Sinus rinsing

- MRSA bladder infection treatments

- Decolonization methods for the skin and the nose

- Remedy tips for children

- Diagnosis, treatment and prevention methods for pets

- Controlling airborne MRSA

- Long-term maintenance

CAUTION: Consult with your doctor before using the techniques described in this chapter. If there are any contradictions between the techniques detailed here and the directions from your doctor, then either follow the directions from your doctor or enlist your doctor's support in using the techniques of your choice.

Wound Dressing

The two main reasons for dressing a wound are to keep germs out and to protect other people from your infection. Dressings can also create a micro-environment next to the wound to promote the healing process and to focus the effects of topical remedies applied to the wound.

There are many kinds of dressings and different materials to make them with. Ask your doctor which type of dressing best fits your needs. Below are steps to take and points to consider when dressing a Staph or MRSA wound.

- **Protect yourself.** Wear disposable latex or nitrile gloves when tending to wounds, especially if the wound is not your own. Handle used dressing materials carefully using sanitary techniques. Dispose of waste to prevent contamination. Never reuse gloves. Wash your hands well with soap and water when you're done.

- **Don't irritate or rip the skin.** The skin surrounding an infected wound can be extra sensitive and easy to damage. Consider using non-adhesive pads and wrapping materials to minimize the risk of tearing, ripping or irritating the skin when the dressing is removed. Non-petroleum jelly may be used to help prevent dressing materials or topical remedies from sticking and ripping the skin when removed.

- **Size it properly and make it secure.** Size the dressing to provide plenty of overlap around the edges of the wound. Include a generous zone of clear skin under the edges of the dressing to provide a wide barrier against bacteria crossing into or out of the wound. Extra room around the edge can also make it easier to apply tape or adhesives to hold the dressing in place if needed. Tape is helpful for securing the edges if the wound cannot be easily wrapped. A roll of gauze works well for securing dressings on arms, legs and fingers that are easy to wrap.

- **Make is absorbent.** A central absorbent pad should be placed under the dressing if oozing of fluids from the wound is expected.

- **Make it breathable.** Wounds that can't breathe lock in too much moisture and heal poorly. Make sure the dressing is well covered but still able to breathe a little.

- **Apply topical remedies.** Dressing changes provide an opportune time to apply a fresh amount of an antibacterial remedy, such as essential oils or manuka honey. See "For Skin Infections" on page 10 for topical remedy guidelines for skin infections. For details on applying a manuka honey wound dressing, see the section "Wound Dressings" on page 98.

- **Seal the edges.** Gaps around a dressing allow infecting bacteria, fluids or cellular debris to escape and contaminate surfaces, objects or other people. Gaps also allow other infectious agents to enter the wound. A poorly applied dressing may also rub and abrade the skin, causing unneeded pain and tissue damage.

- **Keep it moist, but not wet.** A warm, moist environment can help speed the healing of tissues. You want the wound to be kept moist enough so it does not dry out, but not too wet either. Too much moisture can cause tissue damage and promote infections.

- **Keep it water tight when needed.** If you have to shower or expose the dressing to water, then temporarily cover the dressing with an outer layer that will shed water and keep the dressing from getting wet. One option is to tape plastic wrap around the wound.

- **Don't reuse dressing materials.** Always use new dressing or water shedding materials when changing dressings and dispose of all used materials using sanitary techniques.

- **Don't change dressings more than you have too.** Changing a dressing too often causes unnecessary pain and can irritate and damage the surrounding skin. However, not changing it often enough can allow wounds to fester and slow the healing process. Check with your doctor for the proper frequency of dressing changes. A few times per day is not uncommon.

- **Watch closely for changes.** If the wound or the surrounding area of redness grows larger, if stripes begin radiating out from the wound, or if your infection symptoms worsen, be sure to see a healthcare professional immediately.

Sinus Rinsing

Sinus infections are challenging to treat because the sinuses are deep within the body and are encompassed in bone. If you have a MRSA or Staph sinus infection, you may also have painful bumps or boils in your nose. Biofilms are also a common issue for sinus infections which can further complicate treatment.

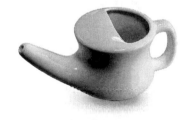

It's important to note that because MRSA and Staph colonize the nose and sinuses of many healthy people, you can be a carrier of these bacteria (a nasal culture test may be positive), but it doesn't mean you have a MRSA or Staph sinus infection, unless you are also showing the signs of a sinus infection.

Sinus irrigation aids, such as the neti pot, are used to rinse the sinuses for infection control.

Nasal irrigation is a popular technique for seasonal allergy relief. Rinsing the sinuses can also help Staph and MRSA sinusitis. There are many irrigation aids on the market, ranging from neti pots (or nose bidets) to pulsating action mechanical devices. For the author, the neti pot was a crucial part of breaking the cycle of antibiotic drugs and her recurring Staph sinus infections.

The neti pot is one of the most versatile sinus rinsing aids on the market and it lends itself to using a range of rinse solutions and liquid remedies. Rinse solutions are typically made using salt or baking soda, or a combination of both, diluted in warm sterile water. Many people find that adding an antimicrobial agent to the rinse solution, such as a mild essential oil, provides excellent infection support. Studies show that people with general sinus problems who irrigated their nose twice daily for three to six weeks saw significant improvement in numerous symptoms. Nasal irrigation can take some getting used to, but once you've done it a few times, the method is quick and easy.

Neti Pot Technique

Below are general steps for using the neti pot, but follow the manufacturer's instructions for any sinus rinse aid you use if they differ from the steps below:

1. **Make the rinse solution.** Bring a few cups of distilled, filtered or purified water to a boil for a minute or so. Let the boiled water cool to a lukewarm temperature. Boiling the water kills potential microbes in the water. Add one teaspoon of non-iodized table salt per cup of lukewarm water. Both too much salt and too little salt may cause burning, so experiment until you find a comfortable amount.

2. **Add an antibacterial remedy (optional).** For added infection support, remedies can be added to the rinse water. Approximately 1/2 teaspoon of manuka honey per cup of the warmed water and salt solution is one option. Be sure to use a high quality UMF 10 to 15+ grade manuka honey for the best results. See the section "Manuka Honey" on page 97 for details. Another option is to add essential oils. One drop of eucalyptus and/or tea tree oil in one cup of solution is generally enough. See the section "Sinus Rinsing Technique" on page 133 for details about sinus rinsing with essential oils.

3. **Start slowly.** If you are not accustomed to sinus irrigation, it can burn at first, especially if your sinuses are inflamed. Most people find that any burning typically gets much better after the first time or two. A pinch of baking soda added to the rinse solution can help squelch any burning, but be sure not to overdo it. Too much baking soda will reduce acidity in the sinuses, which can promote unhealthy microbial growth.

4. **Rinse method:** Stir all ingredients into the warm water in the neti pot. Hold the neti pot in your right hand and bring the spout to your right nostril. Lean over a sink and tilt your head so that your left ear faces down toward the sink. Gently tip the pot so water will flow into your nose. The water will run through your right nostril, into your sinuses and out your left nostril into the sink. Empty the pot halfway then repeat using the left hand and left nostril. Keep in mind if your sinuses are really clogged, the solution may not come out the other nostril. Don't try to force it. You can breathe out of your mouth while you irrigate your sinuses.

5. **Clean the neti pot after each use.** It is very important to clean the neti pot thoroughly to avoid harboring infecting bacteria and contaminating yourself later. Clean and scrub the neti pot with warm soapy water after each use. If your neti pot is dishwasher safe, a dishwasher may be used. Rinse well and allow the neti pot to dry completely to prevent potential germs from surviving.

6. **How often and how long to rinse.** Most people get good results rinsing their sinuses twice per day, reducing the frequency after the infection has cleared. Everyone is different, so start slowly, experiment and find out what works best for you.

Neti Pot Precautions

Tap water should not be used for making the net pot rinse solution without boiling it first. While tap water is safe to drink, using distilled, filtered or boiled water is safer for neti pot use.

Using unboiled tap water introduces the risk of a rare, deadly and easily preventable parasite infection. The parasite *Naegleria fowleri* is commonly found in lakes and streams, and this amoeba can sometimes be found in tap water. While infections are exceedingly rare, this amoeba can enter the body through the nose and lead to a dangerous infection in the brain. These infections commonly happen from splashing, jumping and diving in warm, stagnant water where the amoeba live.

Most neti pots come with instructions on how to use them safely and properly and these directions should be followed. It's also a good idea to talk with your doctor about using the neti pot with your particular needs in mind. The simple precautions below will help protect you from rinse water infection risks and will make sinus rinsing easier and safer:

- Use warmed distilled, filtered or boiled water only to make the rinse solution.

- Clean and scrub the neti pot with warm soapy water after each use.

- Allow the neti pot to dry completely after washing.

- Rinse your sinuses once or twice per day at most. Many people have good results with 2 or 3 rinses per week.

- Start slowly. Irritation and stinging are common when starting out. Reduce the amount of salt, use the neti pot less often, or change the temperature of the rinse solution to help reduce or eliminate stinging or irritation.

Boils and Abscesses

Boils are bumps with a pus filled head that are usually small and near the surface of the skin. The cause can be varied, but can be an ingrown hair or a plugged sweat gland that becomes infected. When more than one boil grows together, they form a multi-headed lump called a carbuncle. An abscess is similar to a boil but is deeper in the skin and usually does not form a puss-filled head. Both boils and abscesses infected with Staph or MRSA can also have biofilms inside. See "Recurring Staph and MRSA" on page 185 for more details.

Sometimes women will report having boils appear in various areas on their body when their monthly menses starts. This is often caused by hormonal imbalances within the body. Be sure to get the boil tested to see if it is MRSA, Staph or another bacteria. Also, help from an endocrinologist (a doctor who specializes in hormones) and/or an integrative MD or naturopath (ND) who is experienced with hormones can help you resolve the imbalance.

Boils and abscesses are often incised or lanced by a doctor and drained of pus to reduce pain and to decrease the number of bacteria in the infected area. The procedure begins with a topical antiseptic, followed by puncturing or opening the skin with a sterile instrument and allowing the pus to drain out. Lancing must be done by a health care professional due to the high risk of spreading the infection internally to the blood stream (such as if the boil is squeezed). Secondary infections and other complicating problems can occur if the procedure is not done properly.

Warm Compresses

Warm compresses are a safe and natural way to bring a boil or abscess to a head and allow it to drain on its own. You can also soak the area in hot water to let the tissue open on it's own. Below is a general procedure for a warm compress, although your doctor may have a preferred method:

1. Moisten a washcloth with hot water and briefly squeeze out the excess water. A heat pack may also be used. Make sure the temperature is not too hot for your skin with prolonged contact.

2. Apply the warm compress over the area of the boil, fixing it in place with some loose wraps if needed. Maintain in direct contact with the affected skin area for about 20 minutes.

3. Reapply a freshly made warm moist compress up to several times per day in 20 minute intervals. Several days of application may be needed to bring the boil to a head.

4. Do not squeeze the pus-filled head as this could push the infecting bacteria into your bloodstream causing a dangerous infection.

5. Avoid shaving near the infected skin area. Small cuts while shaving create an easy route for bacteria to enter the body, allowing the infection to spread.

6. Discard any wraps or cloths that become contaminated with body fluids, or segregate and wash separately according to the chapter "Laundry Precautions & Methods" on page 285.

7. After the boil or abscess comes to a head and drains, you may have a hole in the top. Apply 1-2 drops of the essential oils of tea tree, rosemary, or lavender into the hole if it has one, or on the surface of the boil or abscess. Let it stay open to drain. These oils can be applied morning and night for a few days.

8. Topical antimicrobial remedies may be used along with warm compresses. For additional remedies, see the section "For Skin Infections" on page 10 in chapter 1.

MRSA Bladder and Urinary Tract Infections

A Staph or MRSA bladder infection or urinary tract infection (UTI) is when bacteria travel into the urethra and then to the bladder where urine is stored. For men, the prostate may also be involved. Less commonly, the infection can also spread further upward from the bladder into the ureters and kidneys. While the majority of MRSA bladder infections start at the urethra and work their way upward, it's also possible for infections to move into the kidneys or bladder from other locations, including from the bloodstream. If left unchecked, a UTI can travel into the kidneys and then the bloodstream causing life-threatening infections.

Most UTIs are caused by *E. coli* bacteria that originate in the intestines, but MRSA is becoming a more frequent cause of such infections. An active Staph or MRSA boil or lesion near the groin or buttocks can cause a UTI. People can also get bladder infections after lower abdominal surgeries. However, MRSA UTIs are most common for people who have had a urinary catheter inserted during a hospital stay or for a bladder control issue. Of note, MRSA or Staph biofilms can form in the bladder and may be a factor when dealing with these types of infections.

For those with bladder infections, MRSA or Staph bacteria in the urine can be transferred to other people, so people with this condition should be considered contagious. If infected urine gets onto an open wound or cut, then a MRSA or Staph skin infection can develop. Be sure to use proper hand washing and personal hygiene measures if you're infected, or if you're caring for someone with this condition.

UTI Testing

If you're not sure if you have MRSA in your urine, a simple urine test at your doctor's office will determine if your symptoms are due to MRSA or another type of infection. Below are the most common tests that can be used to diagnose a UTI:

- **Urinalysis.** This is the typical test that is performed that looks at urine color and clarity and may also include a microscopic evaluation to look for bacteria and/or red and white blood cell counts. However, this test alone will not confirm if you have MRSA.

- **Urine culture.** This is the most reliable method to determine if you have an infection. It's important to ask for a urine culture test to determine what specific bacteria is causing the infection.

- **Sensitivity test.** This test can tell your doctor which antibiotic is most likely to work against your particular strain of MRSA or Staph.

UTI Treatment

Antibiotics are the standard protocol treatment for MRSA UTIs. However, many people find that antibiotics do not help due to resistant Staph or MRSA. Part of the problem is that broad spectrum antibiotics are often prescribed for any kind of UTI without first testing the urine to see what's causing the infection. Broad spectrum antibiotics will not help with MRSA and have been linked to antibiotic resistance[70].

There are alternative remedies for UTIs. Some of these remedies kill the infecting bacteria while others help prevent the infection from attaching to the urinary tract so they are voided.

Antibiotics for MRSA Staph UTIs

Antibiotics are the main treatment prescribed by doctors for Staph or MRSA UTIs and oral antibiotics are most common[71]. The prescribed drug depends upon the infection's severity, the age and health status of the patient and other factors. Many of the standard UTI antibiotics are ineffective against MRSA, which is multi-drug resistant[72]. Because of growing antibiotic resistance in MRSA, sensitivity testing is important if MRSA is suspected.

If you are currently using a urinary catheter (which inserts into the urethra to remove urine from the bladder), removal is recommended as catheters are often the source of infecting MRSA or Staph bacteria. Catheter associated UTIs (CAUTI) tend to be more antibiotic resistant, especially for those catheter infections acquired in a hospital. The following drugs are most commonly prescribed for MRSA or Staph UTIs:

- **Trimethoprim-sulfamethoxazole** (also known as TMP-SMX, Bactrim or Setpra) is the most common antibiotic treatment for UTIs. Part of this antibiotic is a sulfa drug in which drug allergies and intolerances are quite common. Trimethoprim alone may also be prescribed.

- **Tetracycline** antibiotics.

- **Nitrofurantoin.**

- **Fosfomycin trometamol** is a single dose antibiotic and is very expensive.

- **Flouroquinolones** such as Ciprofloxacin (Cirpro) and Lefofloxacin are also prescribed for UTI.

  » The 2012 guidelines from the Infectious Diseases Society of America (IDSA) has recommended avoiding fluoroquinolones because of the increased risk of causing antibiotic resistance, MRSA colonization and numerous negative side effects.

- **IV antibiotics:** For severe or complicated UTI infections intravenous (IV) antibiotics such as Vancomycin may be prescribed.

- **Linezolid (Zyvox)** is sometimes used to treat MRSA, but this drug does not get eliminated through the kidneys and bladder in high enough concentrations and is therefore not a good choice for UTIs. The list of successful antibiotics is constantly changing as antibiotic resistance in MRSA grows.

Alternative Remedies for UTIs

Because antibiotics often fail to stop UTI infections, natural remedies are a great alternative[73]. The following remedies work on multiple fronts to combat UTI infections:

- **Garlic extracts**. Allicin extracts from garlic have been proven to fight MRSA. See "Stabilized Allicin" on page 95 for details.

- **Essential oils.** Essential oils effective against Staph or MRSA can be massaged into the skin over the bladder area, applied to the bottom of the feet, added to baths, or added to a sitz bath to target the genital area. Some oils may also be taken internally, including oregano, rosemary, thyme and the Spice Blend. See the chapter "Essential Oil Protocols for Use" on page 137 for details.

- **Uva ursi.** *Arctostaphylos uva ursi* or bearberry is one of the most commonly used antibacterial remedies for UTIs. It has antibacterial qualities and has been used successfully against recurrent bladder infections caused by *Staph aureus, E. coli* and others. This is an herb and can be found as capsules and liquid tinctures.

- **Oregon grape.** *Berberis aquifolium* contains a substance known as berberine which can stop bacteria from adhering to the walls of the intestines and urinary tract. It is available as a tea, in dried capsules or in liquid tincture formulas.

- **Cranberry extract.** Cranberry extracts have been proven to inhibit the growth of both *Staph aureus* and MRSA bacteria[74]. These extracts have also been proven to inhibit production of biofilm structures which protect the bacteria from antibiotics and other treatments. While cranberry extracts inhibited Staph and MRSA biofilms, they did not eradicate them. Adding cranberry extracts to your treatment regimen may shorten your infection regardless of which treatments you use. Cranberry extracts can also be considered for prevention as they support the body against biofilms, which can cause recurring outbreaks.

✧✧

Note: cranberry juice is not a substitute for the extract as it contains too much sugar.

✧✧

Holistic UTI Support

Your natural ability to ward off bladder and urinary tract infections can be enhanced or weakened in different ways. One example is the acidity level inside the urinary tract. When the acidity level drops (becomes more acidic), you become more prone to bladder infections. Many older women become more prone to UTI's because their acidity is altered by menopause. Menopause causes a reduction in estrogen levels and reduces the urinary tract acidity level. Hormone balancing can be helpful for UTIs. The steps below can help make you less prone to infections:

- **Probiotics.** Beneficial bacteria are crucial for support with all kinds of infections. Lactobacilli are normal and beneficial bacterial residents in the urinary tract and help protect your system from invading bacteria. See more about probiotics in the chapter "Probiotics: The Good Bacteria" on page 209.

- **Drink the right fluids.** Drinking lots of fluids, especially water, helps flush bad bacteria out of your system.

- **Be sure to avoid** alcohol, citrus fruit juices and caffeinated beverages, including common brands of cranberry juice. While cranberry can be helpful for bladder infections, most juice products contain sugar, which feeds bacteria and helps them grow even more. Cranberry extract capsules is a better option.

Decolonization of MRSA and Staph

People who are colonized with MRSA or Staph have the bacteria living on their skin or inside their nose but are otherwise healthy and do not have an active infection. People who are colonized carry a higher risk of getting infected and they can pass the bacteria to other people. Being colonized with MRSA or Staph is the same as being a carrier, as described in the section "Staph and MRSA Carriers" on page 27.

Colonization is typically confirmed by collecting a swab sample from inside the nose and sending it to a laboratory where the sample is cultured and examined for the presence of MRSA or Staph bacteria. Test samples may also be collected from the armpits or areas around the groin. The throat may also be sampled for testing as many doctors now consider the throat a better indicator of colonization than the nose. Testing is also performed to gauge the success of a person's decolonization efforts or the effectiveness of an infection treatment. Testing is most often performed for people who have a high risk of colonization, including people who have had a recent infection, people with an infected family member, healthcare workers, or people scheduled for surgery.

Decolonization is defined as the elimination of MRSA carriage, but definitions differ in how long the bacteria are eliminated in order for the therapy to be considered successful. Recolonization of MRSA bacteria is fairly common in the long term. Failure to decolonize is due to many factors, which include a history of MRSA infections, family members with infections, and resistance to chlorhexidine or the antibiotic mupirocin. In addition, MRSA colonization in people is much more common in the community now, so re-exposure is a continual risk. Decolonization is often prescribed for people or family members who are caring for those with weakened immune systems like newborns or immune-compromised individuals.

Decolonization Baths

Bathing can help you decolonize from Staph, MRSA or other pathogens on the skin. Bathing also refreshes, cleanses and hydrates the skin and provides a way for you to relax and control stress.

Doctors often prescribe bleach baths or strong antiseptics like chlorhexidine to people with stubborn Staph and MRSA skin infections. While these chemical baths may kill Staph on your skin, they also kill the good bacteria that help protect you. Your skin flora is made up of dozens if not hundreds of different microorganisms that work together to protect your skin from invasion from disease-causing bacteria like MRSA. When you use such heavy-handed and toxic approaches to decolonize, you're killing off your friendly flora and absorbing chemical toxins into your body at the same time. This is how chemical disinfectants weaken your immune system. They can also cause skin irritation, allergic reactions, damage to your eyes and a reduced ability to cleanse and detoxify.

Chlorhexidine Baths

Chlorhexidine is routinely prescribed by doctors for MRSA and Staph decolonization. While it's generally safe, chlorhexidine does have side effects, some are which are serious. Chlorhexidine washes are commonly used in hospitals to reduce infection transmission, as hand scrubs and as part of decolonization procedures used at home. Studies show that chlorhexidine can reduce hospital acquired infections and can eliminate some strains of MRSA bacteria on people's skin[75].

Decolonization procedures typically include skin baths with a chlorhexidine soap product for 3 days as well as nasal application of the topical antibiotic cream mupirocin for 5 days. Sometimes antibiotics are also prescribed. Skin and/or nose cultures are taken after the decolonization procedures to see if the MRSA or Staph bacteria are still present. If they are gone, decolonization is considered a success.

While chlorhexidine can be effective for decolonization, there are also risks and dangers associated with its use. Studies show that MRSA is becoming resistant to chlorhexidine[76]. Resistance has been growing over the years and may eventually render chlorhexidine unusable against some strains of MRSA and cause decolonization failure[77,78].

Chlorhexidine is generally well tolerated when applied to the skin. However, there can be some serious side effects. Chlorhexidine can be a skin irritant causing itching, irritation, redness and sometimes pain and skin peeling. Severe side effects can include allergic reactions such as hives, rashes, blisters, trouble breathing, and swelling in the tongue, face, mouth or feet. Chlorhexidine should never be used near the eyes or ears as permanent eye damage can result.

Natural Remedy Bathing Options

There are alternatives to bathing with harsh chemicals that can aid decolonization without all the negative side effects. Not only are these alternatives non-toxic, they can promote tissue healing, reduce stress and help bolster the immune system.

Your skin is the largest organ of your body and it excels at absorbing anything it comes into contact with. That includes any products you put on your skin. Your skin's absorbing power is a great advantage for getting beneficial remedies into your body through bathing. Unfortunately, your skin will also absorb toxins and artificial chemicals found in most skin care and beauty products. Because what you put on your skin goes within your body, using natural, non-toxic and health-supporting products is always preferable.

Bathing with natural mineral salts and bacteria-fighting remedies is a non-toxic alternative for Staph and MRSA decolonization. Essential oils provide antibacterial as well as soothing and calming benefits for you and your skin. Bath salts can provide further benefits, including skin hydration, softening and rejuvenation. See below for natural product and remedy options:

- **Bath product quality, purity and toxicity are crucial.** The key is to go as natural as possible and to avoid artificial ingredients, impurities, additives and fragrances from absorbing into your body. There are many different kinds of bath salt products. A few good quality brands can be found at Whole Foods, Vitamin Cottage and other natural product dealers. Himalayan sea salts in particular lacks modern contaminants, toxins and heavy metals found in man-made salts. Dendritic sea salts and finely crystallized salts dissolve more quickly and completely in water.

- **Bath time.** Most bath salts come with a scoop and instructions for how much to use. A 20 minute bath is typically long enough to enjoy the benefits to your skin and get some good relaxation. As for frequency, daily baths are excellent if you have the time.

- **For decolonization support**, tea tree oil is a good option to start with because it's mild yet strongly antibacterial. Other oils that can be beneficial in the bath are lavender, eucalyptus and rosemary. While oregano and thyme oils are also strongly antibacterial, these oils are very hot, irritating and sensitizing to the skin and are poor bath choices. For details on bathing with essentials oils, see the section "Bathing With Essential Oils" on page 134.

- **Spot bathing** can work well for trouble areas. Be careful using oils around the eyes and face as they can burn. See "Essential Oil Protocols for Use" on page 137 for details.

Keep the Bathtub Clean

If you have an active infection, be sure to clean and sanitize the tub before your friends or family use it. After the water drains, some of your skin bacteria are left behind on the bottom and sides. For the same reason, don't bathe in a dirty tub, as you don't want to make your skin infection worse. It's also best if you don't share your personal items like your bath towel, razor, or wash cloths.

Nose Decolonization

A favorite place for Staph and MRSA bacteria to live and grow is in your nose. Staph bacteria love moist and warm places like the upper respiratory system. Staph and MRSA can live in your nose and not cause a nose infection (this means you are a carrier), however many people get painful sores or boils in their nose from these bacteria.

A nasal swab culture test is commonly performed by doctors or hospitals to determine if a person is colonized with MRSA or Staph. If you have an active infection anyplace on your body, chances are the bacteria are living in your nose too. Decolonization procedures often include the skin and/or nose. The following are points to consider when dealing with either nose colonization or nose infections:

- **Sensitive areas.** The skin in and around the nose is sensitive, especially if you have an active infection there. Most remedies should be diluted before applying inside the nose to guard against burning and stinging.

- **Sinus infection risk.** Staph nose infections can become sinus infections. Clearing nose infections is important as it can prevent the infection from spreading.

- **Internal support.** Be sure to support your body with internal infection support if you have a nose infection.

Antibiotics for the Nose

Decolonization procedures typically include nasal application of the topical antibiotic cream mupirocin for 5 days. But mupirocin resistance in MRSA and Staph has been growing and may eventually lead to decolonization failure. See "MRSA Antibiotics for Skin Infections" on page 75 for details on mupirocin.

Nose cultures are taken after the decolonization procedures to see if the MRSA or Staph bacteria are still present. If they are gone, decolonization is considered a success.

Natural Remedy Protocol for the Nose

The following recipe is an alternative to using antibiotic creams in the nose and has been effective in decolonizing the nose from Staph and MRSA. It's also helpful when dealing with a nose infection. For details on essential oils, refer to "Essential Oil Protocols for Use" on page 137

- Mix together the following essential oils: two drops of tea tree oil, two drops of rosemary oil, one drop of lavender oil, and one to two drops of carrier oil.

  » Use additional drops of carrier oil to start out with, especially if your nose is extra-sensitive or if you find the mixture burns.

  » You can mix the oils in the palm of your hand, or the oils can be pre-mixed in a glass bottle.

- Dip a cotton swab or Q-tip in the mixture and swab your nose. Use a clean Q-tip for each nostril. Swab inside each nostril two times a day until infection is gone.

A Balanced View of Decolonization

Some people test negative for MRSA or Staph after following skin and/or nose decolonization methods. However, a negative test does not mean the bacteria are totally gone from your body. If you test negative in your nose, the bacteria may still be colonized on other parts of your body. It's also common to become colonized again after a successful decolonization. If you've been previously infected, Staph and MRSA can form biofilms and L-forms that hide inside the body and will not be visible with standard tests. Therefore, testing negative is no guarantee that you will not become colonized again, or that you will never get infected again.

While total elimination of MRSA from the skin or nose may be possible, a better goal is to restore balance to the protective bacteria inside your gut and on your skin and restore the health of your immune system. Because everyone comes into contact with bacteria in the community, building and maintaining your natural defenses is the most important long-term goal. Resisting infection is easier if your immune system is strong and your protective bacteria are in place. While decolonization is a helpful technique, it should be viewed as part of a larger infection control plan, as outlined in chapter 1 of this book.

Remedy Tips for Babies and Children

Many of the same remedies and natural methods used for adults can be used with children, with some adjustments. Importantly, the usage amounts must be reduced for babies and small children. Also, some of the diet recommendations in this book are not appropriate for infants and babies who are not yet on solid diets.

Many herbal products have limited or no safety information for use with children. Some natural products are best avoided for babies and small children due to known risks. Some products may be too strong for children, especially on their sensitive skin. Below are general guidelines and tips for using supplements and natural products with children. Always follow the directions on the product label if they differ from the guidelines below. And always consult with a natural-minded physician before using natural remedies or supplements with children.

- Look carefully on the label or product instructions for the **proper usage amounts for children**. Also make sure the label has no special warnings for children. Usage amounts for babies and children are usually much lower than for adults.

- Some products spell out a **body weight adjustment** for children. For example, if a product says to use 1 drop for every 10 pounds of body weight, then a 50 pound child would take 5 drops.

- Small children are **unable to swallow pills**. If the supplement can be taken with food, you can often break pills up or empty a capsule, hiding the contents in food or a drink. For older children, a smoothie is an excellent place to hide supplements.

- Only **mild remedies** should be used on babies and small children. Manuka honey is very mild and gentle on the skin. Tea tree oil is mild but needs diluted for babies. Eucalyptus oil, though fairly mild, should never be put near the eyes, nose or face of infants or babies. Applying essential oils to the bottom of the feet is a milder and safer alternative to using oils internally.

- **Raw honey** should not be eaten by babies less than one year old due to risk of botulism. Honey can contain botulism bacteria and babies under one year of age lack the intestinal flora (good bacteria) to prevent botulism sickness. Raw manuka honey is safe for adults and older children, but **sterilized honey** is a better option for small babies.

- Babies and small children have **sensitive skin, stomachs, intestinal flora** and mucous membranes. Products that are especially strong, spicy or irritating should be avoided, including raw garlic and oregano, thyme, clove and cinnamon essential oils.

- Essential oils should be **diluted before use** for children. As a general rule, for children less than two years old, dilute essential oils 75% (1 drop of oil plus 3 drops carrier oil) for skin application protocols. For children 2 to 3 years old, a 50% dilution of essential oils is commonly used. For children over 4 years old, undiluted essential may be used if well tolerated.

- For skin decolonization with small children, use **spot bathing** rather than a bath. Spot bathing with a basin and wet cloth makes it easier to keep remedies in the water away from the face, groin and other sensitive ares of baby's skin.

Infection Control for Pets

Common signs of MRSA in pets include infections of wounds caused by trauma or operations, infections from IV catheters or orthopedic implants, or other skin infections that just don't get better. The majority of MRSA and Staph bacteria isolated from infected pets are actually human strains of bacteria. This means that these infections originate from people, or are passed on from people to pets, rather than originating from pets. Like people, pets can also carry MRSA bacteria without becoming infected.

Pets have a higher risk of catching an infection if any of the following are true:

- The pet has been infected with Staph or MRSA before.

- The owner has a MRSA or Staph infection.

- The owner is a MRSA or Staph carrier.

- The pet has had a recent visit to a vet clinic experiencing an outbreak of the infection.

For additional resources on pets, antibiotics and MRSA, check out the Bella Moss Foundation which promotes prudent antimicrobial use and hygiene in human and veterinary medicine. This foundation was started by Jill Moss following the death of her dog, Bella, from a badly managed MRSA infection. They help link pet patients and veterinary clients with best practice resources and access to good advice. You can find out more here: www.thebellamossfoundation.com

MRSA Diagnosis in Pets

MRSA cannot be identified by symptoms alone. A MRSA culture test is needed to confirm what bacteria is causing the infection. Another test, called a antimicrobial susceptibility test, can help your vet choose the right antibiotic, if antibiotics are needed. Fortunately, most MRSA infections in pets are not severe and tend to be limited to the skin. Mild and moderate infections often respond well without antibiotics by using good wound management and diligent hygiene and prevention techniques. There are also alternatives to antibiotics that work very well for animals.

Pet Treatments

Antibiotics are the standard treatment for MRSA or Staph. But many of the same natural remedies that work for people can also help with pets, especially dogs and horses. In fact, essential oils like lavender, geranium, eucalyptus or rosemary can be used with dogs and horses just as they can for people with skin infections. Below are tips for controlling MRSA or Staph in pets:

- **Antibiotics.** MRSA and *Staph aureus* infections in pets are also antibiotic resistant. If you choose to use antibiotics, ask your vet to perform a susceptibility test to determine an effective antibiotic. Using an antibiotic that is ineffective can make their infection worse and promote antibiotic resistance.

- **Cats** are very sensitive to some natural remedies, including essential oils and most garlic preparations. As a general rule, essential oils should be avoided with cats. If you are using essential oils yourself, keep your cat in another room while applying them, especially when using an air diffuser. See the essential oil "Pet Precautions" on page 126 for more.

  » Homeopathic remedy formulations can be a good choice for cats, along with herbs like echinacea and goldenseal that help support the immune system and enhance the ability to fight infections.

- **Size matters.** Because cats and small dogs are so small, natural remedy usage amounts must be greatly reduced relative to people. Always read the remedy instructions for details about small pet usage amounts. It's important to remember that animals are small and much more sensitive to medicinals than people are.

- **Essential oils** must be diluted when used on smaller dogs before applying to the skin. For details about essential oils and dilutions, see the section "Essential Oil Protocols for Pets" on page 164. See the section on essential oil precautions "Pet Precautions" on page 126.

- **Do your research.** Some foods, herbs and alternative remedies that are safe for people are dangerous for pets. Be sure to do your research before using a natural remedy with your pet. Always talk with your vet about proper usage amount and method of use for your pet.

- **Immune support.** If your pet has been treated with antibiotics, use pet formulated probiotics to help replenish their healthy gut bacteria. There are also supplements available that support your pet's immune system with vitamins, antioxidants, herbs or mushrooms.

- **Holistic veterinarian.** Alternative or holistic vets are educated about non-antibiotic choices as well as immune support techniques to fight infections. The American Holistic Veterinarian Medical Association is a good place to start and has a vet locater here: www.ahvma.org/find-a-holistic-veterinarian/

Pet Preventative Measures

Both pet owners and pets can be MRSA carriers and not be infected, but pets and owners can pass MRSA bacteria back and forth between each other. In fact, recurring infections in people have been linked to close contact with an infected pet[69]. If you have an infected pet, the following tips can help prevent you from becoming infected or reduce the risk of an infection spreading:

- Wash your hands often and keep high-touch surfaces regularly cleaned and disinfected.

- Keep open wounds on your pet covered and well treated.

- Wash your pet with natural antibacterial products to help decolonize the bacteria from their skin. Avoid antibacterial hand or dish soaps as they have been linked to antibiotic resistance.

Just as hospitals are the most common place for people to get MRSA, vet clinics have the highest risk for pets to catch the infection. Most MRSA infections in cats and dogs occur at surgical sites and open wounds. Vet clinics can lower the risk of MRSA spreading with the following practices:

- Good hand washing by staff and cleaning of examination surfaces between pet patients.

- Vet staff can wear disposable gloves, plastic apron, mask and cap when working with an infected patient to reduce MRSA spreading to other pets or people in the clinic.

- Using antibiotics sparingly and prudently helps prevent the spread of resistant infections like MRSA.

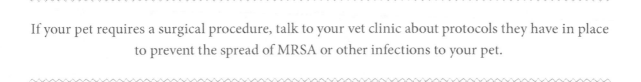

If your pet requires a surgical procedure, talk to your vet clinic about protocols they have in place to prevent the spread of MRSA or other infections to your pet.

Pet Food and Nutrition

Just as with people, diet plays a crucial role in warding off infections for pets. The more natural and less processed your pet's food, the stronger their immune system and the easier it is to recover and prevent infections. At a minimum, your pet's food should meet AAFCO requirements to ensure that basic nutritional needs are met. Because the word *natural* is not regulated, you need to look beyond the food's label and marketing materials to judge its true quality.

For both cats and dogs, look at the list of ingredients for lots of real meat (beef, turkey, chicken, etc) and preferably no corn, soy or wheat or any artificial ingredients. Quality wet food is always better than quality dry kibble. Kibble dehydrates animals and can cause kidney disease. As with people, nutritionally balanced raw food and raw food blends can be an excellent choice, though there is a transition period if your pet is not accustomed to raw food.

Always transition to new pet foods slowly. Be sure to consult with your vet before making any new food choices as it may not be advisable to change food, especially if your animal is sick.

Controlling Airborne Bacteria

Most people overlook the risks of airborne bacteria. Skin flakes shedding from the skin of infected people is a common way for MRSA or Staph bacteria to become airborne. While cleaning, disinfecting, and other preventative measures are important, controlling bacteria in the air is equally important. Specific techniques are needed to control these airborne bacteria to reduce the infection risk.

The techniques outlined below can reduce the number or airborne disease-causing bacteria in your home, office or hospital room. Some of these techniques are preventative, in that they help prevent bacteria from physically getting into the air. Other techniques are antibacterial as they actively kill bacteria after they become airborne. One of the most versatile antibacterial techniques is to air diffuse essential oils.

Essential oils are ideally suited for controlling airborne bacteria for three main reasons: 1) the oils are volatile and easy to diffuse into the air, 2) some oils are highly antibacterial, 3) and oils lack the toxicity or hazardous disinfectants. In 1955 Keller and Kober found essential oils to be effective in controlling a number of bacteria in room air, including Staph bacteria[79]. They found twenty-one different essential oils that reduced or eliminated Staph bacteria when sprayed in an enclosed area.

Several essential oils can be used with cold-air diffusers to control bacterial aerosols in the air, including hospital rooms[80]. Be sure to use a cold air diffuser as heating essential oils destroys their therapeutic value. Below are techniques to help reduce the risk of airborne Staph and MRSA:

- **Keep open wounds covered** per the section "Wound Dressing" on page 190. Open MRSA or Staph wounds are a potent source of bacteria. Skin flakes and particles are the biggest source of dust throughout the home or hospital room. When skin particles are shed, they lift into the air bringing along bacteria from the open wound.

- **Practice good hygiene.** Good personal hygiene is crucial for the infected person, any caregivers and anyone else living with or in close contact with the infected person. See the chapter "Hand Washing and Hygiene" on page 269 for details.

- **Cold-air diffuse essential oils.** Tea tree and eucalyptus oils are ideal choices for air diffusing. The Antibacterial oil blend may also be used, although it may be too spicy or hot for some people. Refer to the section "How to Air Diffuse Essential Oils" on page 132 for details on how to diffuse these oils.

Lymphatic Drainage

The lymphatic system is like your body's garbage disposal system. It eliminates toxins such as bacterial waste products and trapped blood proteins. Infections can cause a buildup of dead bacteria and bacterial toxins in the lymph. A backed up lymph system can cause pain, inflammation, energy loss, obesity and can even lead to chronic diseases.

Bay laurel essential oil can speed the lymph transfer process when applied topically over areas of the lymph nodes[34]. Bay Laurel is most helpful when combined with active physical lymphatic stimulation as detailed in the steps below. The following activities performed daily can help stimulate and support lymphatic drainage.

- Aerobic exercise stimulates lymph movement for much of the body. Note that aerobic exercise is not efficient at moving lymphatic fluids in the areas under the arms, in the groin area and on the feet. Horseback riding is an excellent way to aid the movement of lymphatic fluids, especially after applying bay laurel to the body.

- A brief massage over four different areas with bay laurel oil is a great way to move sluggish lymph. See the *lymphatic drainage stimulation* protocol in the section "Bay Laurel Oil" on page 154.

Maintenance and Preventative Remedies

Using maintenance levels of infection support remedies can help the body guard against bacterial, fungal and viral infections over the long-term. Such maintenance remedies are different than taking supplements. While supplements are taken for general immune and nutritional support, maintenance remedies such as the ones described below specifically target infections and are tailored to reduce the risk of recurring outbreaks.

Note that taking maintenance remedies is not a substitute for an immune-boosting diet and proper supplementation. However, long term use of infection-fighting remedies can help support your body against biofilms and L-forms. The key to success with maintenance remedies is to use them as an add-on along with the immune support methods inside the Action Steps in chapter 1 (see "Action Step 3: Immune Defense" on page 16.)

Below are three protocols that use antibacterial remedies for long-term preventative maintenance. It is not necessary to follow all three protocols at the same time. Most people who choose to use a long-term maintenance remedy select just one protocol.

Botanical Blend Protocol

The maintenance level usage amount of the "Botanical Blend Protocol" on page 106 can be used for long-term maintenance for adults. The protocol combines two broad-spectrum herbal formulations with a probiotic formulation developed specifically for infection support. The protocol can be adjusted for children per the details in the "Botanical Blend Protocol" on page 106, which requires reducing the usage amounts according to the child's age. However, the protocol is not recommended for infants and small babies.

Essential Oil Maintenance Protocol

The life cycles of disease-causing microorganisms living in your body can vary throughout the day. The best time of day to strike at a pathogen is when their metabolism is slowest and they are most vulnerable. Bacteria like Staph tend to be least active at night. Viruses are less active in the morning. And fungi are slowest mid-day. The protocol below takes advantage of these pathogen life cycles to hit the disease-causing organisms when they are most vulnerable.

The adult protocol uses the lowest (mild or maintenance) usage amount of the "Broad-Spectrum Internal Protocol for Adults" on page 156. The oils can be taken orally using an empty vegetable capsule along with several drops of carrier oil. Alternatively, some people use the *lick trick* by placing the drop of essential oil on the back of the hand and then using the tongue to lick the oil into the mouth. This regimen can be followed by most adults for long-term prevention, so long as no negative side effects are experienced. For children and the elderly, the usage amounts and the method of use must be adjusted per the "Children, Babies and Elderly Protocols" on page 160.

Stabilized Allicin Maintenance

For adults and children age 12 and older, stabilized allicin can be used for long-term preventative maintenance as detailed in the section "Using Stabilized Allicin" on page 95. For long-term use, the lowest maintenance level of the protocol is appropriate.

16 Probiotics: The Good Bacteria

Did you know that the average healthy person has over 100 trillion microorganisms in their digestive system? That equals 3 to 4 pounds of bacteria that people carry around with them every day. In fact, in the human body, microorganisms outnumber human cells by 10 to 1. Your health is dependent upon this *microbiome* in ways scientists are just beginning to understand.

Your microbiome is made up of some 10,000 different species of microorganisms that protect your skin, aid digestion, enhance nutrient absorption and produce of significant amounts of B vitamins and enzymes. Some of the enzymes kill off harmful bacteria which help prevent infections. Gut microbes also appear to influence the function of T and B immune cells. The bottom line is that these healthy microbes are a major factor in the overall health of your immune system and protection of your body against invading microorganisms.

Modern society has waged a *war on germs* with disinfectants, sanitizers and antibacterial soaps and toothpastes. But little thought is given to understanding how these products affect your beneficial microbiome. And, when infection strikes, people normally reach for antibiotics. But an unfortunate consequence of taking these drugs is that they kill the good microorganisms on your body and inside your intestines (aka your intestinal flora). While antibiotics may stop a Staph or MRSA infection, they leave behind weakened gut flora and therefore a weakened immune system. This disruption of the intestinal flora makes room for disease-causing microorganisms to grow, often leading to secondary infections like *C. difficile* and yeast infections.

As many as 70 million people in the U.S. have some type of digestive disease, according to the National Institute of Diabetes and Digestive and Kidney Diseases. If you want a healthy immune system, faster infection recovery and reduced risk of digestive diseases, then restoring the balance of good bacteria in your gut is essential. The best way to restore that balance is to take *probiotic* bacteria contained in either supplements or naturally fermented foods.

How Probiotics Work

Your digestive system works side-by-side with the foods you eat to provide your body with all the energy and nutrients it needs. So it's no surprise that your digestive system is a critical factor in the strength of your immune system.

60% of your immune system is located inside your intestines[81].

Properly fortified skin and intestinal flora are among your body's strongest lines of defense against bacterial, viral or fungal invaders. In your intestines, there's a continuous *cross-talk* between the tissues in your gut and your friendly bacteria. This constant communication tells your immune system what is *self* and what is not, allowing your body to fight invading bacteria and other disease-causing organisms[82].

One of the best ways to nourish your digestive health is to take probiotics regularly. Probiotics are good bacteria and other flora that replenish your gut, thereby crowding out the harmful disease-causing bacteria. Probiotics also help keep the gut flora in a healthy balance for optimal immune system performance.

Probiotics do more than boost the immune system. Probiotics can also help with lactose intolerance, diarrhea, constipation, colon cancer and many other diseases. In fact, probiotics are a major area of research and even obesity and depression have been linked to the health of your gut microbiome. Most probiotics come from one of two groups of bacteria, including Lactobacillus (found in the small intestine) and Bifidobacterium (found in the large intestine).

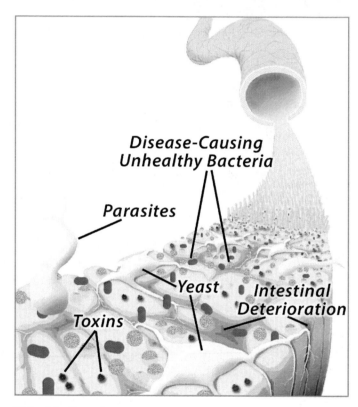

Unhealthy Intestines
Without healthy bacteria, disease-causing unhealthy bacteria, plus yeast, parasites and toxins can accumulate, damaging the intestinal wall and producing poor intestinal health.

What Disrupts Gut Flora?

The word probiotic in Greek contains *pro*, which means supportive or promoting, and *biotic*, which means life. Probiotic literally means *supporting of life*. You can guess what the word *antibiotic* means: *against life*. Factors that can throw off the healthy balance of your gut flora include:

- Antibiotics

- Over the counter and prescription medications

- Sugar

- Highly processed low-nutrient foods

- Residual pesticides and food toxins

- GMO foods

- Stress

- Unfiltered, chlorinated tap water

- Chemical antibacterial soaps, toothpastes and mouthwashes

What Restores Gut Flora?

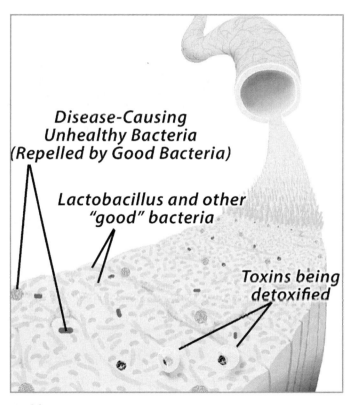

Healthy Intestines
Beneficial or *good* bacteria coat and protect the intestinal wall, inhibiting and repelling unhealthy bacteria and contribute to maintaining bacterial balance and optimal intestinal health.

Most of the factors listed above that kill your gut flora can be avoided or minimized by eating an immune-boosting diet . GMO foods and immune-boosting foods will be covered in detail in the chapters "GMO Foods, Glyphosate & Immune System Stress" on page 259 and "Foods and Your Immune System" on page 237.

Besides taking a daily probiotic supplement, another way to replenish your intestinal flora is to eat healthy fermented foods. Yogurt and other cultured foods have live beneficial bacteria. However, the number of living bacteria in yogurt is often quite low. And most yogurt products also contain processed dairy ingredients and a lot of sugar, both of which make yogurt a poor option. In contrast, unprocessed fermented foods such as fermented vegetables, kefir and sauerkraut are a healthy and rich source of probiotics and vitamins, as detailed in the section "Fermented Foods" on page 242.

Finding Effective Probiotics

- **Look for spore forming strains.** Spores are analogous to a seed. Spores are tough and protect the bacteria within. Most strains that don't produce spores don't survive the acid in your stomach and never make it into your intestines. All strains of Lactobacillus and Bacillus species produce spores.

- **Prebiotic or supernatant.** Look for probiotics that contain a *supernatant* (*prebiotic* is another term for supernatant). The supernatant is the food source that provides the nutrients the probiotic bacteria need for maximum shelf life and potency. Fructooligosaccharides, abbreviated as FOS, is often used as a supernatant. FOSs also support the growth of healthy gut bacteria.

- **Bifidobacterium breve and MRSA.** A combination of the bacteria *Bifidobacterium breve* and it's prebiotic galactooligosaccharides provided a synergistic anti-MRSA effect greater than either component alone. The combination showed both preventative and curative effects against multiple strains of MRSA in mice[83].

- **S. boulardii.** *Saccharomyces boulardii* is a probiotic yeast and is the focus of scientific studies showing favorable results against many infections, including *C. difficile*[84].

- **B. coagulans.** A resilient probiotic is the *Bacillus coagulans* strain, also called *Lactobacillus sporogenes*. This species of bacteria is stable and maintains its potency well.

- **Lactobacillus strains.** Other good choices include Lactobacillus strains such as *Lactobacillus acidophilus* and *Lactobacillus salivarius*.

  » The *Lactobacillus paracasei* species has shown strong antibacterial activity against 32 human strains of disease-causing bacteria, including MRSA[85].

  » Another study showed that *Lactobacillus acidophilus* eliminated 99% of MRSA bacteria after 1 day of exposure[86].

- **Bifidobacteria.** Bifidobacteria consume old fecal matter and have been shown to remove cancer-forming elements, including the enzymes that can lead to cancer formation. Bifidobacteria also protect against the formation of liver, colon, and mammary gland tumors.

- **Multiple strain probiotics.** You gut is diversified, so look for probiotics with multiple types of bacteria. Everyone is different, and some strains may be more or less beneficial than others on an individual basis.

- **Packaging.** Look for moisture and light barrier packaging. Light and moisture greatly reduce the potency and shelf life of most probiotic supplements.

- **Power in numbers.** Look for an indication of the number of bacteria within the product. Bacterial counts are typically measured in Colony Forming Units (CFU) per gram. Look for probiotic products that guarantee billions of CFU/g at the time of manufacture. This will help maximize the number of microorganisms that make it into your intestines. Heat, moisture and light reduce the number of bacteria over time, so refrigeration is important for most products.

Probiotics Protect Your Skin from Attack

Your gut isn't the only part of your body where beneficial bacteria live and ward off infections. Your skin is your largest organ and is your first line of defense against many infections, especially Staph and MRSA. Your skin harbors hundreds of kinds of beneficial microorganisms that actively crowd out and prevent disease-causing bacteria from gaining a foothold.

One study showed that the predominant skin bacteria *Propionibacterium acnes* competes against MRSA bacteria for space on your skin and suppressed the growth of community acquired MRSA[87]. Another study examined three species of Lactobacillus probiotic bacteria commonly found in fermented foods and supplements. The results show that two of the probiotics protected human skin cells against Staph skin infections[88].

Steps to Maintain Healthy Skin Flora

Disruption your skin flora gives Staph, MRSA and other dangerous microbes a foothold to colonize your skin and potentially cause an infection. Supporting your healthy skin flora is therefore an important part of any infection control strategy, especially if you've struggled with recurring skin infections or are a MRSA Staph carrier. Probiotic supplements for your skin are uncommon, but the actions listed below can help you support your skin flora.

- **Minimize antibiotic use**, both topically and internally. Disrupting your protective skin microbiome allows for easier entry for skin infecting bacteria. For details, see the chapter "Hand Washing and Hygiene" on page 269.

- **Avoid chemical antibacterial soaps.** Studies show that they are no more effective than simple soap and water. As you'll learn in the hand washing chapter, most common soaps, personal care products and skin remedies prescribed for decolonization of MRSA can destroy the delicate balance of your healthy skin flora.

- **Avoid contact with bleach** and other harsh chemicals. Consider carefully before using bleach or other harsh chemicals for bathing or cleaning. Wear protective gloves when using any disinfecting agents. The chapter "Cleaning and Disinfecting" on page 275 will give you tools to minimize the health risks and find healthy alternatives for cleaning and disinfecting.

Getting The Most From Your Probiotics

Using Probiotics With Antibiotics and Other Remedies

Some mainstream medical resources recommend against taking probiotics with antibiotic drugs, even if they have no specific reasons or evidence to support this stance. However, there is evidence that taking probiotics with antibiotics supports the health and balance of bacteria in the intestines and supports the immune system. As a rule of thumb, it's typically best to take probiotic supplements 2 hours apart from any antibiotics to avoid potential interactions and to maximize the potency of the probiotic.

Because natural remedies work on many different levels, they are thought to be much safer on flora than antibiotics. Probiotic support is a helpful and integral part of your total infection control program. Just like antibiotics, be sure to take probiotics at least 2 hours apart from any internally used antibacterial remedy.

It's important to understand the contraindications of any drugs you take. For some drugs and circumstances, probiotics may be in appropriate or contraindicated. If you have questions about specific antibiotics and probiotics, or specific probiotics and alternative remedies, consult with a naturopathic doctor or other healthcare professional with specific probiotic experience and training.

Change is Good

Some holistic healthcare professionals recommend changing the type or brand of probiotics from time to time. Occasionally changing probiotics gives your gut a wider range of flora and may reduce the risk of having an unknown imbalance involving a particular species of flora. As mentioned earlier, augmenting probiotic supplements by eating a variety of fermented foods is another excellent way to expose your gut to a broad range of beneficial flora.

Probiotic Flora Blend

One particular probiotic is formulated to promote natural intestinal bacteria as well as healing of the GI tract. This blend contains live cultures of *Lactobacillus acidophilus*, Bifidobacterium and *Lactobacillus salivarius* as well as the medicinal plants dandelion, viola, chlorophyll, peppermint, aloe vera and ginger. This combination of probiotics and medicinals helps the body to restore healthy flora in addition to soothing and restoring intestinal tissue.

This blend is more like a live fermented food than a traditional probiotic. Rather than being dried, processed and coated like most probiotics, this blend is a living culture in a native supernatant. This supernatant increases the effectiveness of other probiotic products if used along with this probiotic blend. This probiotic blend is part of the "Botanical Blend Protocol" on page 106.

Probiotic Precautions

If after starting a probiotic product you have any discomfort reactions such as gas or bloating, reduce the amount of the product you are taking. Once the symptoms subside you can increase again. Discomfort is typically the result of bad bacteria in your digestive system dying off as the new good bacteria are replacing them.

Children and Infants

If you are a nursing mother and you take probiotics, your baby will receive the beneficial probiotics through your breast milk. Young children and babies can not take capsules in which most probiotics are sold. Be sure to look for probiotic formulations designed specifically for use with infants and young children.

NOTE: See the section "Michelle's Recommended Products" on page 303 for product resources.

17 Healing Crisis and Detoxification Support

Many people who start a natural healing program are unfamiliar with what is known as a *detoxification reaction* or a *healing crisis*. While one expects to start feeling better immediately with improvements to one's health, sometimes just the opposite happens. Starting a healthier diet or a new supplement can cause an excess of old toxins to be flushed into the body resulting in a temporary detoxification reaction. In the same way, taking an antibiotic or antimicrobial remedy can cause a die-off of bacteria or yeast which creates an overload of microbial toxins and debris that require cleanup by your body.

While some people may never experience a detoxification reaction, most find they get a mild to moderate increase in symptoms that can include fatigue, nausea or a headache. While you may temporarily feel worse, these reactions can indicate your body has started *cleaning house* and is on its way to better health. This clean up process is something the body must go through, but it can be uncomfortable and worrying, especially if you are not expecting it or if you are not familiar with how to minimize the symptoms.

Many safe methods that promote natural healing can result in a detoxification reaction. Some examples include:

- Starting a probiotic supplement or fermented food

- Using a healing herbal remedy

- Eating better quality and healthier foods

- Eating fruit smoothies or raw juices

- Initiating a liver cleanse or bowel cleanse

- Taking an antimicrobial remedy

The reason people feel worse is because of the sudden release of toxins from body tissues and the resulting toxin backup in the body. This detoxification reaction is usually a sign of a liver that's a bit sluggish and not fully doing it's job. Because of the ever-growing presence of toxins in foods and the environment, most people already have a significant amount of toxin buildup in their body.

Overloaded detoxification organs (like the liver) sets the stage for a healing crisis to happen. Below is a review of why people are over-loaded with toxins and how your body normally deals with toxins.

Toxins, Toxins Everywhere

Every day, the cells within your body create metabolic toxins as a byproduct of making energy. Detoxifying just the toxins your own body makes takes a significant amount of energy, let alone additional toxins you may be exposed to. On top of your body's own toxins, there are now at least 100,000 different industrial chemicals in production that people are exposed to through the environment. Examples include: dioxins, PCBs, flame retardants on furniture, heavy metals like mercury, pesticides, non-stick coatings on pans, fluoridated water and the list goes on. People are also exposed to many toxins in food, water and the air. And if you're dealing with an infection, there are different kinds of bacterial toxins you can be exposed to when bacteria die off.

What is Detoxification?

The process the body uses to clean house is called detoxification, or *detox* for short. This process plays a pivotal yet often unnoticed role in your daily activities as well as the ability to heal from and prevent infections and other diseases. Detoxification is always occurring in your body, 24 hours a day. The liver is a major detoxification organ, as are the lungs, kidneys and skin.

In a healthy person, the body manages to eliminate more toxins than it creates or absorbs from the environment. But when the detox process is thrown out of balance by poor diet, stress, or infection, toxins begin to back up.

One way the body deals with excess toxins is to store them in fat cells until they can be eliminated at a later date. However, unless the detox process is fixed, that later date may never come, leading to continuing toxin buildup in the body. Poor detoxification can set the stage for chronic diseases to develop later in life. Doing what you can to minimize the toxins you are exposed to as well as supporting your detoxification system are important actions that support your best health.

Where Do Toxins Come From?

As mentioned above, everyone is exposed to many different toxins on a daily basis that are a natural part of life. Many of these toxins can be avoided or minimized through awareness and making adjustments to your lifestyle. For example, drinking purified water or eating organic foods are ways to reduce your exposure to toxins.

Bacterial Toxins

For those dealing with skin or internal bacterial infections, when the bacteria in your body are killed by your immune system, antibiotics or other remedies, your body's lymphatic system has to get rid the pieces of bacteria that are left behind. Bacteria like MRSA can also create toxins as part of their metabolism that remain inside your body after the bacteria are killed. These metabolism products and pieces of dead bacteria are toxins and they must be removed for your body.

Chemical-Laden Foods

Many of today's processed foods are laden with pesticides, preservatives, artificial colors and flavors and artificial sweeteners that behave like toxins in the body. Because these chemicals are artificial and not found in nature, the body does not recognize them and sees them as toxins. This extra load of toxins puts stress on your body's ability to detoxify. Anything that puts extra burden on your detoxification systems makes it harder to recover from an infection or maintain optimal health.

GMO Foods

A very common yet largely overlooked source of food toxins comes from GMO foods. GMO stands for Genetically Modified Organisms. The DNA of some types of GMO foods has been artificially changed in ways that cannot happen in nature. While several GM foods have been approved by the FDA, their long-term health risks are a major source of controversy. Emerging science has raised some significant red flags about the long-term safety of several types of common GM foods.

Personal Care Products

One of the biggest ways toxins get inside your body is through your skin via personal care products. From soaps to lotions to makeup, nearly all of these products have many different chemicals, additives and impurities that can build up inside the body and require extra energy to detoxify. This is why using natural plant-based and organic products is so important.

Environmental Toxins

The water your drink, the air you breathe and objects you touch every day are sources of many different kinds of toxins. These include fluoride and chlorine in tap water, nitrogen and sulfur compounds in the air, and flame retardants and plasticizers in the home, just to mention a few. All these sources contribute to the mounting load of toxins that accumulate in your body that must be removed.

Detox and Healing Crisis Symptoms

Surprisingly, when starting a new food, you may start to feel tired for awhile. Ingesting good friendly bacteria in a new probiotic supplement or a fermented food can kill off bad gut bacteria causing an influx of toxins in the body, possibly resulting in abdominal cramping, headache or gas. Both are examples of positive steps you can take for better health, but both can also cause you to not feel as well as you normally do.

Detox symptoms occur when more toxins are released into your body than your body can eliminate. All these backed-up toxins moving around the body can cause some temporary yet unpleasant side effects. These side effects are called *detox symptoms* or *reactions* or a *healing crisis*. Some common detox symptoms include:

- Low energy and fatigue

- Headaches and muscle aches

- Nausea or flu-like symptoms

- Skin rashes and eczema (toxins coming out through the skin)

Is it Detox, an Allergy or Infection?

Some common detox symptoms like skin rashes or nausea can easily be caused by infections or antibiotics. These same symptoms can also be caused by a detox reaction due to eating healthier. It can be hard to tell if these symptoms are due to a detoxification, a drug side effect or an allergy to a drug.

The most important thing for you to know is that a detoxification reaction is possible when you start any new health related program, food, supplement or remedy. And if you believe your body is going through a detoxification process, it's helpful to assist the process gently without pushing your body into a rigorous detoxification. Because it may be hard to tell if you're detoxing too quickly, it's best to take a conservative approach, especially if you have an active infection or you are new to detoxification. If the symptoms are concerning, be sure to notify your doctor.

Detox Dos and Don'ts

There are several ways you can gently support your body's ability to detoxify when you're dealing with infections. Helping detox from microbial toxins can speed the recovery process for infections. The sections below will highlight the most effective and supportive ways to help your body detoxify.

A Balanced View

Some people become obsessed with environmental toxins, living in fear of them and becoming too focused on avoiding them. Remember that exposure to toxins is a normal part of everyday life. Your body is inherently designed to get rid of toxins and to keep you healthy. Obviously, it's helpful to avoid those toxins that you reasonably can. But it's much more helpful to remain focused on supporting your body rather than focusing on avoiding every single toxin in the world. Maintaining a balanced view and avoiding obsession with toxins is the healthiest and most productive way to approach detoxification.

Be Conservative with Detox Programs

Starting a rigorous or assertive detoxification program is generally not appropriate if you're in the midst of a severe infection. There are many detox programs available and some really put your body through its paces. Doing a rigorous detox program will put a drain on your body's resources necessary for fighting an infection. Your body only has so much energy to devote to daily living activities. Adding the extra strain of a strong detox program may not be best, at least initially, unless your doctor advises it.

After your infection clears, you may have the desire to try a more robust detoxification program to help your body remove stored, excess toxins. However, when dealing with an active infection, it's best to detoxify gently to reduce the risk of detox symptoms. If you're having more than mild symptoms, drink more water and back off on the amount of the new food or supplement you are taking for awhile. Once you feel better, you can slowly work up to your desired level of food or supplement again.

Talk to your doctor (preferably a nutritionally minded doctor) before beginning a detoxification program, especially if you have an active infection.

Gentle Detoxification Support

The following actions are great ways to assist your body's natural detox ability with little risk of negative symptoms. These simple detox aids may also be used along with more assertive detox protocols to improve detoxification results.

- **Drink plenty of water.** If you're experiencing a detox reaction, drink water. Remember the saying *dilution is the solution to pollution*. Proper hydration will dilute and help flush toxins through the kidneys and is important when dealing with any detoxification symptoms. See the section "Water, Water Everywhere" on page 247 for suggestions on how much water to drink.

- **Start slowly** with any new remedies, supplements or diet changes. Some natural remedies encourage the body's detoxification processes. This means that starting with too much of a natural remedy, or taking too much too fast, may cause a detox reaction. The same holds true for adding healthy foods to your diet. Eating more healthy foods too quickly can sometimes push your body into detox. While detoxing is helpful, keeping it at a moderate pace will minimize the risks of negative symptoms. So make healthy diet additions slowly and start slowly with any new supplements or remedies to minimize healing crisis reactions.

- **Avoid adding toxins.** If you're trying to detox, it's best to reduce the number of new toxins you're putting into your body. Since food is one of the biggest sources of toxins, it's important to avoid foods that have the most toxins or that are unhealthy. See the chapter "Foods and Your Immune System" on page 237 for suggestions on which foods to minimize or avoid.

- **Slow down or stop if needed.** As mentioned above, the best way to avoid the negative side effects of detoxification is to start slowly and be conservative. If you experience negative symptoms, back off on your detox efforts (or the food or supplement) or give them a break for a while. Stopping any detox supplements or programs usually brings a swift stop to the negative symptoms.

Lymphatic Toxin Drainage

The lymphatic system helps the body to rid itself of bacterial waste products from nearby infections, cellular debris and many different toxins. This system can become backed up, sluggish and overworked, especially if you have an infection. There are some simple methods to support and stimulate your body's lymph to get toxins from nearby infections moving out of the body. One of the simplest methods uses bay laurel essential oil applied topically, combined with a simple form of lymphatic massage. Applied over lymph node areas, this method can help in evacuating toxins from the lymph system. For details on using bay laurel for lymphatic support, see "Bay Laurel Oil" on page 154.

Liver Cleanse

Just like the lymphatic system, the liver plays a key role in dealing with toxins. All of the body's blood passes through the liver and it filters out toxins to be excreted. This organ becomes overtaxed when the amount of toxins are too much for it to handle. The liver also can be overburdened by breaking down and removing prescription medications like antibiotics, as some can be especially hard on the liver.

Sometimes stimulating and helping the liver to cleanse can provide an extra measure of detoxification support. You can help support your liver by using a gentle *liver cleanse* as detailed in the section "Liver Cleanse" on page 178. Several other general liver support techniques are detailed in the section "Liver Support" on page 176. These techniques are also helpful for relief of infection symptoms and antibiotic side effects.

18 Boosting Your Immune System

Your body's first line of defense against an infection is your immune system. If properly strengthened and supported, your immune system can resist and surmount infections much more easily and quickly.

It's amazing that one of the most effective ways to repel infections is something simple that you can do yourself at home. All it takes is a little knowledge and practice to develop the necessary skills and habits.

How to Boost Your Immune System

Thinks you can do to boost your immune system are listed in the bullet points below. Several of the techniques below are covered in detail in other chapters of this book. This chapter is focused on pH balance, nutritional supplementation and stress reduction as they pertain to immune support.

- **Eat immune enhancing and alkaline foods.**

  » Diet is often the biggest factor when it comes to having a strong immune system. To learn about healthy and supportive foods as well as foods that can hamper your healing, refer to "Foods and Your Immune System" on page 237 and "Green Smoothies" on page 253 for immune health.

  » Eating a proper balance of alkaline and acidic foods is one of the easiest, safest and most effective methods of immune support. See "pH Balance" on page 224 for details.

- **Take care of your healthy bacteria.** Most of the function of your immune system is regulated by the beneficial flora in your gut and on your skin. Read the chapter "Probiotics: The Good Bacteria" on page 209 for more details.

- **Get proper nutrition, hydration and supplementation.**

  » Refer to "Foods and Your Immune System" on page 237 for healing foods. See "Vitamins and Minerals" on page 167 for the most important vitamin supplements for natural infection support, as well as the supplementation section in this chapter.

- **Minimize toxins, prescription drugs, and unhealthy foods.** Minimize environmental contaminants and unhealthy processed foods and use prescription and over the counter drugs as conservatively as you can. Toxins, gentle detoxification and liver support are covered in "Healing Crisis and Detoxification Support" on page 217.

- **Reduce your stress levels.** Managing your stress level is one of the most overlooked aspects of immune system health. See "Stress Management" on page 233 for helpful stress reduction techniques.

Immune Health is Largely Ignored

A combination of poor diet, stressful lifestyle, over-reliance on pharmaceutical drugs and a lack of knowledge has left most people's immune systems weakened and vulnerable to disease.

You may ask yourself, if boosting your immune system is so simple and effective, why don't you hear more about it? And why isn't your immune system the primary focus of your doctor's prescribed treatment regimen for an infection? The answer is quite simple. Mainstream medicine pays much more attention to treating and managing symptoms than to addressing the root cause of your infection. If you want real, long-lasting results, it's up to you to take charge of your health and make it happen.

Antibiotic treatments can quickly and effectively kill the bacteria causing your infection. But when your treatment is done, the underlying conditions that helped cause the infection in the first place are still there. On top of that, the same antibiotics you take to treat the infection also weaken your immune system. The effects of these drugs include killing your good gut and skin bacteria, creating an acidic environment in your body and adding an additional toxic burden to your liver and detoxification systems. All of these effects leave you more vulnerable to future bouts of Staph or MRSA.

You can break the cycle of reinfections by boosting your natural immunity with the tried and true methods outlined in this and other chapters of this book. Some of these methods can help fairly quickly while others will take some time and effort. The goal is to permanently change your body's environment so it is harder for infections to get a foothold. While this process can take some time, it's an effective long-term solution to recurring infections.

pH Balance

There are several schools of thought on diet and immune support. One of the most useful and easy ways to gauge your immune support efforts is to measure your body's pH (not your blood pH)[89]. Many different factors contribute to your pH levels. Your diet is perhaps the most important factor, but stress level, your attitude, exercise, your relationships, and environmental factors all play significant roles too.

Your pH levels can be quite variable throughout the day; therefore, measuring pH properly is important. While not a foolproof system, many people find that monitoring their urine pH is an effective way to assess their health.

The concept of pH is especially useful for planning what foods to include in your diet and how much of them to eat[90]. There are specific foods that directly benefit your immune system and others that actually weaken it. High pH or alkaline foods generally boost your immune system and improve your general health. These foods tend to be higher in minerals and vitamins and lower in sugars. Using the simple principles of food pH, you can easily recognize the best food choices and successfully keep your overall diet in a healthy balance.

◇◇◇

NOTE: Within the context of health and wellness, pH only refers to salivary (saliva) and urine pH, not blood pH. Blood pH does not change much and is not relevant to diet pH balance.

◇◇◇

What is pH?

pH stands for *potential hydrogen* and it is a measure of how *acidic* or *basic* something is. If something is in acid/base balance, it is said to be *neutral*. The pH scale starts at 0 and goes up to a maximum value of 14, with a pH value of 7.0 being neutral. Anything from pH 0 to 7 is called acidic, and anything from pH 7 to 14 is called basic or alkaline as shown in the figure below.

When you eat, the food is broken down and changed inside your body as you digest and absorb it. This process is called metabolism. If food produces acidic byproducts when metabolized, it is

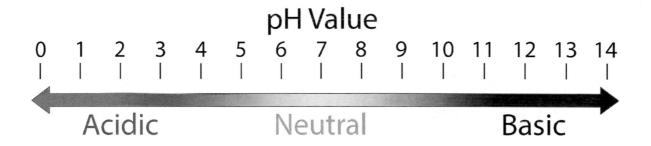

called an *acidic food*. If food makes basic byproducts when metabolized, it is called an *alkaline food*. Eating alkaline foods helps create a more alkaline pH environment inside your body's intracellular fluids, which enhances your immune system and inhibits disease.

It is crucial to understand that some foods have an acidic pH if you measure them directly, but when you eat them, they form alkaline products in your body. Good examples include balsamic vinegar and lemons, both of which are very acidic if measured directly. But when you eat them, they form basic or alkaline metabolic products in your body.

Just as foods produce byproducts that affect your pH, many other things cause bodily responses that change your pH level. Stress, for example, quickly causes your body to produce chemicals and many complex reactions that leave acidic residuals in your body. Likewise, exercise, though good for you, naturally produces acidic byproducts in your tissues.

It's both natural and healthy to have a balance of acidic and alkaline influences or events in your life. The problem is, if you have too many acidic influences relative to alkaline influences, your body will be chronically acidic, the exact conditions in which infections and other diseases prosper.

pH and Your Health

High pH or alkaline foods make your body higher in pH level. Likewise, acidic low pH foods make your body more acidic. If your body is chronically acidic, the condition is called acidosis, a condition which favors the growth of infections and disease. On the contrary, infections and diseases cannot gain a foothold, grow, or thrive easily if your body is alkaline, or high in pH.

A chart listing the most common acidic and alkaline foods is in "Acid/Alkaline Food Chart" on page 305. All the foods on the left side of the chart are alkaline foods and all the foods on the right are acidic. Use this chart to make the best food selections when shopping or planning your meals, selecting a balance of foods from both sides of the chart.

As a great starting point, try the "Super pH Salad Recipe" on page 307. It's delicious, simple to make, great by itself or as a side dish and is loaded with alkaline ingredients. Another super pH (and super nutrition) recipe is in "Green Smoothie Recipes" on page 309.

Staying Balanced

Just because a particular food is on the acidic side of the chart does not mean you should avoid it. There are many acidic foods that contain beneficial nutrients that your body needs. If your body is too high in pH (too alkaline), that is not healthy and can cause problems too. The key is a healthy balance.

*Balance your acidic and alkaline foods so that overall,
your body stays slightly on the alkaline side*

A good rule of thumb is to follow the *80/20 rule*. Try to eat approximately 80% alkaline foods and 20% acidic foods to create an alkaline body pH. With the proper balance of alkaline and acidic foods, you'll get to eat nutritious foods from both sides of the pH chart and your average dietary pH will still be on the alkaline side. There's a simple way to measure your body's pH as detailed below.

How to Measure Your pH

By monitoring your body's pH on a regular basis, you can track how well your diet is working and make adjustments as needed. There's a quick and easy way to measure your body's pH at home. All you need is a simple pH test kit and a sample of either your urine of saliva. For an accurate, easy to use, economical, and respected pH test kit, try the pHydrion kit from www.MicroEssentialLab.com, catalog #067 (pH 5.5 – 8.0).

Urine pH

The urine pH test is a measure of your cellular metabolic health. Test your urine pH first thing in the morning before you eat, drink or exercise. Here's how to perform the test:

1. Urinate into a cup.

2. Remove a piece of pH test paper from the test kit.

3. Dip the piece of paper into the cup.

4. Remove the piece of paper from the cup and shake it off.

5. Immediately compare the color of the paper to the test kit color chart.

6. The color on the chart that most closely matches the paper's color corresponds to your urine pH at that point in time.

The optimal pH range for your urine is 6.5 to 7.1. If your urine pH is less than 6.5, your body may be acidic. If your urine pH is higher than 7.1, it may be too high, which is also not healthy. pH varies considerably depending on what you eat, your stress level and other factors. Measure your pH frequently to approximate its average value over time. Pay attention to long-term trends over time and avoid putting too much stock in any single individual measurement.

> Urine pH values vary day to day and hour to hour, so looking for trends over time is more important than paying attention to one or two isolated measurements.

If your pH is low, adjust your diet by increasing alkaline foods and/or reducing acid foods or reducing your stress level. Be patient. Changing your pH can be quick, or it can take a bit of time. Be aware if your urine pH is less than 5.5, you should not engage in strenuous exercise. With such a low pH, you risk cardiac problems if you exert yourself. Also be aware of the other mentioned factors besides diet that can affect pH and make adjustments to them if needed.

Saliva pH

Saliva pH is a measure of your emotional health and stress level. Test your saliva pH first thing in the morning before you eat, drink or exercise. Here's how to perform the test:

1. Spit into a cup.

2. Remove a piece of pH test paper from the test kit.

3. Dip the piece of paper into the cup.

4. Remove the piece of paper from the cup and shake it off.

5. Immediately compare the color of the paper to the test kit color chart.

6. The color on the chart that most closely matches the paper's color corresponds to your saliva pH.

The optimal pH range for your SALIVA is 6.8 to 7.0. If your saliva pH is outside this range, you may have a lot of negative thinking or emotional stress going on. As with urine pH, this measurement can vary, so measure frequently and average your results over time to look for trends. As with urine pH, trends over time are much more important than one or two measurements by themselves.

A big factor that influences your pH and your immunity is stress. The significance of stress is frequently overlooked or taken too lightly when it comes to immune system health. You'll find out how stress affects your immune system and learn step-by-step tools to manage your stress later in this chapter.

Alkaline Water and pH Solutions

Alkaline water, home water ionizers and high pH solutions are popular health products and many claims have been made about the dramatic health benefits they provide. Despite their purported benefits, drinking alkaline water and other solutions can potentially cause problems, especially if used long-term.

Drinking alkaline water can offset the natural stomach fluids that should be acidic for the breakdown of food you eat. Having too alkaline a stomach may lead to digestive problems. The prominent natural doctors Joseph Mercola M.D. and Andrew Weil M.D. agree that ingesting alkaline fluids over time may be harmful to your health. Your body's cells can be hurt if conditions are too alkaline. Conditions that are too alkaline can also disrupt the delicate balance of beneficial bacteria in the body. While the benefits or alkaline water products are open to debate, if used, they should be used for short time periods only and not relied upon as a miracle cure.

Supplementation

Supplementation can be divided into two main areas for the purposes of dealing with infections:

1. Nutritional supplementation

2. Immune system supplementation

According to Dr. Linus Pauling, two-time Nobel Prize winner, "Every disease is directly linked to a nutritional deficiency." Your body's immune system needs many different minerals, vitamins and other nutrients to work properly and provide optimum resistance and defense against infections. The best way to meet your nutritional requirements is to eat a diet rich in all of the nutrients your body needs. However, eating a nutritious diet is probably not enough to supply most people with all their nutritional needs.

An important property of many supplements is the ability to strengthen or stimulate your immune system. These immune supporting supplements may not directly kill infecting bacteria or treat your infection, but they can help your body to do a better job of ridding itself of infections. There are many different parts to your immune system, and some supplements help different parts. One supplement may help stimulate your white blood cells while another helps balance your intestinal flora. Yet another supplement may aid your body in eliminating toxins and bacterial metabolic byproducts.

The Need for Nutritional Supplementation

Eating an optimal and healthy diet can be challenging, to say the least. And even if you do eat the healthiest whole food diet, you still could be missing out on key nutrients. Therefore, nutritional supplementation is very important. And if your immune system is stressed or has been neglected, there are supplements specially formulated to give your immune system an extra boost. Below are the main reasons most people need nutritional supplementation:

- **Soil nutrient depletion.** The widespread use of industrial farming and agriculture causes soils to become depleted in minerals and other nutrients over time. Most industrial fertilizers replenish only the major nutrients (potassium, phosphorus, nitrogen and others) in the soil but don't replenish the minor and trace nutrients. This leaves most farming soils depleted of vital nutrients. If the nutrients are not in the soil, they will not be in the food grown in the soil.

- **Soil sterilization.** Beneficial bacteria, fungi, worms and other types of living organisms in the soil form a complex biological web that generates nutrients for plants and protects plants from diseases. The widespread use of pesticides in industrial agriculture (non-organic farming practices) often kills more than just insects and pests. Pesticides upset the balance of the biological soil web, and essentially *sterilize* the soil over time. Dead soils depleted of microorganisms will yield malnourished crops.

- **Missing nutrients.** Even if you have an unlimited variety of self-grown foods and eat a very healthy diet, there's a good chance you are still not getting a few key vitamins and minerals. As stated above, missing only a few vitamins or minerals can potentially cause health problems over time, even if you don't have any symptoms right now. Supplementation with a quality multi-vitamin is the easiest way to fill in any potential gaps in your diet.

- **Specific medical conditions.** One of the most important reasons to supplement is to address specific medical conditions. Many vitamins and nutrients have been shown to help fight off infections and boost your natural defenses. Getting increased amounts of specific antibacterial or immune-boosting supplements can give you an added edge in healing from infections.

Supplement Quality

The quality of your supplements is very important. Your body can best recognize and use nutrients which are natural and that are in natural proportions with other nutrients. Unnatural nutritional supplements that are not recognized by your body simply pass through your system unused and are a waste of your money. Below are some of the most important quality factors to look for in good supplements:

- **Plant-based.** Look for supplements that are derived from plants and not made synthetically in a laboratory. Plant-based vitamins and immune boosting supplements have nutrients in the right natural ratios and of the right chemical makeup that your body can recognize and use. Unnatural and synthetic supplements are not recognized by your body and often pass through your system without being utilized.

- **Correct chemical form (not synthetic).** The synthetic versions of most supplements are very commonly used, however, they are not chemically the same as what is found in nature. In some cases, the synthetic version of a vitamin can be hundreds of times less potent than the natural form. Many supplements can also be purchased in more than one form. For example, Vitamin C is available in three forms: 1) ascorbic acid, 2) buffered Vitamin C, and 3) Vitamin C complex. The buffered and complex forms of Vitamin C are the best for your body. Make sure that supplements are in the proper form that is most safe and effective and avoid synthetic versions.

- **Bioavailable.** In addition to the form of the supplement, the other ingredients inside the supplement are also important. Make sure supplements can be easily absorbed by your body. Low-quality supplements often contain poorly formulated binders, fillers and bulking agents and are in a physical form that makes it harder for your body to digest. High quality supplements are usually easier to digest, more potent and more effective. Supplements in powder form usually have fewer binders and fillers, but are a little less convenient to take.

- **Raw and minimally processed.** Look for raw supplements processed with low heat or cold pressed with minimal processing steps. Heat and processing cause delicate nutrients to break down. Pasteurization also can reduce the potency of vitamins and other nutrients due to heat.

- **Complexes and formulas.** As a general rule of thumb, when you buy a vitamin, mineral or herbal supplement, look for complexes rather than isolated nutrients. For example, you can get vitamin E as a single isolated nutrient, or you can get it in a complex along with tocopherols and other biochemicals that make the vitamin E more potent and balanced inside your body. Complexes are closer to what is found in nature than single isolated ingredients and are often safer and more effective to use. Likewise, supplements that contain a well-crafted formula or blend of different ingredients are often better for your body than single-nutrient products. For example, while olive leaf extract by itself can provide infection support, adding other synergistic ingredients, such as garlic, goldenseal and milk thistle, can crate a formula that works better then the sum of its parts.

- **Free from unnatural preservatives, colors and flavors.** Avoid unnatural preservatives such as sodium benzoate, BHA and BHT, and other artificial preservatives. Also avoid artificial colors, sweeteners, and flavors that have dubious long-term safety. 100% natural preservatives and other inert ingredients can be beneficial to help improve digestion and to protect the potency and purity of the supplement.

- **cGMP.** If possible, choose supplements made by a company that follows current Good Manufacturing Practices (cGMP). Following these practices help ensure that raw material sourcing, manufacturing steps and product testing and distribution are all tracked, well documented and done reproducibly by trained employees. cGMP compliance does not guarantee that a product is safe, effective or of the required quality to meet your needs. However, compliance indicates a responsible company with good systems and controls to make its products.

- **The cost of quality.** When it comes to supplements, you get what you pay for. The cost of a high quality and potent herbal extract can be two or three times higher than a low quality version of the same herb. While higher quality ingredients cost more, they usually have much higher levels of the bioactive chemicals. Products made with low quality herbal extracts or other ingredients may be cheap, but they may not work and they often contain contaminants and impurities that can make them unsafe for demanding medicinal uses.

- **Be wary of RDA values.** U.S. RDA (Recommended Daily Allowance) values for nutrients and vitamins are typically the bare minimum level to prevent nutrient deficiency. However, RDA levels are not necessarily the best levels for optimal health. For many nutrients, there's a big difference between the level of nutrient deficiency and the level you need for optimal health. Ideal levels of many vitamins and minerals are much higher than the U.S. RDA values, especially if you are trying to counteract a nutrient deficiency. For multi-vitamins, it's usually better having all of the ingredients in the correct natural ratios (plant derived) rather than looking at the RDA values alone.

Immune Boosting Supplements

When handling infections naturally, the line between supplements and remedies can be a little blurry. Many natural products that have strong therapeutic and natural antibiotic properties also support your immune system. It is useful to consider supplements as playing a secondary or supporting role in treating infections rather than being the primary or lead remedy.

Supplement advice and recommendations abound from many different sources. All of the opinions and advice can be overwhelming and confusing. Keep in mind that while supplements are very beneficial, the most effective way to boost your immune system is with a healthy, immune boosting diet. Therefore, supplements are not a replacement for an proper diet.

Be sure to discuss with your physician any questions or concerns you have before starting on any new supplement. The following list of supplements is by no means complete, but it is a good place to start for most people with Staph or MRSA.

- **Daily multi-vitamin.** The use of a high quality, plant-based multi-vitamin can provide a broad spectrum of required vitamins, minerals and other key nutrients in relatively large amounts. Multi-vitamins are usually taken along with meals. Follow the serving recommendations on the bottle or as directed by a natural-minded physician.

- **Superfoods.** The term *superfood* describes a natural food source with a very complete spectrum of nutrition. Superfoods contain a large number of the major, minor and trace nutrients that your body needs for optimum health. The amount of any single nutrient in a superfood may be comparatively low, but the presence of all required nutrients can fill in the nutritional gaps that other supplements cannot easily fill. Foods such as chlorella, spirulina, blue-green algae and marine phytoplankton are often referred to as superfoods and make a good addition to one's supplement regimen.

- **Sea salt.** Replace your table salt with natural sea salt. Celtic sea salt and Himalayan salt are excellent choices. Sea salt has hundreds of minor and trace minerals in natural ratios without the silica binders, chemical additives and toxins found in regular table salt. Sea salt also has a much better flavor than table salt.

- **Zinc.** Zinc supplementation can help ward off infections and support the immune systems. A common zinc regiment is 20 to 30 milligrams per day for adults, or 10 to 15 milligrams per day for children, for a three month period. For details see "Zinc" on page 171.

- **Omega-3 oils.** Omega-3 oils are very important for your immune system and for proper cellular nutrition. Omega-3 oils are discussed in detail in the section "Get Good Fats" on page 244. A quality *molecular distilled* cod liver oil or krill oil is one of the best sources of Omega-3 oils. A tablespoon of cod liver oil each day is a typical serving size for most adults.

- **Vitamin C.** 1000 milligrams twice a day of buffered vitamin C is a customary serving size for immune support during an infection challenge. See "Vitamin C" on page 169 for details.

- **Vitamin D**. It is best to get your Vitamin D levels tested before starting vitamin D supplements. The correct type of vitamin D to take, along with usage amount and testing recommendations, are detailed in the chapter "Vitamins and Minerals" on page 167.

- **Echinacea.** Echinacea is an herbal supplement that boosts the immune system by enhancing the activity of macrophage white blood cells that fight infections in your body. One of the best ways to get Echinacea is in concentrated liquid extract or tincture form. Follow the directions on the bottle for serving sizes and usage. Echinacea is often combined with the use of myrrh oil for immune support. Echinacea should not be used if you have an autoimmune disorder. You can learn more about this herb in the section "Echinacea" on page 105.

- **Garlic, turmeric and ginger.** Garlic is a powerful immune system booster, in addition to its natural antibiotic properties. Turmeric and ginger also help support the immune system and have other beneficial properties. See the chapter "Alternative Remedies" on page 91 for details.

- **Essential oils.** Many essential oils have immune boosting effects in addition to their natural antibiotic and therapeutic effects. This illustrates the synergy and the beauty of natural remedies. See the chapter "Essential Oil Protocols for Use" on page 137 for more details.

Caution With Iron

Iron is an important nutrient for your body, however, taking iron supplements during an infection may make your infection grow worse. Many infectious organisms use iron for growth. Therefore, consider stopping your iron supplements during an active infection. Only take iron supplements if you have a proven iron deficiency (you can get your iron blood levels tested first) and stop taking iron after your deficiency is corrected.

Stress Management

Perhaps no other factor affecting your immunity is underestimated as much as stress. No matter how devoted you are to proper diet and a healthy lifestyle, infection recovery can be made more difficult if emotional barriers stand in your way. Stress has a powerful ability to lower your immune system and leave you open to sickness and disease. The majority of people say they have stress in their lives and this stress may be the root cause of serious health problems. The sections below will give you some techniques to reduce and control stress.

Sleep

The quality and amount of sleep you get is one of the biggest factors affecting your stress level. The daily stresses that comes from work, family, finances, being infected, and other sources are easy to take to bed with you. Eight hours of sleep per night is a good general guideline. Below are some important recommendations to get a good night's sleep:

- Do a relaxing activity before bed, like a hot bath, reading a book, prayer, meditation, etc.

- Have your last food at least 2 hours before bedtime.

- Avoid caffeine and other stimulants (chocolate, sugar, etc.) as well as alcohol and other depressants at least 4 hours before bed.

- Keep on a regular bedtime schedule.

- Avoid watching the news, or a disturbing movie, or TV in general before going to bed.

- If you can't get to sleep, get up and do a relaxing activity for a while before going back to bed.

- Keep your bedroom comfortable, restful and peaceful. Keep TV's, work desks, computers and other distractions out of your bedroom.

Exercise

One of the best and most healthy stress reducers is exercise. Exercise releases endorphins in your body that gives you a natural high and makes you feel good. Exercise is also a great way to release tension, aid detoxification and increase energy. Even a quick five to ten minute walk to get outside and change your pace can greatly reduce your stress.

Doing some exercise when you feel stressed is great, but having a regular exercise plan scheduled every week will have a bigger effect on your overall stress level and on your health. If you're not accustomed to exercising, start with something low impact like walking, yoga, gentle swimming or light weight lifting and do it for 30 minutes 3 times a week. As your fitness increases, you can slowly increase the duration and frequency of your workouts. Always check with your doctor before beginning a new exercise regimen.

EFT

Emotional Freedom Technique, or EFT, is a powerful acupressure technique based on the same energy meridians of your body used in traditional acupuncture for over five thousand years. Instead of using needles like acupuncture, you simply use your fingertips to tap specific locations on your body. You can perform EFT on yourself anywhere and it only takes about one minute to do.

The tapping puts kinetic energy into specific meridians of your body. While performing the tapping, you think about a specific problem you are having or a specific thing causing your stress and your say positive affirmations about it. Basically, all you have to know to get started are the tapping locations, the correct technique, and the positive affirmations.

For a full step-by-step guide to performing EFT, see "Emotional Freedom Technique (EFT)" on page 311. If you don't get the results with EFT that you would like, consider consulting with an

EFT professional (many offer a free initial phone session). Guidelines on selecting an EFT therapist and listings of EFT practitioners can be found by searching the web.

Tai Chi

The roots of tai chi are a Chinese method of self-defense, but tai chi has also been shown to boost the immune system and improve overall health. Research shows that this ancient martial art helps people lessen the activity of hormones that suppress immunity and beat out infections caused by the shingles virus. According to a recent study by Michael Irwin, M.D., tai chi increases T-cells in the body, an important component of the immune system. The combination of exercise, group practice and a synergistic mind/body experience is especially beneficial for the immune system.

Yoga

Yoga is not only beneficial for your physical health, but also your emotional health. Besides toning your muscles, increasing your flexibility and strength, and giving you a whole body workout, yoga removes stress and anxiety, is calming and improves your mood. Even most mainstream medical doctors recognize the benefits of yoga on both physical and emotional health.

There are several different styles of yoga, and although they are all similar in many ways, each style focuses on a different aspect. For example, some yoga styles focus more on postures and breathing while others focus on meditation and spirituality.

Many health and wellness centers and gyms offer yoga classes for free with membership. Many towns also have dedicated yoga centers to choose from as well. Try out a few different classes to see which one you are most comfortable with. And don't worry about how you look or if you can do the postures as well as someone else. Yoga is for anybody and for any experience level.

Prayer and Meditation

Next to yoga, prayer and meditation are perhaps the most effective ways to reduce stress. Not only are prayer and meditation relaxing, mentally leveling and self-confidence building, research shows that prayer and meditation directly strengthen your immune system.

Prayer and meditation can greatly affect your stress level and overall health, even if you are new to it. And as with many things, the more you practice, the greater the benefits will be. It takes consistency and some time to learn to quiet your mind and begin to discover the greatest rewards from prayer and meditation.

Prayer

You may prefer prayer over meditation depending on your beliefs and what you are most comfortable with. The methods and goals of prayer are usually different from meditation, though they share many commonalities.

- Morning is a great time for prayer and a good way to start out your day. Set a time for prayer and avoid distractions from the outside or from within your own mind.

- Prayer can include reading, memorizing and meditating on scriptures or it can include personal conversation with God.

- Be very open, honest and personal in your prayer time, just as you would be with a close friend.

- Practice humility and surrender by letting go of the need to control the future.

- Give thanks for God's blessings in everything big and small, even your infection and the unseen opportunities that it can create in time through God's grace.

Meditation

Meditation was originally a spiritual component of yoga. To make the most of meditation, schedule and practice it daily with focus and intention and without distractions.

As with prayer, morning is a great time for meditation, setting the stage for the rest of your day. Meditation creates the opportunity to separate yourself from all the fears, stresses and judgments of your mind to find peace, perspective and clarity. There are many different styles of meditation, each differing slightly in focus and method as described below (more details can be found online):

- In Transcendental Meditation (TM), your focus comes from repeating a serious of words called a mantra.

- Mindfulness Meditation focuses on breathing and being in the present moment.

- Another type of meditation is called no-mind or non-duality. In this meditation, you practice being an observer of the thoughts going through your mind without trying to change them, anticipate them or cling to them. Like watching the landscape from the window of a moving car without focusing on any of the content, only perceiving the surrounding context of the view. One seeks to perceive that your true self is not your body, thoughts or emotions, but rather you are simply a witness to them. You are consciousness itself as a creation of God. This *no mind* method is described in detail in two books by David R. Hawkins, M.D. Ph.D.[91]

With either prayer or meditation, don't worry about doing it right or how it looks or even trying to follow the directions above. Just *be* and relax and consistently do something to quiet your mind. These practices will help you reduce stress in your life, and you'll begin noticing the rewards sooner than you think.

19 Foods and Your Immune System

ood, diet and nutrition is a broad topic that can easily fill the shelves of an entire library. Even something more specific, such as how to eat a so-called *healthy diet*, is a topic that produces thousands of new books every year. Each book, website or diet regimen on this topic has its own unique goal, opinions and twist on nutrition. This chapter will help you to make better food choices and improve the nutrition you get from your food for the specific goal of overcoming Staph and MRSA. As you read this chapter, take what you learn with a grain of salt. Everyone is different and food tolerances, allergies, taste preferences and nutrient deficiencies vary significantly from person to person. However, the overall principles in this chapter apply to most everyone.

Why Diet is Important

As you've learned in the chapter on immune support, there are many factors that affect your body's infection-fighting abilities. But the single most powerful way to boost your immune system is through your diet.

What you eat has a dramatic effect on health and disease, an effect that is usually ignored, underestimated or downplayed by mainstream medicine

Consider how your car works. By design, your car only works properly if a particular type of fuel is used. What happens if you put diesel fuel into a car made for unleaded fuel? At best, it will belch black smoke and lurch around making weird noises. What would happen if you put substances into your gas tank such as water or sugar that your car was not designed to process? You'd be lucky if your car even started, and the damage done to the engine would be difficult and expensive to fix.

The example of a car and its fuel is exactly how your body works. Some foods can be safely and effectively used by your body as fuel and these fuels will help keep your systems running smoothly. On the other hand, there are other foods and a host of substances that your body was not designed to process. These foods will compromise your body's functions on many different levels, including your immunity.

What a Healthy Diet Really Means

The biggest obstacle to enjoying a robust state of health is the *Standard American Diet* (appropriately abbreviated SAD). The SAD diet is very acidic, high in refined and processed foods and low in nutritional value. All these attributes conspire to lower your immunity and make you predisposed to many disease conditions.

There's a lot of conflicting information from the media, the Internet, the medical community, and the health and wellness industry on what constitutes a so-called *healthy diet*. The dietary focus of this chapter is not on weight loss, anti-aging or any other popular or trendy *healthy diet* goals. The main focus here is immune support and infection control. While there's a lot of overlap between the diet ideas in this chapter and other healthy diet plans, there are some key differences too.

The dietary principles in this chapter can have an immediate and noticeable impact on your infection and how well you feel. The recommendations you are about to discover can literally change your life, if you pace yourself, set realistic goals and stick with it for the long term. Adopting an immune-boosting diet is a lifestyle change with bigger payoffs than you have probably imagined.

Take It Slow

Trying to follow all of the food ideas in this chapter all at once will probably doom you to failure. Start with the first section and work your way through the chapter and integrate each section into your diet one at a time. For example, start with the next section on sugars first, then add the section that follows it about raw food. Some of the sections below can be challenging for some people, so allow enough time to get accustomed to each change in incremental steps. Always consult with your doctor if you have any questions or concerns before implementing a new dietary program.

Choose Your Sugars Wisely

Of all the food ingredients, sugar has the biggest impact on your immune system. Did you know that the average American eats over a third of a pound of sugar every day? The amount of sugar in the standard American diet adds up quickly because of sugar-laden soft drinks, juices, candy, ketchup and the majority of processed foods, which contain large amounts of refined sugar.

Not all sugars are bad for you and healthy sugars are essential to your body. In fact, the messengers of your immune system that are responsible for its basic function are glycoproteins (the Latin root *glyco* means sugar or sweet). These messengers cannot function properly if they are stuck with the wrong sugars[92].

Good forms of sugar come from healthy complex carbohydrates. Healthy sugars have a low *glycemic index* and improve your general health as part of a balanced diet. The best sources of complex carbohydrates include the following:

Healthy Carbohydrate Sources
Brown rice and wild rice
100% whole grain pasta or bread
Yams and sweet potatoes
100% whole grain millet, quinoa (pronounced *keen'-wuh*), buckwheat, oats and barley
Legumes (peas, beans, soy products)
Most raw fruits (in moderation)

On the other hand, eating refined sugars is the quickest way to depress your immunity. In fact, drinking two cans of regular Coke will suppress your immune system function by 92% for up to five hours[93]. Refined sugars have been processed to strip away the nutrients, fiber and minerals, making them sweeter and prolonging their shelf life. Eating these unnatural products will quickly elevate your blood sugar, stress your body and shock your immune system. Also, in order for your body to process these unnatural sugars, minerals from your bones and other tissues are stripped away to aid digestion. The continual cycle of shocking your system with a diet high in refined sugar takes a big toll on your natural defenses, your energy level and your health over time.

The FIRST THING you should do to reduce reinfections is to stop eating refined sugars

Minimize or eliminate the following refined sugars and replace them with healthier substitutes:

Type of Sugar	Healthier Substitute
Sugar (white sugar)	Raw evaporated cane juice
Corn syrup	Raw Agave nectar & Yacon
High fructose corn syrup	Raw Yacon or Agave nectar
Hydrolyzed or modified cornstarch	Raw Yacon or Agave nectar
Enriched flour	100% whole grain flour
White pasta	100% whole grain pasta
White bread	100% whole grain bread
Honey (the clear generic stuff)	Raw unfiltered honey (local is best)
Soda, Pop, Cola	Water, tea

Kicking the Sugar Habit

Sugar is very addictive. Most people have cravings for sweets when they begin to reduce or eliminate them from their diet. It is therefore important to learn ways to relieve your cravings and get them over with as quickly as possible. You can reduce your sugar craving in the following ways:

- Go **cold turkey**. This is important due to the addictive nature of processed sugar.

- Substitute a healthier alternative. At times when you normally eat dessert, eat berries or another healthy option instead.

- Use the Emotional Freedom Technique (EFT) for stress reduction and reducing addictive food cravings. See "Emotional Freedom Technique (EFT)" on page 311 for details.

Reducing the Negative Effects of Sugar

Below are ways you can help counteract the effects of sugar if you do decide to eat sweets:

- Eat sweets with other foods, especially foods that have lots of fiber. Fiber helps sugar enter the body more slowly and cause less shock to your immune system.

- Eat dessert before the main meal, not after it. This slows down sugar's metabolism in your body.

- Have some cinnamon with your sweets. Cinnamon helps counteract the effects of sugar, so have a little cinnamon or a drop of cinnamon essential oil along with sweets.

- Keep your diet clean. An occasional dessert or sweet is better handled by your body if you are already eating a healthy and immune-boosting diet.

Eat It Raw

When food is cooked, the heat breaks down some of the nutrients so that your body no longer can use them. Cooking foods also produces acidity in your body, the perfect conditions for infections to take hold (see the section "pH Balance" on page 224). If you choose to cook your food, lower temperatures and shorter cook times preserve more nutrients and enzymes. Steaming is the least-damaging way to cook. Deep frying and grilling both produce high temperatures that can actually cause toxins and carcinogens to form from the overheated food.

The more raw foods you eat, the stronger your immune system will be. Here are some specific raw food suggestions (keep in mind organic is always best):

- Salads and greens

- Non-roasted, non-irradiated raw nuts

- Uncooked or lightly steamed vegetables

- Uncooked non-canned fruit

Raw Dairy

Raw milk contains many components that kill pathogens and strengthen the immune system. However, most dairy products are pasteurized to kill possible dangerous bacteria. While it's beneficial to destroy dangerous germs, pasteurization also has unhealthy effects on dairy. Pasteurization kills off the beneficial bacteria along with the bad ones. The naturally-occurring lactic acid bacteria in milk are killed. Therefore, pasteurized milk cannot become sour and quickly decomposes, letting undesirable germs multiply very quickly. In contrast, sour raw milk is widely used as an easily digested laxative and is not unpleasant to eat.

By subjecting dairy products to high temperatures, pasteurization destroys many nutrients and makes calcium less soluble. The homogenization process used in dairy products produces undesirable and unhealthy byproducts due to high shear forces breaking down the delicate proteins. The allergies people have to dairy products can come from allergens created during the homogenization and pasteurization processes which do not occur naturally in raw dairy products.

If you choose to eat dairy products, eating them raw is much healthier and is quite safe for most people

In some states, stores are not allowed to sell raw milk and/or cheese, so you may have to go to a local farm. Raw dairy products, especially raw milk, do have the potential to harbor pathogenic bacteria if they are not processed, packaged and distributed with care. However, the same is true of many other products, including spinach, almonds and other raw food products. Like any other raw food, it's best to buy organic and buy locally. Large-scale industrially-produced dairy foods should be avoided. And just because a food product is labeled as organic, it doesn't mean it's raw. Most organic milk is not raw and has the same drawbacks as regular pasteurized milk.

Raw dairy is actually very safe when compared to other foods in an unbiased way. Large industrially produced dairy products found in most stores increase your risk of illness, have fewer nutrients and contain toxins and allergens.

CAUTION: A small percentage of raw dairy products can contain dangerous bacteria and may not be appropriate if you are immune-compromised. If you want more information about the safety of raw dairy or how to find a reputable source, the following website will answer many of your questions: www.realmilk.com

Amazing Greens

Of all the raw foods that benefit your immune system, the most nutritious are edible leafy green plants. In fact, of all the food groups available, greens most completely match the nutritional needs of humans.

Calorie for calorie, the vitamin and mineral contents of greens are unmatched by any other food

Each type of green has its own unique nutritional profile, so eating a variety of greens in abundance provides nearly every nutrient your body needs. See the chapter "Green Smoothies" on page 253 for delicious recipes and details about this important addition to an immune-boosting diet.

Fermented Foods

In the last few years probiotics and healthy gut bacteria have been the latest popular trend in the health and wellness industry. But long before probiotic supplements were invented, people got their daily probiotics from the foods they ate. In fact, traditionally fermented foods can be packed with literally trillions of beneficial, immune-boosting probiotic bacteria, many times more than the strongest probiotic supplements.

Yogurt is probably the best known food that can contain live probiotic cultures. The trouble is, store-bought yogurts are highly processed, artificially sweetened, contain minimal probiotics or contain large amounts of sugar. But traditional, non-pasteurized yogurt can be an excellent source of probiotic cultures.

Traditional yogurt is not the only probiotic food. Traditional unpasteurized versions of butter, cottage cheese, buttermilk, kefir, miso, tempeh and kombucha tea are other probiotic foods making a comeback in natural grocery stores. Traditional sauerkraut is one of the best known and easiest to make fermented foods.

Fermented Foods Forgotten

Historically, fermented or cultured foods were a common part of most people's diets. In fact, for thousands of years fermentation was one of the best ways to preserve foods before the advent of refrigeration. Until recent decades, probiotic-rich fermented foods provided huge numbers of beneficial bacteria to reseed people's gut flora. In modern times, the healthy heritage of eating fermented foods has been nearly forgotten.

Almost everyone has been programmed to believe that all bacteria are bad and that all bacteria in food must be killed. So modern foods are processed and pasteurized to remove all the bacteria, including the good bacteria people need to be healthy and fight off infections. To add insult to injury, processed foods are full of harmful, probiotic-killing ingredients, such as artificial dyes, flavors, preservatives, and sweeteners.

The recent popularity of probiotic foods has lead processed food companies to jump on the band wagon. Many a food label can be found at the grocery store touting that they contain *probiotics* and *live cultures*. However, most of these popular foods are relatively low in probiotic content and high in sugar and other processed ingredients that offset the probiotic benefit of these foods.

Fermented Food Benefits

Fermented foods are easy to find in a good health food store and they are often not very expensive. Fermented foods are also easy to make, requiring inexpensive ingredients and basic kitchenware. Below are some benefits to adding minimally-processed traditionally fermented foods to your diet:

- Trillions of beneficial probiotic bacteria in every tablespoon, many times more than any probiotic supplement.

- Wide range of different beneficial bacteria for maximum biodiversity of your gut flora.

- More economical than buying probiotic supplements, especially when homemade.

- Wide range of health benefits, including weight loss, mental clarity, and increased energy. Many chronic diseases conditions also respond by eating fermented foods.

- Serve as delicious side dishes or condiments at meal time.

While the health benefits of fermented foods are many, it's best to start slowly if your body is unaccustomed to fermented foods. Changing your gut flora too quickly can trigger a microbial die-off of unhealthy gut bacteria. These symptoms can be uncomfortable and prolonged if you make healthy diet changes too quickly.

It may take a while to begin seeing the full benefits of eating more fermented foods. While it's common for people to experience more energy and other positive results soon after adding fermented foods to their diet, it may take several months to begin seeing major shifts with a long-standing health condition.

Maintaining optimal gut flora is one of the most important steps you can take to improve your health. If you aren't eating fermented foods, you most likely need to supplement with a probiotic on a regular basis, especially if you're eating a lot of processed foods, taking prescription medications or antibiotics or drinking chlorinated water.

Get Good Fats

The adage *you are what you eat* is especially true of fats and oils. Fats are essential for your body and are the very building blocks of your body's cellular walls. In fact, roughly 50% of your cell walls are made of saturated fats. Fats also play a vital role in the detoxification pathways in your liver, among a myriad of other important bodily functions.

Be aware that the terms *fat* and *oil* are essentially the same thing. The main difference is that fats are usually solid at room temperature, whereas oils are usually liquid.

There are many different fats and oils used throughout the food industry, spanning the entire gamut of the health scale. Some fats are healthy and even essential to your health, while others are unhealthy and downright toxic. There are two basic types of fat: saturated and unsaturated. Both types of fat play a vital role in your health.

Unsaturated Fats

Olive oil is probably the best known unsaturated fat. Most unsaturated fats and oils are easily damaged by heat or cooking. Only certain unsaturated fats and oils should be used for cooking. Here are some general recommendations for using unsaturated fats.

- These low-temperature oils are delicate and go rancid quickly, so store them in your refrigerator or in a cool place away from sunlight.

- Beware labels touting high levels of omega-6 and omega-3 oils. Although essential for your health, omega-6 and omega-3 oils must be in a one-to-one ratio. Most so-called *healthy* unsaturated oils have far too much omega-6 relative to omega-3, so check carefully before you buy.

- Make sure you purchase your unsaturated oils as *cold pressed* or *expeller expressed*. Cold or expeller expressed oils are extracted from their source fruits, nuts and seeds using a low temperature process that protects the oil from heat damage. Large scale extraction processes use 230 degree F heat and chemical solvents, usually hexane, to speed up the extraction. These toxic chemical solvents used in the extraction process can never be totally removed.

- Avoid the chemical preservatives BHT and BHA as both are suspected of causing cancer and brain damage. They are often added to cheap, refined oils to replace vitamin E and other natural preservatives destroyed by the heat.

The bottom line: pay as much attention to how an oil is processed as to what type of oil you buy. Below are several healthy unsaturated oil choices:

- **Flaxseed oil:** Flaxseed oil is very high in healthy ALA omega-3 oil. Most unsaturated oils have too much omega-6. Flaxseed oil is very effective at reversing the omega-6/omega-3 imbalance that plagues most other unsaturated oils. Flaxseed oil also contains lots of fiber (nearly 30% by weight) and all of the essential amino acids the human body needs. This is a delicate oil that must be kept refrigerated and never heated or used for cooking. Use alone as a supplement (one teaspoon per day is a common usage amount) or add it to shakes or smoothies. It can also be mixed with olive oil as a salad dressing.

- **Cod liver oil and krill oil:** These marine-based oils are very high in vitamin D and omega-3. In particular, they contain two beneficial types of omega-3 only found in marine based oils: EPA and DHA (flaxseed oil only contains ALA type omega-3). These perishable oils must be refrigerated and never heated. Krill oil is also high in beneficial antioxidants. Buy only high-quality marine oils that are tested to be pure and free of all toxins. Take a half ounce per day as a supplement or as directed. These oils are also a great source of vitamin D.

- **Olive oil:** Great for salads, pasta, bread, and many general uses. The best olive oils are slightly cloudy (unfiltered) and golden yellow in color (indicating it was made from ripe olives). Olive oil is the safest vegetable oil you can use and is OK for limited moderate temperature cooking. Virgin olive oil is best. Because this oil contains more omega-6 that omega-3, use it in moderation.

- **Sesame oil:** A relatively stable oil good for stir fry and moderate cooking. Due to its high percentage of omega-6 relative to omega-3, use this oil sparingly.

- **Peanut oil:** Same recommendations as sesame oil, use sparingly.

Saturated Fats

Despite the vilification of saturated fats by the media and the mainstream health industry, just because an oil or fat is saturated does not automatically mean it's unhealthy. One of the most pervasive health myths is that all saturated fats are bad for you. Virtually every major study describing the dangers of saturated fats makes no effort to differentiate between saturated fats and trans-fats (or hydrogenated oils). The recent Strong Heart Study funded by the National Institutes of Health made no differentiation between saturated fats and trans-fats, using either or both interchangeably[94].

Saturated fats are actually necessary for your body and are nutritious additions to your diet in moderation. In fact, healthy saturated fats are the best choice for frying and other higher temperature cooking techniques. Some healthy saturated fat and cooking oil choices include:

- **Coconut oil:** This is the premier oil choice for cooking due to its good heat stability and numerous health benefits. This is a tropical oil that was commonly used for cooking prior to World War II and it is solid at room temperature. Coconut oil is full of healthy medium chain triglycerides (MCT's) and medium chain fatty acids (MCFA's), including lauric acid. The only other known high concentration of lauric acid is in breast milk. Coconut oil is also an antibacterial and antifungal oil. Lauric acid is one of the most potent antimicrobial lipids, making coconut oil a helpful immune system booster.

- **Palm oil:** This is another healthy tropical oil that's also stable at high temperature. Palm oil has a stronger flavor than coconut oil unless it has been clarified. Palm oil was the most common commercial frying oil before the saturated fat scare in the 1980s which forced manufacturers to abandon this safe oil in favor of hydrogenated oils. Be sure to look for brands that harvest the oil in a sustainable fashion to help reduce deforestation.

Trans-Fats and Hydrogenated Oils

Trans-fats are synthetic, chemically created saturated fats that were developed to increase the oil's shelf life. These unhealthy fats contribute to many chronic degenerative diseases, even though they are widely used by the food industry. Trans-fats are also called hydrogenated oils or *plastic fats*.

Trans-fats are made with high pressure and temperature in the presence of hydrogen, nickel catalysts, chemical emulsifiers, starch, and bleach. The resulting product is an unnatural saturated synthetic fat that has a long shelf life and won't go rancid, an ideal ingredient for use by the industrial food industry. In fact, the resulting chemical structure is almost the same as plastic. These trans-fats are common in a wide array of processed food products including margarine, shortening, baked goods, fast food, and most prepackaged foods.

The big problem with trans-fats is that the chemical changes that occur during the hydrogenation process make them toxic to your body. When you eat trans-fats, your digestive system treats them just like normal saturated fats and incorporates them into your body's cell walls, effectively wrapping your cells in a layer of plastic. Once these plastic fats are in place in your cells, they interfere with cell metabolism and cellular communication, resulting in a long list of health challenges.

The good reputation of natural saturated fats has been marred by their erroneous association with unnatural trans-fats. The take home message is this: avoid trans-fats and don't worry about saturated fat when used in moderation, especially fats from healthy, minimally processed, whole-food sources. Below are some fats and oils to avoid:

- **Trans-fats.** Avoid these fats completely. You'll generally find trans-fats listed on food labels, but be careful: trans-fat free or *0 gram trans-fat* products may still contain hydrogenated oils because of a loophole in the labeling laws. And be aware that canola oil contains trans-fats too.

- **Hydrogenated oils** (hydrogenated corn oil, hydrogenated soybean oil, hydrogenated safflower oil, hydrogenated safflower oil) are the same as trans-fats. Avoid them totally.

- **Partially hydrogenated oils** (partially hydrogenated corn oil, partially hydrogenated soybean oil, partially hydrogenated safflower oil, partially hydrogenated safflower oil). These are the same as hydrogenated oils, avoid them totally.

- **Vegetable oils** – minimize or avoid. They contain an excess of omega-6 with very little omega-3 (omega-6 and 3 should be in equal portions). Avoid the use of corn oil, soybean oil, safflower oil, sunflower oil and cottonseed oil if possible.

- **Canola oil:** Avoid this oil. This very popular and widely used oil contains trans-fats which are created as a byproduct of refining and heating the oil during it's manufacturing process. Most all canola oil is now genetically modified (GMO). Canola may also be linked to certain vitamin deficiencies and health problems.

U.S. Bans Trans-fats

In 2015 the FDA finalized a plan to phase out all trans-fats from U.S. foods. The ban's main purpose is to reduce fatal heart attacks that have been linked to these unnatural hydrogenated oils. While trans-fat information has been required on food labels since 2006, the ban will eliminate trans-fats from U.S. foods by 2018. While the ban is a step forward toward more healthy foods, many other potentially toxic and unhealthy ingredients are still allowed in the foods you eat. Therefore, it's still important to read the list of ingredients and know which ingredients to avoid as part of a healthy, immune-boosting diet.

Water, Water Everywhere

Water is the single most important nutrient. The vast majority of your body's weight is actually water. Of all the food recommendations in this chapter, staying properly hydrated is the easiest to do. Staying hydrated costs nothing and is crucial to your immune system, yet most people don't drink enough water for optimal health.

Nearly all of your body's functions and systems require water. Water carries nutrients to your cells, transports waste and toxins out of your body, maintains your body temperature, provides cushioning for joints and organs, and performs thousands of other vital functions. You lose water constantly throughout the day from sweating, breathing and eliminating waste. That's why staying hydrated is a continuous need throughout the day.

It's important to understand that *water means water*. While there's water in soda, coffee, tea, juice and many other drinks, these drinks are not meant to keep you hydrated. Enjoy a cup of coffee or a soda if you really must, but make the following distinction in your mind: most drinks are simply a treat, not a substitute for hydration throughout the day with pure water.

If you are not accustomed to drinking plain water and you find it unpalatable, you can improve the flavor and make it healthier with the following two suggestions:

- **Filter your water** to remove chlorine and odor-causing compounds found in some municipal water supplies. This will make a huge improvement in the taste and remove many toxins from the water. By the way, chlorine in your water kills both good and bad bacteria in your digestive system. Removing chlorine is a great way to boost your immune system.

- **Liven it up.** To spruce up the taste of your water, **add some fresh cut lemons or limes** or fresh lemon juice. You can also use a little natural unsweetened cranberry juice. These additions support your body's detoxification processes and also alkalize the water (see the section "pH Balance" on page 224 for details).

The easiest way to stay hydrated is to keep a water bottle at your side throughout the day, sipping it often. As a good rule of thumb, always drink water if you are thirsty. But don't wait until you are thirsty before you drink enough water. The guidelines below are a general rule of thumb on how much water to drink.

Circumstances	Quarts (liters) per day
Minimum for a healthy adult	2
Moderate exercise or hot or dry environment	3
Prolonged exercise, excessive sweating	4
Extreme exertion at high altitude or in desert	6 or more

Toxic Food Additives

The push to make foods taste better, last longer and survive the effects of food processing have led to the addition of many chemical additives to processed foods. Many of these additives are becoming widely recognized as being hazardous to your health. Many others have a long history of suggestive evidence linking them to numerous diseases and health problems. Anything that taxes your health will draw your body's resources away from your immune system.

Most safety studies required by the FDA before the approval of new food additives are relatively short in duration and focus on acute effects, or effects from high exposure levels over a short period of time. Long term safety studies to look at the chronic health effects at low levels over many years are lacking.

Fortunately, the vast majority of food additives are not added to fresh, whole natural foods. Artificial food additives appear mostly in processed foods, which require additives to create a long shelf life, to replace the beneficial components that are stripped away during processing, and to minimize costs and maximize profits. The following are food additives to avoid when possible:

- **Trans-fats (hydrogenated oils)** as described earlier in this chapter.

- **Aspartame, Equal, Splenda or NutraSweet** (aspartame) along with MSG, have been implicated in endocrine imbalance and act as excitotoxins in the brain, killing neural cells.

- **MSG** (monosodium glutamate, hydrolyzed vegetable protein) is rampant in fast foods and increases food addiction. It is sometimes called hydrolyzed vegetable protein and has excitotoxic effects in the brain, killing brain cells.

- **Carrageenan** (linked with digestive upset). Carrageenan is extracted from red seaweed and used as a food emulsifier. It's a common additive in dairy products such as milk, cheese, ice cream and yogurt, as well as baby formulas and some processed and canned foods. It's also common in non-dairy drinks like soy, rice, almond and coconut milks. Animal studies have repeatedly shown that carrageenan causes G.I. inflammation and higher rates of intestinal ulcerations.

- **BHA and BHT** are preservatives used in many oil-containing products to prevent rancidity. The World Health Organization lists BHA as a possible carcinogen and California lists it as a cancer causing agent. BHT has been implicated as a carcinogen in some studies.

- **Artificial colors.** Most synthetic dyes serve no purpose other than appearance. Many have been banned, and others have been linked to cancer and hyperactivity in children.

- **Sulfites** are used to keep vegetables and fruits looking fresh and to prevent fermentation and bacterial growth. The FDA has banned sulfites from use in many products due to numerous asthmatic fatalities. Sulfites are still approved for use in potatoes, wine and dried fruit.

- **Nitrite and Nitrate.** Nitrates are used to preserve processed meat products. When heated while cooking and then ingested, nitrates can form powerful cancer causing compounds in your body.

- **GMO foods and ingredients**. Genetically modified organisms, or GMO's, are now in the food supply in the USA and many other countries around the world. These foods have higher herbicide concentrations, are linked to cancer, organ damage, antibiotic resistance, and have also been found to cause stomach and gastrointestinal inflammation in animals. See more in the chapter "GMO Foods, Glyphosate & Immune System Stress" on page 259.

Spice Things Up with Herbs

Several popular herbs and spices used for cooking also have antibacterial and antioxidant activity and immune boosting properties. As a general rule, fresh and organic herbs and spices are healthier than generic dried herbs. For example, the antioxidant activity of fresh garlic is 1.5 times higher than dry garlic powder. Eating 3 cloves of freshly crushed garlic with your meals throughout the day is an excellent herbal remedy and preventative for infections.

Use the following high-antioxidant herbs and spices liberally as part of a balanced diet:

- Oregano
- Raw garlic
- Thyme
- Rosemary

- Turmeric
- Cloves
- Cinnamon
- Sage

- Basil
- Parsley
- Cayenne pepper
- Mustard (dried)

Some spices may irritate your stomach if you are not accustomed to them or if you eat a lot of them. So pay close attention when first using spices and start slowly. Discontinue use if they cause discomfort or an increase in infection symptoms. Below are a few words of caution about salt, a common flavor enhancer:

- Avoid regular *table salt*. It is unnatural, has been stripped of valuable minerals and nutrients and is often adulterated with silica and unhealthy sources of iodine.

- The best salt is natural sea salt. Sea salt has a complex mix of many minerals in natural ratios that are beneficial to your body. If you are concerned about heavy metals and modern day ocean toxins, consider sea salt from ancient land-based sources, such as Himalayan sea salt.

Antioxidants

A few years ago antioxidants were the big health rage and became a popular marketing focus for foods, supplements, superfood drinks and even personal care products. The antioxidant band-wagon made fruits like mangosteen and noni into household words. While there can be a lot of hype surrounding the topic of antioxidants, there are also some health and immune system benefits to using antioxidant foods and supplements prudently and in moderation.

Free radicals are produced in your body from normal metabolic processes, toxins you absorb from the environment, and even from some of the foods you eat. These free radicals are extremely reactive compounds that move throughout your body causing damage to your cell walls, DNA, proteins and just about anything else they come into contact with.

Your body uses antioxidants to neutralize these dangerous free radicals and keep them under control. Your body makes a number of different antioxidants, but the food you eat is another very important source of antioxidants. Antioxidants come in two main types: water-soluble and fat-soluble. Each type works best in different parts of your body and your cells. Also, each type of antioxidant neutralizes it's own unique type of toxin, so no single antioxidant can do it all.

ORAC Values

The Oxygen Radical Absorbance Capacity, or ORAC, is a measure of the antioxidant capacity of foods. ORAC values are used extensively in marketing materials for foods and supplements and for implying that one antioxidant is stronger than another. The ORAC test can be used to compare one antioxidant to another but the test has many limitations.

The ORAC test can only be used for water-soluble antioxidants. The test is standardized for laboratory uses and does not reflect how effective an antioxidant will be for a particular use inside the human body. For example, mangosteen may have a higher ORAC value than noni, however, noni can raise nitric oxide levels to combat inflammation and viruses whereas mangosteen does not effect nitric oxide levels. However, mangosteen produces different antioxidant effects, including immune system support, because it contains xanthones, which are not found in noni. Xanthones have been found to have the following qualities: antioxidant, anti-tumor, anti-inflammatory as well as antibacterial, antifungal, and anti-viral.

Therefore, ORAC values by themselves are of limited use outside of the laboratory. It's much more important to get a well-rounded mix of different antioxidants with different properties than to simply pick supplements with high ORAC values.

Helpful Antioxidants

The following is a list of helpful antioxidants to include in your diet. While the list is not complete, it's a good place to start. As you learn more about antioxidants, you can add to and subtract from the list of foods and supplements below to best fit your needs.

- **Raw berries.** Many common berries, especially blueberries and cranberries, have high ORAC values ranging from 1,000 to 2,400 per 100g. Berries are a great substitute for sugary desserts and they contain many beneficial nutrients, especially inside the skin of the berry.

- **Vegetables.** Many vegetables are high in antioxidants, especially if raw, fresh and unprocessed.

- **Vitamin C.** Also called ascorbic acid, this important water soluble antioxidant cannot be produced by your body and must be ingested in food or as supplements. This important vitamin is detailed in the section "Vitamin C" on page 169.

- **Vitamin E.** This fat-soluble antioxidant is also an important dietary component.

- **Dark chocolate.** With and ORAC of 13,000 per 100g, chocolate is the highest antioxidant common food. Chocolate in moderation is a very healthy addition to an immune-boosting diet. Because chocolate is bitter, it is usually sweetened with sugar. Therefore, it's best to limit chocolate to one ounce per day. Organic chocolate with a natural sugar source is best. Of course, if you are currently battling an infection, avoid chocolate and other sweets. And avoid unhealthy chocolate with artificial sweeteners, trans-fats, high fructose corn syrup, lard, waxes and unhealthy fillers.

- **Astaxanthin.** A very powerful red-colored fat-soluble antioxidant, astaxanthin has 400 times the antioxidant capacity of vitamin E. Astaxanthin is usually extracted from algae and is what gives wild salmon its red color (farmed salmon are colored using synthetic dyes). Many people take between 4 and 16 mg of astaxanthin per day with excellent results. Find astaxanthin extracted using a low temperature, non-chemical process such as supercritical CO_2 extraction, to ensure maximum antioxidant content and a safe product.

- **Turmeric.** This common eastern herb contains curcuminoids which are powerful phytonutrients with antioxidant properties. Turmeric also supports the gastrointestinal system and liver. Turmeric with Meriva is a patented processing method that makes the beneficial phytonutrients up to 10 times more easily absorbed by the body.

- **Green tea.** Green tea contains multiple antioxidants with cancer prevention properties, alzheimer's protection abilities and blood sugar regulation effects. Green tea can also support healthy brain cells and help prevent brain cell death. The benefits of green tea can be blocked by casein, a component in dairy products. Therefore, green tea should be enjoyed without dairy products.

Buying Healthy Foods

Once you start shopping for truly healthy foods, you'll soon discover that refined sugars, transfats, artificial sweeteners and other toxins are listed on the vast majority of packaged food labels. In fact, it can be difficult to find foods that don't have these unhealthy ingredients in them. That's why it's important to pay close attention to food labels on every item you buy. With a little practice, you'll quickly learn to identify the good and the bad ingredients on any food label.

Read food labels carefully, especially the list of ingredients!

Where can you find foods without all the unhealthy ingredients? Many grocery stores now have natural or organic sections which stock products containing healthier options. Natural food stores can provide even more healthy choices and selections. But still be careful. You still have to read food labels, even inside the health food store. Remember that the words *healthy* and *natural* are used for marketing purposes only and that legally they don't mean anything. Any number of unhealthy ingredients can be added to foods with healthy and natural on the label.

There are no regulations that govern what the words *healthy* or *natural* mean on food labels

The word *organic* is regulated in its usage. However, even organic foods can contain unhealthy ingredients. The bottom line is that no matter where you shop, read food labels carefully and follow the suggestions in this chapter on what to look for and what to avoid.

20 Green Smoothies

You've probably heard that greens are good for you. A key benefit of eating greens is the enhancing effect on your immune system. This is because greens are high in vitamins and minerals, protein, fiber and they are highly alkaline. In fact, more than any other addition to her diet, Michelle Moore achieved the greatest benefit to her heath, vitality and immunity by adding green smoothies.

Green smoothies are a new way to eat greens without the bitter taste and unpleasant texture that many people find unappetizing. Blending greens, bananas and other fruit together provides a satisfying and nutritious meal. Unlike eating cooked greens, this method unlocks the immune-supporting nutrients inside the greens and makes them readily available to your body. On top of that, green smoothies can be a delicious start to you day.

Calorie for calorie, greens are the most concentrated source of nutrition of any common food

3 Green Misconceptions

1. **Greens are vegetables.** Greens are in their own food group and they are not vegetables at all. Greens (aka *leafy greens* or *vegetable greens*) include kale, Swiss chard, collard greens, spinach, mustard greens, arugula, lettuce and other green leafy plants. The vegetable group includes root vegetables (like beets, carrots, turnips etc.), flowers (broccoli, cauliflower, etc.) and non-sweet fruit (tomato, cucumber, etc.).

2. **Greens aren't nutritionally important.** Greens are actually the only food group that most completely matches the nutritional needs of humans. But most diet plans and food pyramids hardly mention greens. Even vegetarian and raw food diets give little attention to greens.

3. **Greens are unpalatable.** Surprisingly, greens can be enjoyed without cooking them or eating the well known yet unpopular recipes they are known for. As you'll see below, there is a more nutritious and better tasting way to enjoy the health benefits of greens.

The Health Benefits of Greens

Greens are nutritional powerhouses that supercharge your immunity. Below are some of the amazing health benefits that adding more greens to your diet can bring:

- **Lean, mean protein.** Contrary to popular belief, greens are one of the best sources of protein available. Amino acids are the building blocks of proteins, and they are abundant in greens. In fact, eating a variety of greens in your diet will cover all of your essential amino acids in abundance.

  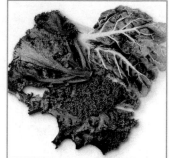

  Greens are the food group that most completely matches the nutritional needs of humans.

  » For example, one pound of kale contains similar or larger amounts of protein and essential amino acids than the Recommended Daily Allowance (RDA). Because greens contain all the amino acids you need, it's much easier for your body to build proteins by using these basic raw materials.

  » In contrast, the complex proteins found in meat and animal products are harder to break down into amino acids and harder to digest, which can actually contribute to food allergies, immunological disorders and other health problems.

- **Fabulous fiber.** The abundant insoluble fiber found in green leafy plants is critical for your body's waste and toxin removal system. Insoluble fiber acts like a sponge that can absorb many times its own weight in toxins making it supportive for your body's detoxification processes.

- **Packed with vitamins, minerals and antioxidants.** Greens are rich in vitamins, including vitamin K, E, A, C, and B vitamins. Greens also contain a wide variety of minerals and important phytonutrients.

  » Calorie for calorie, greens are the most potent source of nutrition of any common food.

  » The greens of plants usually have much higher vitamin and mineral contents than the roots. Carrot top greens, for example, have several times more nutrition than carrot roots, yet the tops are usually thrown away.

  » Each type of green has its own unique nutritional profile. If a nutrient is low in one type of green, it is usually abundant in another. Therefore, consuming a variety of greens is the best way to maximize the nutritional benefits.

- **Superior nutrient absorption.** The most unique advantage of green smoothies is their ability to supercharge your nutrient absorption. Even people with digestive challenges can absorb surprising amounts of key nutrients. The key to superior absorption is to break up of the raw greens during the blending process, as you'll read more about below.

- **Enzymes to ease digestion.** Unlike vegetables, which can cause fermentation and gas if eaten with fruits, greens actually aid digestion by stimulating your body to secrete digestive enzymes. Greens can be successfully combined with any other food, including fruit.

- **Infection fighting immunity.** It you take a look at any acid-alkaline food chart, you'll see greens are one of the most alkaline of all foods. Raising your body's pH by eating an alkaline diet is one of the best ways to support your natural immunity, raise your energy levels and support the beneficial bacteria in your gut. So adding more greens to your diet will do more than elevate your nutrition. Greens can also boost your immune health, speed your body's healing response and ramp up your resistance to infection.

The Most Nutritious Greens

Organic foods are always best, and the same is true for greens. Organic greens have the highest nutrient content and lowest level of toxins like pesticides. Fresh non-wilting greens are much more nutritious than greens that are past their prime. Growing your own greens or buying locally is the best way to ensure freshness and maximize nutrients.

Raw greens are always best as the cooking process breaks down and destroys nutrients. The higher the cooking temperature, the more nutrients are lost. That being said, low temperature cooking like steaming preserves much of the nutrition in greens. Adding greens to soup or stews toward the end of cooking is another great way to preserve more nutrition. While eating greens uncooked is more nutritious than cooked greens, enjoying a green smoothie provides even more nutrition and they taste great too.

The Green Smoothie Superfood

Green shakes and raw juices require less energy from the body to be digested. The superior nutrition of smoothies also gives your body more energy and resources to help heal and fight off an infection. But to get the most benefit from greens, a key challenge must first be overcome in order to unlock their full nutritional value.

The Biggest Challenge With Greens

Leafy greens are made up of tiny plant cells that are made of cellulose, a hardy and difficult material for your digestive system to break apart. This tough cellulose wall has to be ruptured in order to get the nutrients out so they can be digested. While you rupture some of the cellulose cell walls when you chew greens, the majority are left intact, locking in the nutrients so your body cannot digest and absorb them.

Getting all the nutrients from greens is even more difficult because most people have weak chewing muscles and chronically low stomach acid from eating processed foods. The combination of tough cellulose cell walls, reduced ability to chew and low stomach acid means that most of the nutrients inside normally-prepared greens are never absorbed by your body.

Squeezing More Nutrition Out of Greens

The key is to blend the greens so that the cellulose walls get broken apart and all those beneficial nutrients get squeezed out. While blending ruptures the cellulose cell wall, it leaves all of the cellular nutrients intact and readily available, making them much easier for your body to digest.

The best way to enjoy blended greens is to add some banana and other fruit together with the greens to create a smoothie. This combination of greens and fruit creates the perfect balance of taste: not too sweet, not too bitter, with the pleasant smell and taste of freshness.

It's important to use a powerful blender to break the greens into very small particles (less than a millimeter). High power blenders specially designed for making smoothies work best. An ultra-high speed blender called a Vitamix is ideal for making smoothies and is worth every penny it costs. A Vitamix produces the smoothest, tastiest

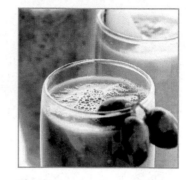

Blending greens into a delicious smoothie unlocks the full nutritional benefits of the greens.

and most nutritious smoothies, plus they are easy to clean and can last for decades. The Vitamix blades actually come dull as the motor blends so fast, sharp blades aren't even necessary. You can get acceptable results with other blender brands such as Cuisinart, so long as the blades are kept sharp and you finish blending with the highest speed setting.

Detox Precaution

Green smoothies provide many times more nutrients than simply eating raw greens. Because smoothies are such a powerful source of nutrition, it's important to start out slow and give your body time to adjust. If you begin eating too many greens too often, the bacteria in your gut can produce extra gas until they get used to the changes. Your body may also begin to detoxify by releasing long-held toxins when you begin getting better nutrition (see "Healing Crisis and Detoxification Support" on page 217 for details). Feeling tired or having a headache after beginning to drink smoothies is a sign that your body is starting to clean house and detoxify. So start out with a small green smoothie each day or every other day. After a few weeks, slowly increase the size or frequency if you like.

Don't Forget to Chew

An important part of the entire digestion process actually occurs in your mouth. The act of chewing releases enzymes that start the breakdown of food inside your mouth. Chewing also sends chemical signals to your stomach to produce more acid and to get ready to digest the incoming food further. Without these chemical signals and enzymes, your body cannot properly digest your food, leading to poor nutrient absorption and unhealthy fermentation in your stomach.

Because green smoothies are liquid and they don't require chewing, drinking smoothies by themselves can cause incomplete digestion, gas, bloating and reduced nutrient absorption. The best way to avoid these problems is to eat something crunchy or chewy right before or when drinking a green smoothie. Eating a few crackers or apple wedges will help get the digestion process started and minimize the chances of unpleasant gas and bloating.

Delicious Smoothie Recipes

To learn more about green nutrition and green smoothies, including many health testimonials, recipes and green smoothie case studies, the book Green For Life[95] is highly recommended. Also, see "Green Smoothie Recipes" on page 309 for some simple, great tasting recipes.

21 GMO Foods, Glyphosate & Immune System Stress

Genetically modified foods have been widely touted as the foods of the future, and foods that will feed the world. Short for Genetically Modified Organisms, GMO (or GM) foods have been prominent in the media and in recent political battles.

Genetically modified foods have potential health risks, both direct and indirect, that you may not be aware of. Because the majority of your immune health is dictated by the health of your gut, anything that damages your GI system and gut bacteria is a barrier to healing from infections.

You are probably eating GMO foods and don't even realize it. Dr. Oz reported that more than 80 percent of the foods Americans eat every day contain one or more types of GM foods[96]. Some types of GM foods are the result of unnatural genetic modification, where the food is designed to tolerate the herbicide glyphosate. Unfortunately, GM foods are housed in secrecy and the food companies who own them won't allow any independent studies. However, animal studies performed using GM foods are producing results that are extremely concerning.

"Several animal studies indicate serious health risks associated with GM food."
- The American Academy of Environmental Medicine

Aside from major health effects like cancer, kidney and liver damage, animal studies have found an increased incidence of stomach and intestinal tract inflammation from ingesting GM foods and the herbicide glyphosate. Other studies show glyphosate encourages the growth of disease-causing bacteria in the gut. GM foods are also linked to an increase in antibiotic resistance. In March 2015, the herbicide glyphosate was classified as "probably carcinogenic to humans" by the International Agency for Research on Cancer, an agency of the World Health Organization[97].

There are enough studies and scientific evidence to raise major red flags about the safety and environmental effects of growing GMO crops and eating GM foods with glyphosate residues. Unfortunately, there is heavy resistance to evidence supporting the dangers of GMOs in government, media and industry circles.

Science, Politics and Profits

GMOs are big business. And where the money flows, politics usually follows. As with many things backed by a lot of money and political pressure, studies and other scientific information that call GMO safety into question faces an uphill battle to be taken seriously by the media, the public and ultimate by policy makers.

While there are many studies showing the negative consequences of GMOs, you can also find studies that back the safety and nutritional benefits of GMOs, usually funded by groups with a vested interest in GMOs.

One of the challenges with pinning down GMO health risks is how long-term the risks are. Unlike poisons the cause harm immediately, the health risks of GMOs, including cancer, organ damage and premature aging, accumulate over many years and are not noticeable right away[98]. This makes real-time human studies to gauge the health risks very challenging to perform. Unfortunately, one of the biggest holes in the Food and Drug Administration's approval process is long-term chronic side effects.

The Risks and Dangers of GM foods

Below is a list of concerning facts and potential risks of GM foods and farming practices.

- GMO's are artificially made in a laboratory using methods that are either impossible to duplicate in natural breeding and hybridization, or that would require long periods of time.

- GMO's can be less nutritious than natural varieties of the same food.

- Despite claims to the contrary, GMO's actually promote the use of more harmful pesticides rather than reduce their use.

- GMO growing practices do not improve crop yield, despite claims to the contrary.

- GMO's and their growing practices contribute to *superweeds* that are resistant to herbicides. This is very similar to the problem of antibiotic resistance that is rendering antibiotic drugs ineffective.

- Common growing practices used with GM crops contribute to reduced biodiversity, low soil nutrient quality and food contamination with herbicides and insecticides.

- GMO's are increasingly contaminating natural, non-GM crops and have negative economic consequences, especially for small farms and organic farms.

- Despite claims of reducing world hunger, GMO's fail to address the root cause of world hunger, including loss of irrigable land, poverty and poor food supply infrastructure in third world countries.

- According to many GMO opponents, GMO's are not properly tested or regulated to ensure they are safe for people or the environment, especially after many years of exposure. To date, there have been no long-term safety studies conducted on GMO foods and humans.

- GMOs and their growing practices have been linked to many negative health issues, including: cancer, organ damage, allergies, antibiotic resistance, autism and premature aging.

- Farmers across the world are reporting thousands of sick, sterile and dead livestock related to eating GM feed[99,100].

- The common herbicidal ingredients used to grow GM foods (glyphosate) disrupts intestinal flora and promotes the growth of disease-causing bacteria in the gut (see the section "Glyphosate Promotes Pathogenic Gut Bacteria" on page 263).

- The European Union (EU) does not allow GM foods to be imported and they require GM foods to be labeled.

- At least 60 countries ban or require the labeling of GM foods, including Australia, France, Japan, Italy, Russia and China[101].

- The Department of Agriculture (USDA) and the FDA do not require GMO foods to be labeled in the United States.

- A long term study performed with pigs (which have similar digestive tracts to humans and serve as a good model for people), showed severe stomach inflammation in animals fed GM corn and soy during their normal life span, as compared to pigs who ate a diet of non-GM corn and soy[102]. While one could argue that it may be something to do with eating GM foods and not glyphosate, these GM foods were sprayed with glyphosate.

The Most Common GM Foods

Below is a list of the most common GM foods on the U.S. market today. Keep in mind the certified organic versions of these foods are free of GM genes and ingredients[103].

- Corn
- Sugar beets (sugar)
- Margarine
- Baking powder
- Peanut butter
- Corn meal
- Soy protein

- Canola
- Tofu
- Mayonnaise
- Vanilla extract
- Tomato sauce
- Corn syrup
- Soy cheese

- Soybeans
- Cereal
- Salad dressings
- Powdered sugar
- Tamari
- Soy flour
- Soy sauce

- Soy lecithin (emulsifier)
- Maltodextrin
- Protein powders
- Ice cream & frozen yogurt

- Fructose
- Veggie burgers
- Zucchini squash
- Hamburger & hot dog buns

- Dextrose
- Enriched flour
- Instant infant formula
- Chocolate

How to Avoid GM Foods

The following tips will help you reduce your exposure to GM foods.

1. Eat organic foods. Keep in mind that while organic foods are certified to contain no GMO genes, it's possible for cross-pollination between GMO and non-GMO plants to occur. You can also ask local vendors about their growing practices at your farmers market.

2. Minimize meat, eggs and diary because non-organic livestock may eat GM crops. Organically produced livestock are fed non-GM feeds.

3. Avoid processed foods and the most common GM foods listed above. Processed foods often contain canola oil and many other GM ingredients.

4. Avoid cooking with GMO oils like canola, corn and soy.

5. Look for the Non GMO Project Verified label for foods that are free from GMOs.

Glyphosate Herbicide and G.I. Disruption

While it's likely you've heard of the popular weed killer called *Roundup®* you probably don't know about its active ingredient glyphosate. Besides killing weeds, glyphosate is also a strong antibacterial and has been linked to killing beneficial gut bacteria and causing gut inflammation, as detailed later in this chapter.

Roundup herbicide is being used at an ever increasing rate around the world since its introduction in the 1970's. Roundup's claim to fame is that it's supposed to be safe and non-toxic to people. Thus, Roundup has been used to kill weeds and grasses for many years. More recently, it's been sprayed on GM food crops. These so-called *Roundup Ready®* crops were genetically modified and designed to withstand exposure to the Roundup herbicide. This allows a farmer to spray an entire crop, with only the weeds being killed.

A new independent review which examined more than 300 different studies performed on glyphosate was released in 2013[104]. This review revealed that this weed killer may be linked to many health issues, including birth defects, miscarriages, vitamin and mineral deficiencies, cancer, disruption of gut flora and inflammation of the digestive tract. It also shows a correlation between increasing use of glyphosate and infections.

Finding The Truth

So why do the makers of Roundup say it's safe if so many studies show otherwise? Before a product is released for public use, short-term animal studies are often performed by the manufacturer to demonstrate if a product is toxic or not. However, the review mentioned above was independent and not performed by the manufacturer. The review in question also includes long term studies which indicate many types of problems with glyphosate exposure that were not apparent in short-term trials performed by the maker of the product.

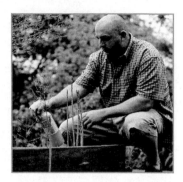

According to review authors Anthony Samsel and Stephanie Seneff Ph.D., a research scientist at MIT, *"glyphosate is likely to be pervasive in the food supply, and, contrary to being essentially nontoxic, it may in fact be the most biologically disruptive chemical in the environment"* and that the *"negative impact on the body is insidious and manifests slowly over time as inflammation damages cellular systems throughout the body."*

Weed killers have been implicated in promoting inflammatory bowel diseases.

Glyphosate Promotes Pathogenic Gut Bacteria

As mentioned in the chapter "Probiotics: The Good Bacteria" on page 209, scientists agree that several pounds of bacteria reside in the gut and make up 70-80% of a person's immune system function. Alarmingly, mounting evidence is showing that glyphosate is altering the normal flora in animals. Not only does it kill beneficial gut bacteria, it also promotes the growth of pathogenic types of bacteria.

A study on poultry gut flora has confirmed glyphosate is toxic to beneficial gut bacteria including Enterococcus, Bacillus and Lactobacillus species[105]. This study shows that the friendly bacteria are the most susceptible to glyphosate, however, disease-causing bacteria are very resistant to glyphosate. When the healthy gut flora are killed, disease-causing flora can overgrow, leaving the door open for overgrowth and gut infections.

Over the last 10 to 15 years, an increase in *Clostridium botulinim* associated with cattle diseases has been seen in Germany. As in poultry, healthy gut flora helps prevent Clostridium overgrowth in cattle because healthy bacteria like Lactobacillus and Enterococcus species produce toxins that inhibit these pathogens. This is part of Nature's checks and balances. The German study also reported that glyphosate disrupted healthy Enterococcus gut bacteria in cattle. The study proposes that glyphosate is a significant factor in the rise of Clostridium infections in cattle[106].

The makers of Roundup assert that glyphosate is nontoxic to mammals, based on a few short-term animal feeding studies, and that it's therefore not a problem for people either. Because GM crops are widely consumed by people in the U.S., there is a great need for long-term studies performed on humans eating GM foods (which contain glyphosate residues). However, such studies have never been performed.

Is Glyphosate an Antibiotic?

With the emergence of animal studies demonstrating disrupted gut flora with glyphosate ingestion, it's easy to deduce that glyphosate is acting like an antibiotic (a substance that inhibits or kills bacteria). However, herbicide industry spokesmen and Monsanto, the maker of Roundup, have denied that glyphosate acts as an antimicrobial, and that it's only an herbicide. However, recent evidence indicates otherwise.

In 2010, Monsanto applied for a patent for using glyphosate as an antimicrobial agent[107]. This patent describes the use of glyphosate against pathogenic infections through a process of microbial enzymatic inhibition. Since Monsanto is claiming glyphosate can inhibit microorganisms, they are in essence saying that glyphosate is an antibiotic. Because of this patent, it's obvious Monsanto is aware of its antibacterial properties.

In summary, glyphosate acts as an antibacterial agent (or antibiotic if you prefer) and it is sprayed on the majority of GM food crops that both animals and people eat. When ingested, this compound can cause an overgrowth of pathogenic strains of Salmonella and Clostridium in animals, and a depression of immune supporting bacteria. With rates of inflammatory bowel disease doubling in people in recent years, gut infection rates rising, and new long term glyphosate animal studies showing similar trends, it appears that the *smoking gun* has been found to what's behind this rise in inflammatory bowel diseases.

Where is Glyphosate Used?

If you're not using Roundup (which contains glyphosate) on your weeds around your house, your neighbor probably is. It's used for grass and weed control along the edges of highways, on railroad tracks, on school playgrounds, on sidewalks, on roads and in parks. This herbicide is also used by farmers around non-organic fruit trees and non-organic fruit and vegetable crops.

Roundup is also sprayed on *roundup ready* crops which are genetically modified to withstand direct exposure to the herbicide. Animals and people consume these crops which include: corn, soybeans, canola, sugar beets and cotton. Glyphosate can enter the human body by either consumption of the GM foods that are sprayed with it, or by direct absorption through the skin if you are near where the product is being used. With such rampant use of glyphosate herbicides, glyphosate has also been found in drinking water[108].

Can You Remove Glyphosate From Foods?

The bottom line is: you can't. Glyphosate cannot be simply washed off of the plants it is sprayed on. After being sprayed on genetically modified plants, the plants pull the glyphosate from both the leaves and the soil, so glyphosate is inside of the plant. When you eat the plant, you eat the glyphosate as well.

Glyphosate residues are now found in many everyday foods. However the foods you should be most concerned with include sugar (sugar beets), corn (including fructose, corn syrup and high fructose corn syrup), soybeans or soy, canola oil and wheat. However, these foods may not be labeled that they contain GM ingredients, glyphosate or pesticide residues.

Recently, several state level initiatives to label GM foods have been initiated, but most have not yet passed. Vermont was the first state to pass an unrestricted mandatory labeling bill for GM foods, and hopefully other states will pass similar bills. While the majority of people in the USA support the labeling of GM foods, such initiatives have failed due to heavy funding against them by chemical companies and large scale food producers.

What Can You Do?

There are several steps you can take to minimize your glyphosate intake and exposure:

- Don't use Roundup or other herbicides containing glyphosate. You can pull weeds or use non-toxic alternatives.

- Talk to your school, church, and city about not using Roundup or glyphosate in public places (or anywhere).

- Eat organic foods. Roundup and other chemical fertilizers are banned for use in or around organic agriculture.

- Demand GMO labeling in your state and at your local stores. GMO foods are built to tolerate being sprayed with Roundup or other chemicals. If food products are labeled, it will help you make educated and informed choices about what you eat.

- Eat whole foods and less processed foods. Most GMO foods that are sprayed with Roundup are processed foods that use corn, soy, sugar, canola oil and wheat. These ingredients make up about 80% of processed foods (foods that are packaged or boxed). Eat more whole foods and organic foods to help reduce your exposure to this antibacterial agent.

- While it's unknown if you can detox from glyphosate, research has shown that eating an all organic diet reduces pesticides levels in the body[109].

- According to the EPA, activated carbon used in water filters can help remove glyphosate from water supplies and according to the ASCE, both chlorine and ozone treatments will destroy glyphosate[110].

What Are Your Glyphosate Levels?

In 2014, Mom's Across America discovered high levels of glyphosate in human breast milk and urine in American test subjects as compared to levels found in people living in the EU. What was alarming about the results was that the majority of people who submitted samples had been trying to avoid GMO foods and glyphosate exposure for some time.

Drinking water samples tested were also found to contain glyphosate. A validated test method was created in order for the general public to test their breast milk, urine or drinking water samples for the presence of glyphosate. Getting the testing done can be especially important if you have a chronic health issue or if you have young children. Testing details can be found at the following website:

http://feedtheworld.info/glyphosate-testing-test-yourself/

More Info

The Institute for Responsible Technology is a world leader in educating policy makers and the public about genetically modified (GM) foods and crops. Find out more here:

www.responsibletechnology.org/gmo-education

The Weston Price foundation has a nice article on the many health effects related to glyphosate. The article's name is *Roundup: "Nontoxic" Chemical that May Be Destroying your Health* and it can be found online here:

www.westonaprice.org/environmental-toxins/roundup-the-nontoxic-chemical-that-may-be-destroying-our-health.

The Non GMO Project is a leader in the field of GMO education and has taken the lead in the labeling and verifying non-GMO food products:

www.nongmoproject.org

22 Hand Washing and Hygiene

Human life is intricately linked with microorganisms, and nobody can live without them. Beneficial or *good* bacteria live on your skin, inside your body and in every environment on earth. They are crucial to the proper functioning of your immune system, and they defend your gut and your skin against pathogenic or disease-causing microorganisms.

Whether you want to prevent getting infected or you're infected and want to minimize spreading your infection, proper hygiene is very important. The goal of hand washing and hygiene is to control just the *bad* bacteria and leave the *good* protective microorganisms alone. With the prevalent mindset that all bacteria are dangerous and the over-abundance of antibacterial soaps and products available to kill bacteria, achieving this balance can be a challenge. However, the methods and protocols in this chapter can help you make healthy, effective and balanced hygiene decisions.

Hygiene and How MRSA and Staph are Spread

In order to have the most effective hygiene practices, it's important that you know how easy and common it is for bacteria, viruses and other infectious pathogens to pass from person to person. Most people outside the microbiology profession have little or no idea of just how easy it is to unknowingly spread bacteria like Staph and MRSA to other people.

The following example illustrates one easy way that people spread germs through simple day-to-day activities. Consider that many people do not wash their hands properly after using the bathroom. When they exit the bathroom, they leave bacteria behind on the door handle. You use the same bathroom, wash your hands and touch the handle on the way out. If you later prepare and eat dinner without washing your hands first, you've likely just ingested some of the germs from that bathroom door knob. Even if you simply touch your mouth, scratch your nose, apply makeup, or scratch at a cut, you can contaminate yourself in the same way. You can easily imagine many other scenarios that would result in contaminating yourself with infectious germs. If you really pay attention, these kinds of scenarios happen many times every day.

Staph and MRSA live on many people and are likely present on any high-touch surfaces. Examples include doors and door knobs, elevator buttons, kitchen surfaces and faucets, exercise equipment, phones, remote controls and keyboards. MRSA and Staph bacteria can also hang out on clothing and even on skin particles in the air. Refer to the chapter "Symptoms, Risk Factors and Carriers" on page 27 for more specific details on how MRSA and Staph spread.

The key to proper hygiene is awareness. Once you know how MRSA and Staph are spread, it's easy to make better hygiene choices by adopting simple practices and precautions to control and minimize the risks.

The Pros and Cons of Hygienic Practices

The use of bleach, chlorhexidine washes and antimicrobial soaps remove good bacteria from your skin that are necessary to ward off disease-causing bacteria. The widespread and uneducated use of toxic chemicals and antibacterial products has been counter-productive to everyone's health. These products indiscriminately kill the good bacteria and put a toxic burden on your body which suppresses your natural immunity.

The media and manufacturers of antibacterial cleaning products have done their best to get people to believe that all bacteria must be killed. Remember, this is not an all-out war on bacteria. Everyone relies on their own personal microbiome for their very survival.

Don't Overdo It

Many people are actually too fastidious about hand washing. For others, their job requires constant hand washing, like those in the healthcare arena. Too much hand washing destroys the natural oils that help defend your skin against infection. This will cause the fatty acids in the skin to become depleted, which leaves you susceptible to skin cracks, open wounds and sores.

These small openings in your skin actually increase your risk of getting a MRSA or Staph skin infection. So, wash your hands, but don't go overboard. If you have to wash your hands frequently or if you suffer from dry skin, moisturizers and lotions will help reduce skin cracking. If possible, use a mild, natural soap when frequent washing is required.

The Limitations of Hand Sanitizers

Hand sanitizers have become quite popular as a substitute for hand washing, both in hospitals and for personal home use. The reasons for this popularity are understandable. Hand sanitizers are fast, convenient, easier to use, don't require sinks or running water, and they can reduce the amount of many common bacteria on your hands. However, as helpful as hand sanitizers are, they are not a substitute for hand washing, especially for MRSA protection.

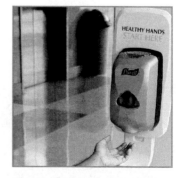

Hand sanitizers provide only partial protection, but they are fast and convenient and don't require a sink or water.

The big drawback of hand sanitizers is that they do not physically remove bacteria from your hands like soap and water do. Sanitizers work by killing some of the bacteria on your hands, but MRSA and other germs will not be completely killed. Also, hand sanitizers aren't effective against *C. difficile* because alcohol can't kill the spore form of this bacteria.

In contrast, properly washing your hands with soap and water actually removes bacteria and germs from your hands. This is why hand washing is very important for controlling Staph and MRSA. Hand sanitizers are still helpful for moderate protection, but they are not a substitute for soap and water.

Best Practices for Hand Sanitizers

If you are going to use an alcohol-based hand sanitizer, look for the following for the best sanitizer and use practices [111]:

- Alcohol based sanitizers should have 60-95% alcohol for best effectiveness against harmful bacteria and viruses. Many sanitizers on the market are actually made with less than 60% alcohol and theses will not provide effective sanitizing properties.

- After rubbing the sanitizer on your hands, don't wipe it off. Allow it to air dry on its own for best effectiveness.

- If your hands are heavily soiled or greasy, hand sanitizers will not work well. Instead use soap and water.

- Washing with natural soap and water should always be your first choice.

The Dangers of Antimicrobial Soaps

Have you been told to use antimicrobial soaps or chlorhexidine body washes for controlling infections? If so, you are not alone. You may be surprised to learn that antimicrobial soaps can actually cause more harm than good.

Antimicrobial agents are added to soaps and cleansers to reduce all of those bad germs in your home. The most common antimicrobial agent used is triclosan, which kills or inhibits the growth of bacteria and was introduced into personal and household products in 1995.

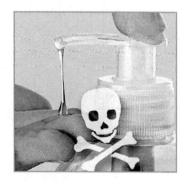

Plain soap and water are non-toxic, unlike antibacterial soap.

A surprising 76% of all liquid soaps sold in the United States now contain antimicrobial ingredients (close to 30% for bar soaps). These antimicrobial agents are in products ranging from toothpaste, mouthwash, lotions, shampoos, baby care products, clothing and even plastic toys.

Triclosan

One recent study has shown that dish soap with triclosan, when combined with normal tap water containing chlorine (typically found in city water), can form significant amounts of chloroform. The EPA has labeled chloroform as a probable human carcinogen (cancer causing substance).

Amazingly, triclosan not only kills bacteria, it also kills human cells, according to a European dental study. And new research shows that another active ingredient in antimicrobial soaps and personal care products called MIT, or methylisothiazolinone, may cause nerve damage.

Triclosan has been linked to causing endocrine disruption in people. It's been shown to decrease thyroid hormones which could lead to infertility. It also can act as an estrogen mimicking chemical and can help promote breast cancer[112] It's also linked to numerous environmental issues.

What the Experts Say

Since 2000, the American Medical Association (AMA) has questioned the use of antimicrobial agents in soaps and cleaners and has been advising the Food and Drug Administration (FDA) to monitor and possibly regulate the home use of such products.

Myron Genel, chairman of the AMA's Council on Scientific Affairs and a Yale University pediatrician has stated that there's no evidence thus far showing antimicrobial cleaners actually help and that there is reason to suspect they can create antibiotic-resistant bacteria. It appears the AMA's concerns about triclosan and other antimicrobial soap agents are justified:

- A study published in the Annals of Internal Medicine showed no better results for antimicrobial cleaners in keeping people healthy. The study evaluated both antimicrobial and non-antimicrobial products that were used in homes for almost one year. The study showed no significant difference in disease symptoms between people who used antimicrobial products and people who did not.

- The AMA's Myron Genel stated that the use of these products may contribute to the well-recognized problem created by excessive use of antibiotics that has led to mutated bacterial strains that are resistant to drugs.

- Microbiologist Dr. Stuart Levy of Tufts University has warned that these antibacterial agents could promote the creation of superbugs, whereas hand washing with regular soap can keep these bacteria in check. Dr. Levy also indicated that using antibacterial soaps upsets the natural balance of microorganisms, leaving behind only the superbugs.

Asthma and Allergies in Children

Recent studies have pointed to the fact that growing up in a so-called *sterile environment* may contribute to the development of allergies and asthma. The vast majority of the bacteria and viruses that kids are exposed to are completely safe and non-pathogenic and may in fact be quite beneficial. Exposure to many different bacteria, viruses, fungi, and other microbes is critical to the proper development of a child's immune system. This is another reason why being a *germ-o-phobe* and trying to create a germ-free environment inside your home is not the best idea.

FDA Warns of Antibacterial Soap Safety

Because of new data that suggests safety and health risks with long term use of antibacterial soaps, the FDA and EPA are now reviewing data on antibacterial soap ingredients.

According to Colleen Rogers, Ph.D., a microbiologist at the FDA, *"there currently is no evidence that over-the-counter antibacterial soap products are any more effective at preventing illness than washing with plain soap and water. Moreover, antibacterial soap products contain chemical ingredients, such as triclosan and triclocarban, which may carry unnecessary risks given that their benefits are unproven.*[113]*"*

As of December 2013, the FDA has required soap manufacturers to prove that antibacterial chemicals are safe, effective, and superior to non-antibacterial soaps in preventing or reducing infections, or else they won't be allowed to market these products. Many other countries are ahead of the United States and FDA when it comes to these risky ingredients. Because of human health and antimicrobial resistance concerns, triclosan has already been banned or restricted in other countries, including the European Union.

Antimicrobial Soaps: The Bottom Line

For your optimal health and minimizing the possibility of antibacterial resistance, stop using antimicrobial personal care products as soon as possible because they:

- Have not been shown to reduce disease symptoms.

- Can produce significant amounts of the carcinogen chloroform when used to wash your hands or dishes with normal city tap water.

- Have been shown to kill human cells.

- Can contribute to allergies and asthma and suppress the immune system.

- Likely contribute to the problem of antibiotic resistance.

- May be causing nerve damage.

- Can cause dermatitis with repeated usage, toxicity with middle ear contact and corneal damage after eye contact (Chlorhexidine washes).

- Decrease your body's good bacteria that aid in your immunity and your natural defenses.

- Are linked to hormonal disruption in people.

Use of antimicrobial soaps, shampoos, toothpastes and mouthwashes can aggravate infections and make your body more prone to new infections. Fortunately, there are better, healthier and more effective ways to control bacteria on your hands, as described below.

Best Hand Washing Practices

Below are three *best practices* for washing your hands and other parts of your body:

1. **Read product labels carefully** and avoid soaps with synthetic antimicrobial agents. Avoid the following:

   » Triclosan

   » Triclocarban

   » Methylisothiazolinone (MIT)

   » Chloroxylenol (PCMX)

   » Chlorhexidine gluconate (CHG)

2. Wash with **regular soap and warm water**. Scrubbing with soap kills or removes germs.

   » Scrub hands briskly for at least 15 to 30 seconds, rubbing soapy water to the front and back of your hands, between the fingers and under the nails. If someone in your house has MRSA or Staph, have them use a separate towel.

   » When away from home, grab a paper towel immediately after you finish washing your hands before turning off the faucet or touching anything. After drying your hands, use a paper towel to turn off the water and to open the bathroom door.

   » Carry a small bottle of a natural hand sanitizer when you don't have access to soap and water. Natural products are a better alternative to alcohol based sanitizers. Many are actually made with antibacterial oils such as thyme oil.

3. For soaps with extra germ killing capacity you can:

   » Purchase natural or organic liquid soaps with essential oils, such as tea tree oil, which is naturally antibacterial.

   » Create your own safe and natural hand and body soaps and sanitizing sprays using your own therapeutic quality essential oils. See the following section for some simple recipes.

Sanitizer and Personal Care Recipes

You can easily create your own hand sanitizer and increase the bacterial control of your soaps, shampoos, body washes and other personal care products with a few simple ingredients. The sanitizer and personal care recipes below will help you control bacteria without the toxicity and health drawbacks found in commercial antibacterial products.

Note that the following protocols are adjustable and the amounts of essential oils may be scaled up or down as needed. You can use more or less of an ingredient or even omit some of the ingredients according to your needs. Ingredients marked with an asterisk (*) are optional and those marked with a plus (+) should be used with caution around the face.

Name	Ingredients	Recipe	Uses
Hand sanitizer	• Witch hazel, 2 ounces • Tea tree oil, 10 drops • Lavender, 10 drops • Eucalyptus(+), 10 drops • Geranium(*), 5 drops	Combine the oils and witch hazel inside a 2 ounce glass spray bottle with cap. Shake well before each use. Spray on and rub over hands after touching any high-risk objects. Use before eating, applying makeup or touching your face.	Keep this with you when out and about in the community, at work or in public places. For use when you can't wash with soap and water. Ideal to replace alcohol gels, synthetic hand cleaners and wipes.
Personal care	• Lavender oil, 25 drops • Tea tree, 20 drops • Rosemary(*), 20 drops • Sandalwood(*), 10 drops	Add oils to about 8 ounces (236 mL) of personal care product. Use the products as you normally would.	For hand soaps, shampoo, body wash, or lotion products, these oils can enhance bacterial and immune support as well and skin health. For best results, use only natural or organic body care products.

For best results with personal care products, be sure to use only natural or organic body care products. Your local health food store will carry natural brands you can choose from. The recipes above are generally safe for children, elderly or for sensitive skin areas as they are diluted significantly. However, always start slowly when trying new recipes and make adjustments to the recipe to best suit your needs if it's too strong or burns. Keep essential oils away from your eyes and see the precautions in the chapter "Essential Oil Safety, Techniques and FAQs" on page 121 for details about using these natural products.

23 Cleaning and Disinfecting

long with proper hand washing, cleaning and disinfecting are an integral part of a complete prevention program for reducing the risk of spreading Staph and MRSA to others. There's a lot of confusion about cleaning and disinfecting and about how to do it properly. There's even more confusion about the differences between cleaning, disinfecting and sanitizing and about the different roles that each play in controlling MRSA and Staph.

Cleaning, sanitizing and disinfecting all have a time and a place when it comes to Staph and MRSA prevention. Few disinfectants have a stated *kill time* for MRSA bacteria. And even if a disinfectant can kill MRSA, it can only do so when it's used properly. Basic cleaning also provides important benefits, as does sanitizing. Even though cleaning may not kill MRSA, it reduces the number of bacteria by physically washing them away.

Cleaning, Disinfecting and Sanitizing

While cleaning, disinfecting and sanitizing are all important for controlling bacteria, they serve different functions and provide different results. Using the wrong method at the wrong time can increase the risk of spreading infecting bacteria and it can also expose your immune system to unneeded risks.

Cleaning

Cleaning simply means to *remove dirt or contamination from a surface*, including some bacteria. It's typically performed using soap and water. Cleaning physically lifts bacteria, dirt, oils and other contaminants off of a surface so that it's easier to wipe them away. Cleaning does not kill bacteria, nor does it remove all bacteria from a given surface. Cleaning a surface first is actually vital to the disinfection process, as disinfectants are not as effective at killing germs if the area is dirty.

Disinfecting

Disinfecting means to *kill bacteria or germs on surfaces*, but it does not physically remove bacteria, dirt or contaminants from a surface. Disinfectants do not always kill 100% of the bacteria on a surface. Because only a few disinfectants have been verified to kill MRSA or *Staph aureus*, it's important to use the right disinfectant product and use it correctly.

There are many kinds of disinfectants on the market and they work against bacteria by destroying their cell wall or interfering with their metabolism. Many have broad-spectrum killing action, but unfortunately most are also corrosive and hazardous to people and pets. High strength disinfectants are used widely in healthcare settings and hospitals. Even with home-use disinfectants, care must be taken when using them as their toxic nature can impact your body and weaken your immune system when inhaled or absorbed through your skin. Fortunately, there are newer, non-toxic disinfectants available that have a tested kill time for MRSA (more on this later).

Because of their health concerns, disinfectants should only be used when and where they are most needed to limit your exposure to their toxic ingredients. High-risk and high-touch surfaces and objects are the best places to use of disinfectants, as detailed later in this chapter.

Sanitizing

Sanitizing means to *reduce the number of bacteria on a surface* or object. Sanitizing is less effective at killing bacteria and germs than disinfecting is. While sanitizing is beneficial for lowering the numbers of bacteria on surfaces, it will not kill or control MRSA completely. For best results, clean up dirt, grime and debris before sanitizing. Some sanitizers can also clean, serving two functions with a single product.

Sanitizers can reduce the risk of many kinds of bacteria and viruses spreading around the home. They are convenient, easy to use and are generally less toxic than disinfectants. Some sanitizers, like hand sanitizers, are ideal for use while traveling or on the go.

There are safe and natural sanitizer products on the market, which can protect your family's health and help safeguard their immune system. For the vast majority of the surfaces and objects in the home, a sanitizer will work just fine, reserving corrosive and toxic disinfectants for the highest-risk areas.

Best Household Cleaning Practices

Cleaning is the best overall option for controlling bacteria on the majority of home surfaces and objects that are low-risk or infrequently used. However, for high-risk, high-touch objects or objects and surfaces near or in contact with an infected person, use of a disinfectant is best after cleaning is done.

What to Clean

- Any household surfaces with visible dirt or debris. This includes surfaces or objects that are not close to or in contact with someone who has a Staph or MRSA infection.

- Any high-risk surfaces or objects that need disinfection that are dirty or soiled.

Household Cleaning Tips

- **Avoid mops and mop buckets.** Mop water containing cleaning solutions will become dirty and contaminated when used. Using a dirty mop smears bacteria all over, increasing the extent of contamination. Adding a sanitizing agent to your cleaning solution will help control bacteria.

- **Avoid kitchen sponges and reusable rags.** These types of cleaning aids are some of the most highly contaminated objects inside your home. If you choose to use a kitchen sponge, then soak it with water until dripping wet and heat inside a microwave set on high for 2 minutes to sanitize the sponge once or twice each week. If you use reusable rags, dry them as quickly as possible after each use. Wash them every few days at high temperatures and add bacterial control aids to the wash water.

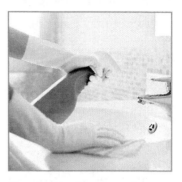

Cleaning is an important first step before disinfecting surfaces. Removing dirt and grime improves the effectiveness of disinfectants.

- **Use a natural cleaning product whenever possible.** Several companies make natural cleaning alternatives, including Seventh Generation, Burt's Bees and others. Such products contain few hazardous chemical ingredients. Avoid chemical antibacterial agents.

A Safe Household Cleaning and Sanitizing Recipe

You can make your own inexpensive and non-toxic household cleaner using soap, vinegar and water. Add essential oils to create a natural sanitizing cleaner. This recipe can be used for surfaces, counters, and floors, and to prepare surfaces for disinfecting. Your home will smell great and it will be healthier without caustic, and dangerous chemicals. This recipe is adjustable and approximate. The amounts may be scaled up or down and some ingredients may be omitted if you prefer (though removing the essential oils will remove the sanitizing ingredients).

Name	Ingredients	Recipe	Uses and Precautions
Household cleaner sanitizer	- Water, 1 cup - Castile soap, 1 squirt - White vinegar, 1 cup - Lemon oil, 20 drops - Thyme oil, 15 drops	Add 1 squirt Castile soap to 1 cup water, or as directed on the soap instructions. Add 1 cup vinegar and essential oils. Shake well before each use, spray onto surfaces, then rinse/wipe off excess. Larger amounts can be made for cleaning floors. Castile soap can be found online or in health food stores.	Ideal for mild to moderate bacterial control and routine cleaning. Keep out of reach of children and away from pets. Do not use thyme oil if you are pregnant. Substitute tea tree oil. Thyme and tea tree may be toxic to pets. Substitute oregano oil for thyme oil if you have pets.

Household Sanitizing

Sanitizing is the safest and best option for reducing bacteria on the majority of home surfaces. However, for high-risk objects and high-touch surfaces, a disinfectant is best.

Some products or recipes combine sanitizing agents and cleaning agents together so that both can be done in one step. The household cleaner recipe in the previous section is an example. This section contains recipes for two natural sanitizers made with essential oils that do not contain soap.

What to Sanitize

- Sanitize any low-risk surfaces or objects that people touch or contact infrequently. Depending on your household, examples may include floors, tables, chairs, low-use counter top areas, and furniture. Low-risk also includes things that are not used by someone with an active infection.

- Avoid reusable cloths, mops and sponges. As mentioned in the cleaning section, reusable cleaning aids just spread bacteria around.

- Replace cloths, wipes and other sanitizing aids before sanitizing each new area of a home. Changing your cleaning wipes often prevents spreading bacteria from one area to another.

- If you choose to use reusable wipes, mop heads, sponges or other sanitizing aids, be sure to disinfect them well after each use. If they are bleach safe, they can be soaked in 10% bleach solution for at least 5 minutes. Cloths and wipes may be disinfected in the same way, followed by laundering according to the highly contaminated laundry methods in the chapter "Laundry Precautions & Methods" on page 285.

- Sanitize while traveling or on the go. When you are away from home, soap and water may be unavailable. Keep a small bottle of natural sanitizer in your purse, vehicle or travel bag while on vacation or running errands around town. Sanitize your hands after leaving public places and before eating, handing food or applying makeup. See "Sanitizer and Personal Care Recipes" on page 274 for how to make your own natural hand sanitizer.

Household Sanitizer Recipes

You can create your own household sanitizer very easily with a few simple ingredients. The following recipes are adjustable and approximate. The amounts may be scaled up or down and some ingredients may be omitted according to your needs.

If you intend to spray furniture or fabric, be sure to test the sanitizing spray on a small, inconspicuous area to make sure it doesn't stain or fade the surfaces or materials.

Name	Ingredients	Recipe	Uses
General sanitizer	• Water, 2 cups • Rosemary oil, 20 drops • Lemon oil, 15 drops • Eucalyptus oil, 3 drops • Lavender oil, 4 drops	Add the oils to water in a spray bottle and shake well before each time you spray. Spray onto surfaces, let sit for a minute or so and then wipe off.	For sanitizing counter tops, sinks, door knobs, floors and other household surfaces. Can even be used for rinsing vegetables.
Potent sanitizer	• Water, 2 cups • Oregano oil, 5 drops • Clary sage, 10 drops • Thyme, 10 drops • Lemon oil, 20 drops	Same as above.	For localized bacterial control of high-risk surfaces or surfaces more prone to contamination. May be too strong for general household uses. Do not use thyme oil if you are pregnant. Substitute tea tree oil. Thyme and tea tree may be toxic to pets so substitute oregano oil for thyme oil if you have pets.

Disinfecting High-Risk Surfaces

Most consumer disinfectants are toxic and hazardous to use. Because of the health risks, strong disinfectants should only be used when needed and only on the highest-risk surfaces. Below are details of two common disinfectant products proven to kill MRSA and most other bacteria, along with detailed steps for using them effectively and as safely as possible. A safer, non-toxic alternative that also kills MRSA is the silver ion disinfectant described later in this chapter.

What to Disinfect

Focus your efforts on the highest-risk surfaces and objects to limit your exposure to harsh products. Below is a list of the surfaces with the greatest chance of being contaminated with MRSA:

- For higher risk (meaning high-touch) surfaces, such as sinks, bathrooms, or surfaces and objects the infected person touches, a disinfectant will provide stronger bacterial control.

- High-risk surfaces and objects, including the infected person's:

  » Toilet seat and toilet handle. Disinfect daily during active infections.

  » Bathroom sink, knobs, shower or tub and floor. Disinfect daily during active infections.

  » High-touch surfaces around the bed (including handrails). Disinfect daily during active infections.

- Surfaces or objects that are close to or in contact with someone who has MRSA or Staph, including the infected person's:

  » Tables, hard chairs, counter tops, dresser tops or other furniture touched by the infected person. Disinfect two or three times per week during an active infection.

  » High-touch surfaces, such as light switches, doorknobs, dresser handles, remote control, phone, computer keyboards and mouse, and medical equipment. Disinfect two or three times per week during an active infection (test disinfectant on an inconspicuous spot first to ensure it's compatible).

  » High-touch objects, such as personal care product containers (deodorant, cosmetics, hair spray bottles, etc.). Disinfect two or three times per week during an infection.

Household Bleach

For many years, household bleach has been the most common disinfectant for kitchens, bathrooms or other high-risk areas of the home. This tried-and-true disinfectant remains one of the most effective and least expensive ways to kill MRSA on surfaces.

Household bleach must be diluted in water to work properly as a disinfectant. 100% bleach will not kill bacteria as well and can destroy surfaces and cause greater health risks to the user, pets and any people nearby.

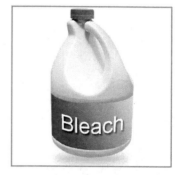

Household bleach is the most commonly used disinfectant, but it must be used properly to be effective and to minimize its health risks.

There are different kinds of bleach, and it can be a bit confusing knowing which one to use. What is called *household bleach* is actually a solution of 5.25% sodium hypochlorite. Note that for the purposes of making a disinfectant solution, you should ignore the hypochlorite concentration and simply consider what's in the bottle as *100% household bleach*. Other types of bleach include germicidal bleach (6.15% or more hypochlorite), laundry bleach (6.0% hypochlorite), and various products containing bleach along with cleaning agents. Concentrated bleach is becoming more common, with hypochlorite concentrations of 6%, 6.15% and 8.25%. Again, for the purposes of this chapter, the term *bleach* refers to the household bleach only with 5.25% hypochlorite.

Bleach freshly diluted in water in a 1:10 ratio (a 10% dilution) is very effective at killing bacteria, including MRSA. However, it can be toxic to adults, children and pets and must be used with caution and care. People have gone as far as washing their walls with bleach. There will be a point of diminishing returns for over-using bleach, which can lead to unneeded health problems and the weakening of your body's natural defense system.

The hazards of bleach are not to be taken lightly. Bleach fumes are highly corrosive and irritating to the lungs, nose and eyes and will burn and damage your skin. Bleach can react with metal surfaces to produce toxic gases. Bleach can also produce dioxin when it reacts with organic materials (such as dirt). Dioxin is a potent cancer-causing chemical and can accumulate in the environment over time and can create endocrine-hormonal problems for both people and animals. Therefore, ensure surfaces are well-cleaned if using bleach, and only use it when absolutely necessary. Consider replacing bleach with a non-toxic disinfectant that's discussed later in this chapter.

How to Make 10% Bleach Solution

A 10% solution of household Clorox bleach in water has a 5 minute kill time for both Staph and MRSA bacteria, as listed on the Clorox product specifications (note that other bleach brands may differ on kill times). The following steps can be used for making a standard 10% solution of household bleach. However, **always follow the directions for use on the bleach bottle label**, especially if the product is something other than 5.25% hypochlorite.

1. Wear gloves and eye protection and ventilate the area when making bleach solutions.

2. Mix 1 part household bleach to 9 parts water. Pour the bleach into the water slowly without splashing. Using squirt bottles or buckets with graduation lines make it easier to measure the right amount of bleach and water.

3. Make only enough bleach solution for one day's use. Discard any left-overs after 24 hours, even if it looks and smells the same, as bleach solutions quickly lose their effectiveness.

NOTE: Always follow the directions on the label if there is a discrepancy with the steps in this book.

Using 10% Bleach to Disinfect Surfaces[114]

1. Follow the directions on the product's label and pay close attention to warnings.

2. Wear gloves to limit your skin exposure. Wear old clothing or a cleaning apron or coat because bleach splashes will permanently discolor clothing.

3. Clean and remove any visible residues from the surface. If residue is noticed, remove with a clean, damp cloth before disinfecting. This is important because disinfectants work best on surfaces without any dirt or visible debris.

4. Ventilate the area well. Open windows or turn on exhaust fans in the kitchen or bathroom if applicable to pull bleach fumes out of the house.

5. Thoroughly wet the surface with the 10% bleach solution using a wiping cloth. If using a bucket rather than spray bottle, change bucket solution and cloth frequently to avoid spreading germs from one surface or household area to another.

6. If the product has a 5 minute kill time for MRSA or *Staph aureus*, allow bleached surfaces to sit wet for at least 5 minutes, rinse with water, and then allow the surface to air dry. Always follow the manufacturer's stated kill times and use directions if they differ from this book.

7. Use a fresh cloth for each room or area to minimize the risk of spreading contamination from the same cloth (such as when moving from the bathroom to the kitchen).

8. After applying the bleach solution and letting it sit for the proper time, rinse the surface with clean water. Use clean water for rinsing, such as in a spray bottle.

9. Change gloves immediately if they are visibly dirty or soiled. Remove cleaning apron or coat and gloves before entering any non-contaminated areas of the home.

10. Wear gloves when disposing of used wipes and dispose with your normal household trash. If you have a dedicated trash for medical waste like used dressings and bandages, the wipes can be disposed of there.

11. Stay out of the area after cleaning with bleach. If possible, keep adults, children and pets out of the area for at least 30 minutes to allow for the fumes to diminish.

12. Do not mix bleach with ammonia, vinegar or other acid-base cleaners. This combination creates a toxic gas called chloramine. Short-term exposure to this gas can cause mild asthmatic symptoms and serious respiratory issues.

13. Wash your hands. After you finish disinfecting and have removed your gloves, wash your hands throughly with soap and water.

Bleach Precautions

Keep bleach away from your children and pets. Use only on hard, non-porous surfaces. Do not use bleach on metal surfaces or fabrics. Use only in well ventilated areas. Follow all safety precautions, directions for use and hazard warnings on the product label.

Clorox Healthcare Bleach Germicidal Wipes

This bleach-containing product made by Clorox has special ingredients to reduce two of the biggest drawbacks of using regular bleach: 1) the strong odor and 2) corrosion of surfaces. This professional-grade product is meant for use in hospitals, but you can also find it online at many outlets, including Amazon.com.

This product has a short 30 second kill time for MRSA and regular Staph bacteria. Few other common disinfects have such a short MRSA kill time. It also kills many other types of bacteria, fungi and viruses. Containing odor-masking ingredients, this formula retains a slight bleach smell that is less strong than regular bleach. These wipes also contain a corrosion inhibitor that makes it less likely to corrode things as much as regular bleach. These wipes can be used on stainless steel, plastic, glazed ceramic, glass and porcelain without causing corrosion. However, the wipes cannot be used to disinfect fabric, wood, natural rubber, painted and paper surfaces. Follow the *directions for use* on the product's label for proper use and safety instructions.

Other Disinfectants

There are other disinfectants that can kill MRSA, along with other disease-causing microorganisms. Many of these products don't have the downsides that bleach has, although they almost always have safety issues of their own.

Disinfectants made by Lysol and Pine-Sol have been used for killing MRSA. However, there are several versions of these products and not all have stated kill times for the bacteria on the label. Therefore, review the product label or their website for the specific product you want to use. Look for stated kill times for either *Staph aureus* or MRSA to ensure they will work.

Keep in mind that most consumer non-bleach disinfectants contain toxic and harsh chemicals, including phenol and cresol. Many products also contain the preservative formaldehyde which is a suspected human carcinogen that can irritate your eyes, throat, skin and lungs. Artificial color and odor enhancing ingredients add further to the health-harming brew found in most commercial disinfectants. Because of the inherent toxicity and safety issues with these phenolic disinfectants, it's best to minimize their use or substitute a safer option, as detailed below.

Safe, Non-Toxic Silver Ion Disinfectants

Disinfectants made with silver ions are very effective against a wide range of bacteria and other pathogens, including MRSA. These disinfectants are economical, very safe and easy to use. Silver disinfectants can be used anywhere you would normally disinfectant.

One of the author's favorite disinfectants contains silver ions (Silver Ion SDC technology), citric acid and water. This disinfectant has a two minute kill time for MRSA. It's safe to use around children and animals too. There are many different silver-based cleaners and disinfectants on the market. Make sure any silver disinfectants you use meet the following criteria:

- Has a stated kill time for the bacteria you want to control (MRSA, *Staph aureus*, etc).

- SDC silver ion technology. Most silver products have a very short shelf life and lose potency over time. SDC (silver dihydrogen citrate) ensures the product is stable and effective over time.

- EPA IV toxicity rating. IV is the lowest (meaning the safest) rating assigned by the Federal EPA.

NOTE: See the section "Michelle's Recommended Products" on page 303 for product resources.

24 Laundry Precautions & Methods

Because Staph and MRSA live on people's skin, they can easily hitch a ride on clothing, towels or sports clothing and gear. Anything that touches someone's infected skin area can become contaminated with these bacteria. Even people who are simply MRSA Staph carriers can transfer the bacteria from their skin to clothing or towels. Contaminated clothing and towels can provide an easy route for the bacteria to travel from one place to another, or from one person to another.

Studies show that the majority of washing machines contain potentially dangerous bacteria, including fecal bacteria from underwear. Contaminated laundry items can easily spread bacteria to non-contaminated laundry and to the inside of your washing machine.

Minimizing laundry contamination is especially important for families, schools, athletic clubs and sports teams where many different people in close physical contact all share the same towels, clothing and/or sports equipment. Laundry is also a major issue for assisted living or nursing homes if different people's laundry are washed together.

Using bleach as a laundry additive to control bacteria has long been a standard practice. However, bleach can only be used with white laundry, and there are other problems with bleach, including toxicity to people and environmental issues. Bleach alternatives are available, but you must weigh the pros and cons of using products with harsh chemical cleaners. More recently, natural alternatives to bleach have become available. They can be effective at reducing bacteria in the laundry without the undesirable properties of bleach and harsh chemicals.

General Household Laundry

Below are some general laundry recommendations for handling and cleaning laundry if it might be contaminated with Staph or MRSA bacteria, or if a person in the house has an active infection. Refer to the next section for laundry that is more heavily contaminated, or if you want to add extra bacterial control.

- For infected family members, use a separate, impervious laundry hamper for clothing and towels. Use a solid plastic container, not one with ventilation holes or made of canvas or wicker. Keep contaminated laundry separate from other laundry to reduce the spreading of bacteria.

- Handle contaminated laundry carefully with minimal agitation.

- Wear gloves to better protect yourself if the clothing was used by an infected person.

- Wash contaminated laundry separately from other laundry to minimize cross-contamination to other people's clothes, towels, etc.

- Use natural, non-toxic laundry detergents to support your immune health.

- Wash laundry in hot water as this will help reduce the amount of bacteria. If the clothes can't be washed in hot water, add extra bacterial control per the next section.

- If possible, set the dryer to its hottest setting as the heat will kill many of the bacteria. If the clothes can't be dried this way, add extra bacterial control per the next section.

Added Bacterial Control for Highly Contaminated Laundry

There are additional steps you can take to further reduce bacteria in the laundry beyond the techniques listed in the previous section. These additional steps will provide added control and are safe for most types of fabrics and colors.

- **Essential oils.** Adding several drops (5 to 15 drops depending on your load size) of medicinal quality tea tree essential oil to the wash water is a natural way of reducing bacteria in your laundry. Adding the oil to the detergent first will help the oil mix into the water. Eucalyptus, orange, lavender, lemon and other antibacterial oils can also help your infection control efforts while also making your clothes smell great. Essential oils are easy to use and work in combination with detergents in any laundry. See "Essential Oil Protocols for Use" on page 137 for essential oil details.

- **Silver ion systems.** Laundry systems utilizing silver ions can significantly reduce bacteria in laundry, though such systems can be expensive.

- **Ozone systems.** Laundry systems using ozone provide excellent bacterial control. An added benefit of such systems is that detergents are not needed. See the section "Ozone Laundry Methods" on page 288 for details.

- **Antimicrobial coating.** A liquid product is available that uses a new technology to chemically bind a very thin layer of antimicrobial coating to fabrics. This coating does not change the feel or color of the fabric, but it does kill bacteria including MRSA that come into contact with the fabric. This technology is not a natural product, but it is inert, long lasting (dozens of washes) and does not leach from the fabric after it is applied. This is an attractive option for athletic teams, hospital workers and nurses, and other high-risk environments.

NOTE: See the section "Michelle's Recommended Products" on page 303 for product resources.

Bleach Laundry Methods

Adding bleach to the laundry's wash water is a tried-and-true way to help control bacteria in highly contaminated laundry. The recommended concentration of bleach in washing machine water for heavily contaminated laundry is between 50 to 150 parts per million (ppm) of chlorine, which is equal to approximately a 1:500 dilution of household bleach in water. For *normal sized* top-loading machines, between ½ and 1 cup of household bleach will be the right amount to add to a load of laundry.

Be aware that there are many different bleach products with different concentrations of chlorine. **Always follow the directions for use on the product label to determine how much bleach to add.** Be sure to check clothing before washing with bleach to make sure it's bleach-safe or white to reduce the risk of discoloration. Note that ozone doesn't discolor clothes and is a safer option for people and the environment.

Washing Laundry with Bleach

The following recommendations can be helpful for washing highly contaminated laundry with bleach solutions:

- Any clothing soiled with body fluids should be bagged or placed in leak-proof containers and should not be mixed with unsoiled laundry.

- Handle contaminated laundry as little as possible with minimal agitation.

- Wear rubber or latex gloves when handling contaminated laundry to better protect yourself.

- Set the washing machine to its hottest water cycle for maximum bacterial control and begin filling the washing machine with water.

- Before adding any clothing to the washer, add the desired amount of detergent, following the directions for heavily soiled clothing.

- Before adding any clothing, add household bleach to the filling wash water to make a 1:500 dilution of household bleach, or as directed on the product's instructions for use. For most family sized top-load machines, approximately 1 cup of household bleach will suffice, or half a cup for smaller loads or machines.

- Add the dirty clothing last, and then wash the load normally.

Ozone Laundry Methods

Ozone is a natural compound found in the air that helps absorb hazardous UV radiation from the sun and regulate the earth's temperature. Ozone is responsible for the crisp, fresh smell in the air after a thunderstorm and is actually made by lightning.

Ozone also has very strong bacterial killing properties. Ozone in various forms has been used for decades for disinfection in medicine, food processing, water purification, chemistry, bioremediation, dentistry and commercial laundry washing. For laundry uses, ozone gas is dissolved into the wash water to make *ozonated water*. One study showed that 30 ppm of ozonated water effectively kills MRSA on contaminated clothing[115].

Commercial grade ozone washing systems have been used by many washing companies, hospitals and hotels for decades. Ozone washing systems are also available for home use. Ozone cleans clothes by oxidation which removes stains and bacteria within the clothing fibers. On top of that, ozone systems actually work better when used with cold water. Home use ozone systems are becoming much more affordable, especially when you account for the energy savings and money you'll save by never buying laundry detergents or fabric softeners again.

Ozone pros

- Studies of commercial ozone systems show very effective results killing MRSA, many times more effective than standard bleach washing methods.

- No detergent residues left on clothing after laundering.

- Is more effective when used with cold water, which reduces energy costs.

- Can be used effectively without any detergent in the wash, which saves you money.

- Not harmful to clothing and safe for people and the environment when used properly.

Ozone cons

- It can be difficult to know which ozone washing systems work best. Some manufacturers of home ozone systems provide unsubstantiated claims about the effectiveness of their products.

- Most studies on ozone MRSA control used commercial and industrial wash systems. There is a lack of scientific studies on home control of MRSA using home ozone systems.

- The cost of home ozone wash systems can be high for people on a tight budget. However, the up-front costs will eventually pay for themselves in reduced energy costs and eliminating the need for detergent.

25 Prevention: Home, Work, Hospitals and Travel

While a large number of MRSA and Staph infections are a result of being hospitalized, this chapter focuses on reducing the risk of catching MRSA or Staph from others who are infected in your community or household. Over the last decade or so, community associated MRSA (CA-MRSA) has become much more common with people getting infected from gyms or going to the beach, or children going to daycare or school. According to the Journal of the American Medical Association (JAMA), CA-MRSA has become the most frequent cause of skin and soft tissue infections (like boils, cellulitis or abscesses), accounting for over 12 million hospital and doctor visits.

This chapter includes simple and effective tips to reduce your risk when visiting people who are infected, visiting healthcare facilities, or when venturing into your community. If a family member is infected, this chapter will help you understand how to help prevent other family members from getting Staph or MRSA. For additional support on how to stay safe when care-giving, refer to the chapter "Caring for Someone with Staph or MRSA" on page 297.

While preventative measures are important, it's best to adopt a balanced approach to avoid becoming overly paranoid about the risks. The tips and methods in this chapter should not be cause for fear of or obsession with germs. In fact, being overly preoccupied with preventative measures can easily lead to becoming a *germaphobe*, which will do more harm than good in the long run. The key to success in preventing these infections is being aware of the risks and minimizing them as much as possible without going overboard.

Hospitals, Nursing Homes and Healthcare Facilities

If you're going to be admitted into a hospital or other healthcare facility, refer to the chapter "Staying in Hospitals: What You Need to Know" on page 51 for actions you can take to reduce your exposure to MRSA, Staph and other infections.

Healthcare environments have one of the highest risks when it comes to exposure to bacteria and viruses. The author's sister-in-law acquired a MRSA skin infection while simply visiting someone in a hospital. One of the best preventative measures you can take is to simply avoid touching high-risk surfaces and objects, or if you do, wash your hands immediately after touching them. Exercise caution and use extra-good hand washing and hygiene after contacting hospital personnel, patients or any surface or object in healthcare settings:

- **Floors and bed rails.** These are the two most heavily contaminated surfaces found in hospital rooms, however, all hospital surfaces and objects are suspect when it comes to MRSA bacteria, even those found in the waiting room.

- **Objects in rooms.** High-touch objects also carry higher risk of exposure and include: toilets, faucets, door knobs, light switches, call buttons, drapes segregating beds, remote controls, waste baskets, etc.

- **Touching others.** This can include someone who's infected or touching or being touched by hospital staff or doctors. Hospital staff are always working with those who are sick, and it's common for some hospital staff to practice ineffective hand washing and hygiene procedures.

- **Avoid touching your face.** This includes you nose, eyes or mouth until you've washed your hands thoroughly.

- **Reduce MRSA or other germs in the air**. Air diffusing essential oils can reduce airborne germs including MRSA. If you need to stay in the hospital, see if you can bring in an air diffuser to reduce germs. Visitor, patient and hospital staff activity in rooms increases the number of particles with bacteria floating in the air. Find out more about "Controlling Airborne Bacteria" on page 206.

- **Cover all open cuts or wounds:** This will keep your cut or wound from being exposed to germs.

- **Wash your hands.** Wash using proper techniques and avoid antibacterial soaps (you may need to bring your own). Be sure to follow the chapter "Hand Washing and Hygiene" on page 269. Use your personal hand sanitizer in a pinch, but wash your hands as soon as possible.

- **Take preventative remedies.** When visiting any high risk environment, it's best to take preventative remedies before and after the visit to help combat any infectious agents you might encounter. Remedies that support your immune system and control infections can be helpful. Some great choices are included in "Alternative Remedies" on page 91.

The section "Steps to Take While In the Hospital" on page 56 contains additional tips that can be helpful in understanding and reducing your infection risk when visiting healthcare environments.

Home and Family Prevention

In addition to the tips below, when taking care of others who have MRSA or Staph, be sure to also read "Caring for Someone with Staph or MRSA" on page 297. The following tips apply if you or a family member has MRSA or Staph.

- **Inform everyone** sharing a home with an infected person of the applicable prevention strategies in this chapter as well as the risk factors and how Staph and MRSA infections are spread. Get everyone's buy-in to follow good hygiene and prevention practices. Make sure everyone knows how to wash their hands properly and to avoid high-risk surfaces, objects and areas of the house if possible.

- **Maintain a strong immune system.** One of your most powerful allies is your immune system. This is important for those who are infected as well as family members who are not. Be sure to bolster your immunity per the chapter "Boosting Your Immune System" on page 223.

- **Wash your hands.** Good hygiene is key. Wash your hands after touching any high-risk objects, contact with an infected person, after treating wounds and before touching your face. Use natural soap, not antibacterial soaps. See the section "Best Hand Washing Practices" on page 274.

- **Maintenance remedies.** Consider putting family members who are not infected on a lower, maintenance level of antibacterial herbs, spices or essential oils to help prevent infections as detailed in the section "Maintenance and Preventative Remedies" on page 207.

- **Disinfect the home.** See the chapter "Cleaning and Disinfecting" on page 275 for disinfection techniques and non-toxic disinfectants. Keep surfaces and high-touch objects used by the infected person disinfected, like telephones, door knobs, refrigerator handles, remote controls, etc. Any home areas used for wound or skin infection management should be disinfected after use.

- **Avoid sharing personal items**, such as towels, washcloths, tooth-brushes, deodorant, clothing or sports gear with someone who's infected.

- **Avoid sharing clothing.** Because Staph and MRSA can shed from infected skin areas onto nearby clothing, avoid sharing clothing with an infected person.

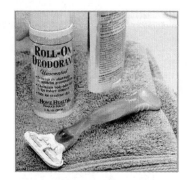

Personal care items provide an easy route for bacteria to spread among family members.

- **Segregate laundry.** Keep the infected family member's laundry separate from other clothing and wash separately. Use hot water and dry your clothes well in the dryer to reduce bacteria. You might consider a laundry system that cleans with ozone as it's superior to bleach. Refer to the chapter "Laundry Precautions & Methods" on page 285 for laundry details.

- **Reduce airborne MRSA or Staph.** Using an air diffuser with medicinal essential oils can reduce

Staph and MRSA in the air. It can be placed in any room and most antibacterial oils have a pleasant aroma. Find out more about "Controlling Airborne Bacteria" on page 206.

- **Keep the bathtub clean.** The bathtub is one of the dirtiest places in your home and contains more than 100,000 bacteria per square inch, some of which have just washed off the last person who used it. Clean the tub well after use by those who are infected. Natural sanitizers or disinfectants will help reduce bacteria in the tub.

- **Keep natural remedies on hand** in case an infection develops, as it's much easier to stop an infection when it's just starting. Refer to "Alternative Remedies" on page 91 for more details.

- **Scratches, cuts and suspicious areas.** Areas of broken skin are at a higher risk for infection. Always have essential oils on hand and use on cuts, scrapes, razor nicks, and burns. Also use essential oils or Manuka honey at the first sign of any suspicious areas on the skin. It's generally much easier to "ward off an infection" then deal with one in full swing. Some great essential oil choices are Tea Tree or the Antibacterial Blend. Refer to "Essential Oil Protocols for Use" on page 137 for more information. Genuine Manuka honey is another great choice.

Prevention in Your Community

The following prevention strategies can help protect you from MRSA and Staph in the community, or protect others if you have an infection. These prevention tips can also reduce the risk of flu and other infectious diseases:

- **If you are infected, stay at home.** If possible, stay home during the worst stage of your infection. Have other people run errands for you and take sick time from work.

- **Avoid touching high-risk surfaces.** Surfaces or objects that many people touch frequently have a high-risk, such as door handles, elevator buttons, shopping carts, keyboards, telephones and gym equipment. Take extra precautions such as using a paper towel to avoid directly touching bathroom stalls and latches, toilet handles, bathroom faucets and paper towel dispensers. Be sure to sanitize or wash your hands after touching high-risk surfaces.

- **Health clubs or gyms.** Be sure to use your own towel. Use a barrier like clothing or a towel, between your skin and shared equipment. Wipe equipment surfaces before and after use (a disinfectant bottle should be available in most gyms).

- **Pools and spas.** Do not enter swimming pools or hot tubs if you currently have an open or draining wound to prevent getting an infection from the water. Improperly maintained spas have been implicated in transferring MRSA. Also, if you are currently infected, do not enter swimming pools or hot tub spas as it's possible to transfer MRSA or Staph bacteria to others through the water.

- **Use hand sanitizers if you can't wash your hands.** Keep a natural hand sanitizer with you when you're out and about. Use after touching any high-risk surface or object.

- **Wash your hands.** Wash your hands after being in public, especially if you've touched high-risk objects. Use natural soap and water. Be aware of everything you put your hands on.

- **Use sanitizing wipes** to sanitize high-risk surfaces before touching them. Surfaces such as shopping cart handles, library computer keyboards, hotel TV remote controls or any other high-touch surface can be easily wiped down with sanitizing wipes that you can carry with you.

School or Professional Athletes

Contact sports like wrestling, football and basketball are avenues to transfer bacteria from one person to another. The following tips will help you stay safe while enjoying your favorite activities:

- **Shower immediately** after practices or competitions. This will help remove any MRSA bacteria that could have been picked up after skin-to-skin contact. Be sure to use natural soaps. See "Sanitizer and Personal Care Recipes" on page 274 for creating a natural antibacterial soap with essential oils.

- **Bring your own towel** and do not share towels, bar soaps or toiletries with others.

- **Wash your hands when possible**, and do not use common antimicrobial soaps (you'll probably need to bring your own soap).

- **Keep any cuts, scrapes or wounds covered** to help prevent infection. If a bandage or dressing falls off, immediately replace it. Depending on the sporting event, it may be wise (or required) to not play until the wound is healed.

- **Do not enter swimming pools or spas** if you currently have an open or draining wound. Improperly maintained spas have been implicated in transferring MRSA to others. Do not enter spas if you are currently infected as it's possible to transfer the bacteria to others.

- **Dry out any equipment or padding after each use.** Antibacterial treatments for uniforms and equipment can help prevent MRSA and Staph (see "Added Bacterial Control for Highly Contaminated Laundry" on page 286 for details). Use a natural disinfectant on equipment between uses. Do not store equipment in a dark or moist environment.

- **Keep essential oils on hand** for use on any skin cuts or scrapes as these are avenues for MRSA or Staph to cause an infection. Be watchful for any suspicious areas on the skin and use essential oils or genuine Manuka honey. Apply these immediately and frequently to help prevent infection from occurring. Some great choices are Tea Tree or the Antibacterial Blend. Refer to"Essential Oil Protocols for Use" on page 137 for more information.

- **Take preventative remedies.** Bolster your immunity with immune support and/or preventative remedies before and after events or practices to help combat any infectious agents you might encounter. Some great choices are included in "Alternative Remedies" on page 91.

Travel Prevention

Summer is the most popular time for travel and vacations. Because Staph and MRSA are contagious and can linger on surfaces for a long time, crowded vacation spots can be a breeding ground for these infections. If you have a history of MRSA, Staph or other infections, or if you have a weak immune system (including children and elderly), then taking a few extra steps to protect yourself while traveling is a good idea.

30% of people in the U.S. carry Staph bacteria on their skin. Carriers can leave behind bacteria in hotel rooms and on surfaces that are frequently touched by lots of people. While the Southern U.S. has the highest MRSA rates, the risk can be found anywhere, especially in crowded public places. Surfaces touched by many people harbor the highest risks of contamination, and many such surfaces are not cleaned or sanitized on a regular basis. Some common high risk surfaces or areas you may encounter while traveling include:

- Hotel elevator buttons, door knobs, light switches, drawer handles, remote controls and telephones.

- Recreational gym and spa equipment.

- Crowded beaches, beach sand, hot tub and swimming pool water.

- Pool chairs and chaise lounges.

- Surfaces inside hotel kitchens and bathrooms like faucets, knobs, and counter tops.

- Steering wheel, door handles and console areas inside rental cars.

You can greatly reduce your risk of picking up unwanted bacteria and disease-causing germs by following a few simple prevention measures. Below are easy ways to reduce MRSA Staph risks in places you'll likely visit on vacation.

Hotel and Motels

- Keep a small container of natural hand sanitizer with you while traveling, or you can use sanitizing wipes. Sanitize high-risk surfaces before use, including the surfaces listed above.

- Avoid skin contact with the top of comforters or bedspreads. Unlike sheets, these linens are infrequently washed and can harbor many bacteria.

- Wear socks, slippers or sandals inside your hotel room. Carpets are frequently vacuumed but rarely cleaned.

- Avoid using non-disposable hotel room cups and glasses.

Swimming Pools and Beaches

- Ask how often chlorine levels and pH in swimming pools are checked. They should be checked twice per day. You can check levels yourself with test strips available at pool supply stores.

- Avoid children's wading pools which often have inadequate cleaning and chlorine levels.

- Always shower before and after using the pool, hot tub, sauna or crowded beach areas. Use natural soap and water. See "Sanitizer and Personal Care Recipes" on page 274 for making your own natural antimicrobial soap.

- Never swim or use hot tubs if you have an open cut, scrape or wound to prevent getting an infection from the water. Improperly maintained spas have been implicated in transferring MRSA to others. Also, if you are currently infected, do not enter swimming pools or hot tub spas as it's possible to transfer MRSA or Staph bacteria to others through the water.

- Clean and cover any scrapes or cuts before playing in the sand. Sand and beach water have been found to contain MRSA bacteria on crowded beaches.

- Keep a towel between you and pool chairs or lounges.

Spas, Gyms and Resorts

- Avoid sharing towels or other personal items with other people.

- Avoid touching your face in gyms, saunas and spa areas. Use a clean towel to wipe off instead.

- Sanitize equipment surfaces before use, especially gym equipment handles, mats and frequently touched surfaces.

- Improperly maintained spas, hot tubs and whirlpools are common and they carry a higher risk of MRSA and Staph. Always ask about maintenance before use.

- Always sit or lay on a clean towel to separate yourself from a sauna, recliner and shared equipment or furniture.

Summary

Your best defense against getting MRSA and Staph is to understand how the infections spread and the best protection techniques, especially how to wash your hands properly. Avoid antimicrobial cleansers and soaps and chemical disinfectants and move to all-natural disinfectants, cleaners and soaps. Use plain soap and water or natural antibacterial products to wash your hands to help support the health of your gut bacteria and your immune system. Only use harsh chemical disinfectants like bleach on the highest risk surfaces to minimize your exposure, or replace with natural disinfectants proven effective against MRSA.

Equally important is to keep your immune system strong as detailed in the chapter "Boosting Your Immune System" on page 223. Getting 15 minutes of unprotected sun on your skin every day will help boost you vitamin D levels and immune strength. Keep a few natural infection remedies on hand to nip potential skin infections in the bud. Tea tree essential oil and botanical herbal blends are great choices to help, as detailed in "Alternative Remedies" on page 91.

26 Caring for Someone with Staph or MRSA

Many people are caring for babies, children, a spouse or elderly parents who have a Staph or MRSA skin infection. Your number one responsibility when caring for others with MRSA or Staph is to protect yourself from also getting infected. As a caregiver, your risk of exposure is greatest during the active infection phase, especially if there are open skin lesions or weeping boils, abscesses or wounds.

Extra precautions should be taken during an active infection, which can include more frequent cleaning and disinfecting, more stringent hygiene and contact precautions. Because MRSA and Staph bacteria can survive on surfaces for days to weeks, continued preventative measures are also important after the infection has cleared.

This chapter works hand-in-hand with techniques found in the chapter on prevention. When caring for an infected family member, be sure to also review "Home and Family Prevention" on page 291 for additional details.

Family Colonization Risks

Because MRSA and Staph are easily spread, the infections often readily pass between family members who live together or spend time together. Family members who are caregivers are more often *MRSA or Staph carriers*, meaning they are colonized with the bacteria but are not infected. See "Staph and MRSA Carriers" on page 27 for details on carrier risks.

A 2012 study showed that family members are nearly 10 times more likely to be colonized by MRSA bacteria if they have a child with a Staph infection in their household. This demonstrates that household members are much more likely to be colonized with *Staph aureus* than the general public. For the household members, 19% were MRSA colonized and 53% were Staph colonized. Nationally, MRSA colonization is only 2% and Staph colonization is only 30%, according to the Centers for Disease Control and Prevention. The study also highlights that for family members who are colonized with MRSA, 53% were parents but only 29% were siblings[117].

The study results above underscore the risk a family is exposed to when a child comes down with MRSA or Staph. Because parents are more likely to be in close contact with an infected child, the risk of colonization appears to be greater for parents.

Infected Infants and Nursing Risks

Infants and very young children are at a higher risk for developing infections as their immune systems are not fully developed. It's possible for newborns to pick up MRSA or Staph bacteria from the vaginal canal during birth. However, babies are more likely to pick up the bacteria from their moms several weeks later due to close personal contact[116]. Infants can also be exposed to these bacteria through contact with hospital staff, catheters and other medical devices, or from contact with contaminated hospital surfaces[118]. Skin infections can later develop due to disrupted skin such as a diaper rash or any kind of skin abrasion.

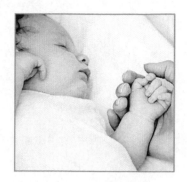

Babies are likely to take on the bacteria that the mother carries within a few months of birth.

Breastfeeding is important for infants and is critical in establishing a strong immune system. Breastfeeding provides important health benefits to both child and mother. Breastfeeding goes a long way toward improving the health, vitality and immune function of the newborn through vital nutrients that are difficult to get any other way.

Keeping Mom Healthy

As a mother, you can reduce your risk of a potential infection if your newborn is infected. It is important to nurture your immune system (see "Boosting Your Immune System" on page 223) as well as the healthy bacteria on your body and in your gut. Probiotics are crucial for the mother, plus avoiding harsh chemical disinfectants and cleaners. It's important for both mom and baby to avoid common antibacterial soaps that disrupt the healthy bacteria on your skin and in your gut. You can learn more about helpful bacteria in "Probiotics: The Good Bacteria" on page 209.

Treatment Options for Babies

Treating MRSA in children, especially infants, requires extra care. While some natural remedies can be used with newborns and babies, the usage amount must be reduced or diluted properly. Milder remedies for external use on skin infections include sterilized Manuka honey (not raw) and diluted medicinal tea tree oil (see "Manuka Honey" on page 97 and "Essential Oil Protocols for Use" on page 137). Antibiotics can help if found effective against the strain of Staph or MRSA causing the infection. However, antibiotics put a big strain on a baby's undeveloped immune system and the good bacteria in their gut, which has been linked to allergies and possible future chronic health conditions. Be sure to work with a well qualified holistic or integrative physician when it comes to naturally treating your child.

Antibiotic Risks for Mother and Baby

It's important to remember that babies, just like adults, depend on many kinds of good bacteria to stay healthy. Anything that changes their natural good flora can compromise their health. It's been well established that antibiotic therapies change the good flora of the mother to unhealthy flora. Since newborns are largely dependent upon the mother for their bacteria, antibiotic use in the mother may put the newborn at a disadvantage.

Research shows that treating newborns with antibiotics can disrupt how they develop their gut flora[119]. In addition, some researchers suggest it may be difficult to normalize newborn gut flora after exposure to antibiotics. Because of the link between antibiotic use and chronic health issues, it's best to use natural alternatives that work with the body whenever possible.

Caregiver Tips and Techniques

In addition to the information covered in "Home and Family Prevention" on page 291, these tips can reduce your chances of becoming colonized with MRSA or Staph, or from getting infected while caring for a friend or family member.

- While not always practical, keeping an infected person isolated to a certain room or part of the house can reduce the risk of others in the home becoming infected.

- Use gloves when handling an infected person's bodily fluids or when directly touching them to provide care, such as dressing wounds or washing infected areas. Change to a new pair of gloves immediately if you touch body fluids or infected skin areas. Gloves must be removed and discarded hygienically without getting any contamination from the gloves onto your skin or hands, otherwise their use is much less effective. Immediately after glove removal, hands should be washed with regular soap and water. The following website has a short video demonstrating the proper way to remove gloves:

  www.procpr.org/en/training_video/glove-removal-and-disposal

- Practice good hand hygiene with soap and water rather than using alcohol sanitizers. Never touch your face, mouth or nose after handling high-risk objects or after working with someone who's infected, until you first wash your hands.

- Follow contaminated laundry procedures for any high-risk clothing, as detailed in the section "Added Bacterial Control for Highly Contaminated Laundry" on page 286. If possible, have the infected person wear bleach-safe clothing to facilitate washing with bleach.

- Disinfect high-risk surfaces and objects daily or after each use and follow good cleaning and sanitizing practices as detailed in the chapter "Cleaning and Disinfecting" on page 275.

- Be aware that jewelry or watches worn by those who are infected can pass the bacteria to others if they are shared.

- Wear a gown or dedicated clothing for providing care to a person with Staph or MRSA. Be sure to segregate these clothes from other clothing and wash according to the chapter "Laundry Precautions & Methods" on page 285.

- If practical, dedicate medical equipment that touches the infected person to that person. Otherwise, these high-risk objects should be cleaned after use to remove contamination.

- If you yourself have a history of Staph or MRSA infections, or if you are in one or more of the high-risk categories mentioned in the chapter "Symptoms, Risk Factors and Carriers" on page 27, take extra precautions when caring for someone with these infections. Better yet, see if someone else can provide care in your place.

Providing Compassionate Care

MRSA and Staph can inflict a huge mental and emotional toll and cause a lot of stress to those suffering from the infection. High levels of stress and emotional turmoil are formidable challenges that can compromise your friendship and render your care less effective. In fact, such challenges are often the most difficult part of being a caregiver.

Dealing with the stress and emotional upsets are an important but often overlooked part of being an effective and compassionate caregiver. Handling such challenges properly is especially important when caring for friends or family members. The tips below will help you side-step the most common emotional challenges that accompany care-giving.

- **Become informed and be a good health advocate.** If you are the primary caregiver, then become informed about your loved one's condition, their doctor, their prescriptions and any other health challenges they may have. Go with them to doctor appointments to help them ask questions and take notes.

- **Do your research.** Find out all you can about the infection and what options exist to control it using both alternative and mainstream medicine.

- **Get permission.** Ask your loved one for permission to help them. People often have trouble being told what to do by friends and family, especially in matters of health. Getting the buy-in of the person you're helping is crucial, especially if they are less open to alternative options than you are. Unless there is mutual trust and openness, your efforts to help could be rejected.

- **Be encouraging and provide hope.** MRSA and Staph can be successfully treated and overcome. However, people with these infections can easily become pessimistic, lose hope and focus on the negatives, especially if they've had a long-standing or recurring infections. It's important to encourage the person that they can and will overcome their infection. Also, encourage the person to be open, honest and candid about their feelings, worries and frustrations.

- **Be open and clear.** Avoid misunderstandings and confusion by being clear and open about what you are doing and why. Practice good communication by being a good listener and explaining things as clearly as possible.

- **Be balanced.** If the infected person is skeptical of alternative medicine, then present alternative options as an add-on or supplement to their mainstream medical treatments, not as a substitute for them. Avoid polarizing conventional medicine against natural medicine. You may also need to expand you own belief system to become more open and willing to acknowledge the validity of approaches you are unfamiliar with.

- **Understand the limits of your responsibility.** Remaining objective can be difficult when a friend, sibling or parent you love is suffering from a dangerous and debilitating infection. Because everyone is responsible for their own health, it's not your responsibility to make them better. Understanding the limits of your responsibility will help you stay more balanced and less stressed and improve the care you provide.

27

Michelle's Recommended Products and Support

What to Do First

For the most important things to do first to control a Staph or MRSA infection, focus on chapter 1 and the three Action Steps. There's a lot of information in this book, and it may seem overwhelming at first. As you read this book, refer to chapter 1 often to keep focused on the most important ways to handle these infections. Use the rest of the book and the other resources to answer your questions and fill in any details you may need.

While some infections are easy to control with just a few key remedies or methods, many others require a more comprehensive strategy, especially serious or chronic recurring infections. Relying on a few remedies by themselves without following a more complete plan will likely provide mediocre results at best. For the best results with an infection, be sure to follow as much of the Action Steps in chapter 1 as possible, rather than relying on a single treatment, remedy or technique.

Additional Resources and the Latest Protocols

There are additional tools and resources available to you at no cost inside Michelle Moore's members only website. These include Michelle's recommended products and resources, the *Infection Care Network* of natural doctors and professionals with chronic infection experience, audio expert interviews, Michelle's 3 Step video series, and detailed printable guides for the methods and protocols in this book.

If you purchased Michelle's book online, please check your email for directions on how to enter the members only website. If you did not get your email invite, be sure to contact us at *Michelle@ Staph-Infection-Resources.com* to get access to these materials.

Michelle's Recommended Products

This book gives you the tools to find safe and effective remedies, supplements and other products for infection support without promoting specific brands. This is by design as products can change and it's difficult to keep a book up-to-date with the most recent and relevant brand information.

Therefore, specific brands are only provided in Michelle's members only website. Refer to the members only website for the latest product details and protocols for using them.

◇◇◇

For specific products and brands that Michelle recommends and uses herself, see the members only website. You can also send a request for Michelle's product resources and members website to *Michelle@Staph-Infection-Resources.com.*

◇◇◇

Support

If you can't find an answer to your question in this book or in the members only website, then feel free to email your question to *Michelle@Staph-Infection-Resources.com.* Michelle's support team will do their best to answer your questions about Staph and MRSA and about the methods and topics inside this book. Please be aware that Michelle and her staff are not doctors and therefore cannot provide medical advice, nor can they treat, prescribe treatments or diagnose a medical condition.

Further Reading

There are several great resources online which provide much more detailed information on many of the health topics covered in this book. You'll also find some helpful support groups. See "Further Reading Online" on page 315 for these helpful resource links.

Appendix A Acid/Alkaline Food Chart

More Alkaline	Slightly Alkaline	Food Group	Slightly Acidic	More Acidic
Leeks, tomato, cabbage, beets, black radish, carrot, horse radish Spinach, celery, wheat grass and most greens	Asparagus, artichoke, cabbage, lettuce, zucchini, peas, chives, red radish	**Veggies, Roots and Greens**	Onion, cauliflower	
Limes, fresh lemon, pineapple, avocado, mandarin orange, papaya, peach, mango	Grapefruit, cherry, unripe banana, raspberry, ripe grapes, pear, apricot, orange, date	**Fruits**	Blueberry, cranberry, plum, currant, cantaloupe, fig, watermelon, fresh coconut	Ripe banana
	Olive oil, flax seed oil, fish oil, borage oil	**Oils and Fats**	Margarine, ghee, corn oil, butter, sunflower oil	
Fresh soy beans, fresh lima beans, fresh navy beans, fresh soy nuts	Fresh lentils, fresh spelt	**Grains and Legumes**	Rye bread, whole grain bread, brown rice	White bread, white biscuit, wheat
	Cashews, almonds, sesame seeds, cumin seeds, fennel seeds	**Nuts and Seeds**	Walnuts, Brazil nuts, hazelnuts, pumpkin seeds, flax seeds, sunflower seeds	Pistachios, peanuts
		Meat and Dairy	Organ meats, oysters, liver, cream, homogenized milk, yogurt	Pork, beef, eggs, freshwater fish, chicken, hard cheeses, ice cream

More Alkaline	Slightly Alkaline	Food Group	Slightly Acidic	More Acidic
	Honey, brown rice syrup, molasses, apple cider vinegar	**Sweets, condiments and drinks**	Evaporated cane juice, fructose, barley sweetener, wine, natural fruit juices	Artificial sweeteners, white sugar, beet sugar, fruit juices with sugar, soda pop, ketchup, mustard, mayonnaise, liquor, beer, coffee, white vinegar
Cayenne pepper, cinnamon, ginger, garlic, some essential oils	Goldenseal, lemongrass, echinacea, many essential oils	**Spices, Herbs and Drugs**	Curry, vanilla, nutmeg	Antibiotics, many pharmaceutical drugs and over-the-counter meds

Appendix B Super pH Salad Recipe

This is one of Michelle Moore's favorites. It can be used as an appetizer or a side dish. It can even serve as a main course, especially with the addition of a protein source (meat or fish) on top.

Salad Ingredients

- 1 bunch organic green or red kale
- 1 bunch organic red chard
- 1 bunch organic collard greens (the big leaf type)
- 1 bunch organic cilantro
- 1 bunch organic parsley
- Handful or two of raw, organic walnuts, chopped

Place leaves from the kale, chard, collard greens, cilantro and parsley into a food processor (stalks can be added too, if you prefer). Run until greens are chopped into smaller pieces (like Cole-slaw consistency). Add all together in a large bowl.

Dressing

Amounts are approximate.

- 1/2 cup organic olive oil
- Raw garlic (1-2 cloves)
- Raw ginger (1 tablespoon chopped)
- Juice from approximately 1 to 2 organic lemons
- Agave nectar or pure maple syrup for sweetness, 1 to 2 tablespoons or to taste
- Himalayan crystal salt or Celtic sea salt to taste

Add all to a small Cuisinart or mixer and blend together. Drizzle dressing over salad greens, add walnuts and mix well. Refrigerate and enjoy! Freshest for a few days, but lasts up to 5 days if sealed well.

Options

You can add curry, soy sauce or other herbs to the dressing for a different twist. You can also add chopped onions, carrots or other veggies to the main salad. Wild caught salmon, organic chicken or other natural meats may be added on top. Be creative!

Appendix C Green Smoothie Recipes

Below are a few green smoothie recipes. You can substitute other greens or fruit to suit your taste. Bananas make the smoothies smoother. You can make your smoothie thicker or thinner by using more or less water. You can add ice cubes to make a cold or frozen smoothie. Add a drop or two of peppermint, lemon or orange essential oils for a twist. Be creative and experiment.

Romaine Green

- 8 leaves Romaine lettuce
- 1 cup red grapes
- 1 orange
- 1 banana
- 2 cups filtered water

Blend well. Makes 1 quart.

Cool Blue Bonanza

- 2 leaves of kale
- 2 leaves of collard greens
- 1 leaf of red chard
- 1 cup Italian parsley
- 1 banana
- 1 cup wild blueberries
- 2 cups filtered water
- 1 cup ice cubes

Blend well. Makes 1.5 quarts.

Wild Banango

- 2 cups chard or spinach
- 1 banana
- 1 mango
- 2 cups filtered water

Blend well. Makes 1 quart.

Appendix D Emotional Freedom Technique (EFT)

Emotional Freedom Technique, or EFT, is a powerful acupressure technique based on the same energy meridians of your body used in traditional acupuncture for over five thousand years. It can be used to help reduce stress or pain and to improve your immune response.

Preparation

- Tap with your fingertips (you may use all of your finger tips or just your index and middle finger). If you have long finger nails, use your finger pads instead of your fingertips.

- Use both hands at once.

- Remove all watches, bracelets or anything else around your wrists.

- Remove your glasses if possible.

The Tapping

- Tap solidly, but NOT hard enough to hurt or bruise yourself.

- Tap on each of the points shown below, about 5-7 times each, long enough for one full breath on each point.

- Tap the points in the order shown below.

The Tapping Points

There are ten tapping points as shown below, each with an abbreviation:

1. Top of your head (TH)

2. The inside of your eyebrow (EB)

3. On the bone on the outside of your eye socket (SE)

4. On the bone under your eyes (UE)

5. Under your nose (UN)

6. Under your mouth, above the point of your chin (Ch)

7. At the junction of your breastbone, collarbone and your first rib. To locate this point, first find the U-shaped notch on top of your breastbone. From the bottom of the U, go down 1 inch and then sideways 1 inch. This point is abbreviated (CB)

8. Under your arms about 4 inches below your armpit, even with the nipple (for men) or the bra strap (for women), abbreviated (UA)

9. The inside of both wrists (WR). Tap with your wrists.

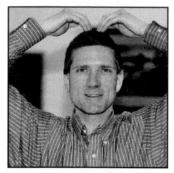

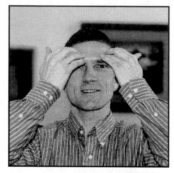

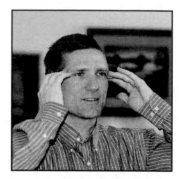

1 TH – Top of Head

2 EB – Inside of Eye Brow

3 SE – Side of the Eye

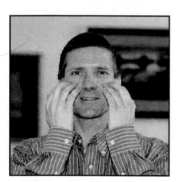

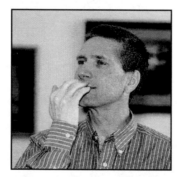

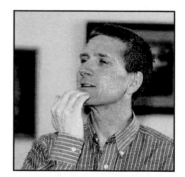

4 UE – Under the Eye

5 UN – Under the Nose

6 Ch – Chin

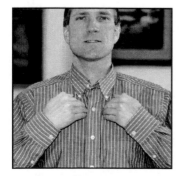

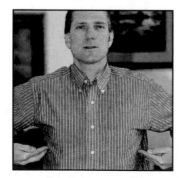

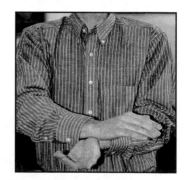

7 CB – Collar Bone

8 UA – Under the Arm

9 WR – Inside of Wrists

1. TH – Top of Head
2. EB – Inside the Eye Brow
3. SE – Side of the Eye
4. UE – Under the Eye
5. UN – Under the Nose
6. Ch – Chin
7. CB – Collar Bone
8. UA – Under the Arm
9. WR – Inside of Wrists

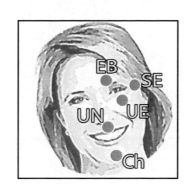

The Affirmation

- There are no limits to the types of issues you can use with EFT.

- It's OK if you don't believe the affirmation... just say it.

- It's best to say the affirmation out loud if possible.

- You must think about and "tune in" to the very specific problem you want to address.

- You repeat the affirmation while tapping, repeating it every time you begin tapping a new point.

- Traditional phrases use the following setup:

"Even though I have this _____,
I deeply and completely accept myself."

- The blank above is filled in with a brief description of the specific issue or problem you want to address.

- Here are some examples:

"Even though I have this infection,
I deeply and completely accept myself."

"Even though I have this anger towards my father,
I deeply and completely accept myself."

"Even though I have this fear of snakes,
I deeply and completely accept myself."

- You can also phrase your affirmation like this:

"I accept myself even though I have this_____."

Performing EFT – One Full Round

1. Select an affirmation based on a very specific issue or problem.

2. Think about and "tune in" to the issue or problem.

3. Tap on each of the points described above while saying your positive affirmation with enthusiasm. Avoid distractions and be present and focused on your affirmation.

4. You repeat your affirmation each time you move to a new tapping point, one with each full breath. One round should take about one minute or less.

After one round of EFT, you'll probably notice a major improvement in the issue that you were addressing while tapping. If new problems related to your original issue come up in your mind while tapping, perform additional rounds of EFT addressing each of the new problems using the following example with the added words "still" and "some":

"Even though I still have some of this _____,
I deeply and completely accept myself."

Want More Help With EFT?

If you don't experience the results that you would like, consider talking with an EFT professional. Many offer a free initial phone consultation, and you find EFT practitioners in your area by searching online. Please note that Michelle Moore does not endorse any particular practitioners.

Appendix E Further Reading Online

Below is a short list of excellent resources online for further reading about MRSA and Staph and related health topics.

- **www.CDC.gov/drugresistance/threat-report-2013/** - This 2013 CDC report about the top antibiotic resistant infections that threaten the United States is informative and easy to read and understand. The title is *Antibiotic resistance threats in the United States, 2013* and it can be downloaded as a PDF file or eBook.

- **GreenMedInfo.com** - This website provides a large collection of scientific article abstracts on the topic of holistic medicine. The abstracts can be searched based on medical condition, natural substances or the actions of substances in the body.

- **www.JonBarron.org** - This is the website of a holistic healthcare expert with many detailed articles on a wide range of health topics focused on a balanced, evidence-based approach to natural medicine.

- **www.Mercola.com** - Dr. Mercola is a practicing doctor and surgeon and his website has many articles on a vast array of alternative health topics.

- **www.ncbi.nlm.nih.gov/pmc/articles/PMC3424311/** - a good article on the use of probiotic supplements for health and support with gastrointestinal challenges and antibiotic associated diarrhea.

References

1. Antibiotic Resistance Threats in the United States, 2013; CDC report

2. Cell wall deficient forms: stealth pathogens, 3rd ed. Lida H. Mattman, 2001 CRC Press LLC

3. Emerging Infectious Determinants of Chronic Diseases, Volume 12, Number 7—July 2006. Siobhán M. O'Connor from the Centers for Disease Control and Prevention

4. Wu SY, Green A. Projection of chronic illness prevalence and cost inflation. Santa Monica, CA: RAND Health; 2000

5. Kung HC, Hoyert DL, Xu JQ, Murphy SL. Deaths: final data for 2005. National Vital Statistics Reports 2008;56(10). Available from: http://www.cdc.gov/nchs/data/nvsr/nvsr56/nvsr56_10.pdf

6. Detection and Identification of Previously Unrecognized Microbial Pathogens, David A. Relma, Emerging Infectious Diseases, Volume 4, Number 3—September 1998; Also, Infectious agents and the etiology of chronic idiopathic diseases, Fredricks DN. Current Clinical Topics in Infectious Diseases. Vol. 18 1998

7. Arch Otolaryngol Head Neck Surg. 2001;127(6):725-726

8. Vanderbilt University Medical Center. "MRSA in pregnancy may be less dangerous than previously thought."; Buddy Creech, M.D., MPH; Pediatrics, April 18, 2012

9. Association for Professionals in Infection Control and Epidemiology (APIC), 2007

10. August 2006 issue of Critical Care Medicine, the journal of the Society of Critical Care Medicine, Lead author Garrett E. Schramm, PharmD

11. Journal of Family Practice 1996; (42:357—361)

12. Science, July 13, 2013, quote by Veysel Berk at California Institute for Quantitative Biosciences

13. Evans RC, Holmes CJ. Effect of vancomycin hydrochloride on Staphylococcus epidermidis biofilm associated with silicone elastomer. Antimicro Agents Chemother 1987;31:889-94

14. Cell Wall Deficient Forms Stealth Pathogens, Lida H. Mattman, 3ed ed. 2001 CRC Press

15. WHO launches the first global strategy on traditional and alternative medicine, World Health Organization website http://www.who.int/mediacentre/news/releases/release38/en/

16. Advanced Aromatherapy: The Science of Essential Oil Therapy, Kurt Schnaubelt

17. Renis HE, In vitro antiviral activity of calcium elenolate, an antiviral agent. Antimicrob. AgentsChemother., 1970; 167-72

18. Antimicrobial activity of commercial Olea europaea (olive) leaf extract., Front Neurol Neurosci. 2010;28:107-12

19. Fitoterapia, Volume 5, 1984

20. Koch and Lawson, Garlic: The Science and Therapeutic Application, 2nd edition, Williams & Wilkins, Baltimore 1996

21. Antibacterial activity of a new, stable, aqueous extract of allicin against methicillin-resistant Staphylococcus aureus. R R Cutler, P Wilson. Br J Biomed Sci. 2004;61(2):71-4

22. A unique natural antimicrobial agent. European Journal for Nutraceutical Research, 30/10/08:1-15

23. Effectiveness of honey on Staphylococcus aureus and Pseudomonas aeruginosa biofilms. Otolaryngol Head Neck Surg. 2009 Jul;141(1):114-8

24. blogs.naturalnews.com/manuka-honey-madness-tale-sabotage-theft-food-fraud/, July 13, 2014, Deane Alban

25. Antimicrobial Effects of Propolis Extracts on Escherichia coli and Staphylococcus aureus Strains Resistant to Various Antibiotics and Some Microorganisms. J Med Food. 2000;3(4):173-80

26. Silver colloid nanoparticles: synthesis, characterization, and their antibacterial activity. J Phys Chem B. 2006 Aug 24;110(33):16248-53

27. *Prescription For Nutritional Healing.* Third edition, 2000. Phyllis A Balch, James F Balch

28. Curcumin Reverse Methicillin Resistance in Staphylococcus aureus. Molecules 2014, 19(11), 18283-18295

29. Quorum quenching and antimicrobial activity of goldenseal (Hydrastis canadensis) against methicillin-resistant Staphylococcus aureus (MRSA). Planta Med. 2012 Sep ;78(14):1556-61

30. Antibacterial activity of Hydrastis canadensis extract and its major isolated alkaloids. Planta Med. 2001 Aug;67(6):561-4

31. Antibacterial and synergy of berberines with antibacterial agents against clinical multi-drug resistant isolates of methicillin-resistant Staphylococcus aureus (MRSA). Molecules. 2012 ;17(9):10322-30

32. Healing with Essential Oils, Kurt Schnaubelt Ph.D., 1999 Frog, Ltd

33. Integrated Use of Essential Oils, Dana Young, 2005 Young Dreams Publishing

34. Desk Reference for Pure Therapeutic Essential Oils, Dana Clay Young PhD, 2009 Young Dreams Publishing

35. Guide to Home Use of Essential Oils, Second Edition, Daniel Pénoël, M.D., 2002 Essentia Publishing

36. Medical Aromatherapy –The Science of Essential Oil Therapy, Kurt Schnaubelt Ph.D., First U.S. Edition, 1998 Healing Arts Press

37. The Healing Intelligence of Essential Oils, Kurt Schnaubelt, Ph.D., 2011 Healing Arts Press

38. The Illustrated Encyclopedia of Essential Oils, Julie Lawless, 1999 Barnes and Nobel Books and Element Books Limited

39. Essential oils found to fight (MRSA) in Hospitals, Feb15, 2002, Dallas – Reuters' Health News

40. The International Journal of Aromatherapy 11(2), Caelli, M., Porteous, J., Carlson, C. F., Heller, R., & Riley, T. V. (2001)

41. What To Do When Antibiotics Don't Work, Dirk Van Gils, 2002 Health Practice Books

42. Belaiche, Paul. 1979. Traite de phytotherapie et d'aromatherapie. Maloine S.A. Editeur, Paris

43. Alternatives to Antibiotics, Dr. John McKenna, 1998 Avery

44. The Fatal Menace of MRSA Suberbug, Maryn McKenna, 2010 Free Press

45. Immunology of Biofilms, Department of Health and Human Services

46. Cell Wall Deficient Forms: Stealth Pathogens, 3rd Edition, 2001, by Dr. Lida H. Mattman

47. J Med Microbiol. 2006 Oct; 55 (Pt 10):1375-80; In vitro activity of tea-tree oil against clinical skin isolates of methicillin-resistant and sensitive Staphylococcus aureus and coagulase-negative staphylococci growing planktonically and as biofilms; Brady A, Loughlin R, Gilpin D, Kearney P, Tunney M

48. J Med Microbiol. 2009 June; 58 (Pt 6):791-7; In vitro activity of carvacrol against staphylococcal preformed biofilm by liquid and vapour contact; Nostro A, Marino A, Blanco AR, Cellini L, Di Giulio M, Pizzimenti F, Sudano Roccaro A, Bisignano G

49. *Over the Counter or Nature's Pharmacy?* Dana Clay Young, 2007 Essentials in Health.

50. *Integrated Use of Essential Oils*, Dana Clay Young Ph.D., 2005 Young Dreams Publishing

51. E.O.B.B.D Certification – from Plant to Laboratory, webpage at Honest-Essential Oils.com

52. Essential Oils, A New Horizon in Combating Bacterial Antibiotic Resistance; Yap, Yiap, Ping and Lim; Open Microbiol J. 2014; 8: 6-14

53. Effect of Essential Oils on Pathogenic Bacteria, Nazzaro, Fratianni, Martino, Coppola and De Feo; Parmaceuticals (Basel) 2013 Dec; 6(12):1451-1474

54. The antimicrobial activity of four commercial essential oils in combination with conventional antimicrobials, van Vuuren, Suliman and Viljoen; Lett Appl Microbiol. 2009;48(4):440-6

55. Tea Tree, lavender, peppermint, oregano, & thyme essential oils showed the strongest killing power against MRSA & VRE resistant bacteria, 1997 UK studies (Dr. D. Gary Young (N.D.), Dr. Carolyn DeMarco (M.D.), & Dr. David K. Hill (D.C.)

56. J Hosp Infect. 2004 Apr;56(4):283-6

57. Antibacterial effect of essential oils from two medicinal plants against Methicillin-resistant Staphylococcus aureus (MRSA). Phytomedicine. 2009 Jul 1. Epub 2009 Jul 1

58. In Vitro Antibacterial Activity of three Indian Spices Against Methicillin-Resistant Staphylococcus aureus. Oman Med J. 2011 Sep ;26(5):319-23

59. Minimum inhibitory concentrations of herbal essential oils and monolaurin for gram-positive and gram-negative bacteria. Mol Cell Biochem. 2005 Apr;272(1-2):29-34

60. Oregano could help eradicate MRSA superbug. Nov 2008. The Telegraph. http://www.telegraph.co.uk/health/alternativemedicine/3516157/Oregano-could-help-eradicate-MRSA-superbug.html

61. Science Daily 10/11/2001

62. The antimicrobial activity of high-necrodane and other lavender oils on methicillin-sensitive and -resistant Staphylococcus aureus (MSSA and MRSA). J Altern Complement Med. 2009 Mar;15(3):275-9

63. Scand J Infect Dis. 2010 Jul;42(6-7):455-60

64. Toll-Like Receptor Triggering of a Vitamin D-Mediated Human Antimicrobial Response, Science 24 March 2006: 1770-1773

65. Calcium and Vitamin D. Diagnostics and Therapeutics. Clin Lab Med. 2000 Sep;20(3):569-90)

66. Vitamin D Council website: http://www.vitamindcouncil.org/about-vitamin-d/how-do-i-get-the-vitamin-d-my-body-needs/#

67. http://articles.mercola.com/sites/articles/archive/2012/12/16/vitamin-k2.aspx?e_cid=20121216_SNL_Art_1

68. http://livertox.nih.gov/Phenotypes_fail.html

69. J Hosp Infec. 1988

70. Effect of antibiotic prescribing in primary care on antimicrobial resistance in individual patients: systematic review and meta-analysis: BMJ 2010;340:c2096

71. Uncomplicated Urinary Tract Infections: A Focus on Women's Health, Kimberly L. Still and Daryn K. Norwood, US Pharm. 2012;37(9):56-60

72. Guidelines (2008) for the prophylaxis and treatment of methicillin-resistant Staphylococcus aureus (MRSA) infections in the United Kingdom, J. Antimicrob. Chemother. (2009)

73. Natural Approaches to Prevention and Treatment of Infections of the Lower Urinary Tract, Kathleen A. Head, ND; Alternative Medicine Review, Volume 13, Number 3, 2008

74. Effects of cranberry extracts on growth and biofilm production of Escherichia coli and Staphylococcus species. LaPlante KL, Sarkisian SA, Woodmansee S, Rowley DC, Seeram NP. Phytother Res. 2012 Sep;26(9):1371-4. http://www.ncbi.nlm.nih.gov/pubmed/22294419

75. Efficacy and limitation of a chlorhexidine-based decolonization strategy in preventing transmission of methicillin-resistant Staphylococcus aureus in an intensive care unit. Clin Infect Dis. 2010 Jan 15;50(2):210-7

76. Limited effectiveness of chlorhexidine based hand disinfectants against methicillin-resistant Staphylococcus aureus (MRSA). J Hosp Infect. 1998 Apr;38(4):297-303

77. Low-Level Mupirocin, Chlorhexidine Resistance Thwart MRSA Control in Hospitals, Dr. Andie S. Lee, The Annual Interscience Conference on Antimicrobial Agents and Chemotherap 2010

78. Longitudinal analysis of chlorhexidine susceptibilities of nosocomial methicillin-resistant Staphylococcus aureus isolates at a teaching hospital in Taiwan. Journal of Antimicrobial Chemotherapy (2008) 62, 514– 517

79. Keller, W., Kober. 1955. *Arzneim. Forsch.* 5, 224

80. *Essential oils 'combat superbug', Tests of new machine at a hospital have found it could be effective in the battle against the superbug MRSA*, BBC NEWS UK

81. J. International Archives of Allergy and Immunology 2002;95:2698

82. Host-Pathogen Interactions: the seduction of molecular cross talk, J. Gut 2002;50:32

83. Anti-infectious activity of synbiotics in a novel mouse model of methicillin-resistant Staphylococcus aureus infection. Microbiol Immunol. 2010 May ;54(5):265-75

84. A randomized placebo-controlled trial of Saccharomyces boulardii in combination with standard antibiotics for Clostridium difficile disease, McFarland LV, JAMA 1994 Jun 22-29; 271(24):1913-8

85. Characterization and purification of a bacteriocin from Lactobacillus paracasei subsp. paracasei BMK2005, an intestinal isolate active against multidrug-resistant pathogens. World J Microbiol Biotechnol. 2012 Apr ;28(4):1543-52

86. Antibacterial activity of Lactobacillus acidophilus and Lactobacillus casei against methicillin-resistant Staphylococcus aureus (MRSA). Microbiol Res. 2010 Oct 20 ;165(8):674-86

87. Fermentation of Propionibacterium acnes, a commensal bacterium in the human skin microbiome, as skin probiotics against methicillin-resistant Staphylococcus aureus. PLoS One. 2013 ;8(2):e55380

88. Applied and Environmental Microbiology, August 2012 vol. 78 no. 15, 5119-5126

89. pH Primer Understanding Your Body's Basic Needs, 2nd edition, Maria Dolgova 2003 Natural Health Consortium

90. The pH Miracle. Balance Your Diet, Reclaim Your Health, Robert O. Young, 2002 Warner Books

91. I – Reality and Subjectivity and Devotional Non-duality, Discovery of the Presence of God, both by David R. Hawkins M.D. Ph.D., Veritas Publishing.

92. Complex carbohydrates are essential in the correct functioning of the immune system, J. Science 2001;291:1237)

93. J. Archives of Surgery 1999;134:1229

94. American Journal of Clinical Nutrition October 2006; 84(4): 894-902

95. Green For Life by Victoria Boutenko, Raw Family Publishing 2005

96. http://www.doctoroz.com/article/genetically-modified-foods-get-facts

97. http://www.iarc.fr/en/media-centre/iarcnews/pdf/MonographVolume112.pdf

98. Food and Chemical Toxicology, Sep 19, 2012

99. Jeffrey M. Smith, Genetic Roulette: The Documented Health Risks of Genetically Engineered Foods, Yes! Books, Fairfield, IA USA 2007

100. Mortality in Sheep Flocks after Grazing on Bt Cotton Fields—Warangal District, Andhra Pradesh" Report of the Preliminary Assessment, April 2006

101. http://www.labelgmos.org/the_science_genetically_modified_foods_gmo

102. Carman, J.A.; Vlieger, H.R.; Ver Steeg, L.J.; Sneller, V.E.; Robinson, G.W.; Clinch-Jones, C.A.; Haynes, J.I.; Edwards, J.W. A long-term toxicology study on pigs fed a combined genetically modified (GM) soy and GM maize diet. Journal of Organic Systems 2013, 8(1), 38-54

103. http://www.nongmoproject.org/2010/10/28/gmo-foods-what-they-are-and-how-you-can-avoid-them/

104. Samsel A, Seneff S. Glyphosate's Suppression of Cytochrome P450 Enzymes and Amino Acid Biosynthesis by the Gut Microbiome: Pathways to Modern Diseases. Entropy 2013, 15, 1416-1463; doi:10.3390/e15041416

105. Shehata AA, Schrödl W, Aldin AA, Hafez HM, Krüger M. Curr Microbiol. The effect of glyphosate on potential pathogens and beneficial members of poultry microbiota in vitro. Current Microbiology, 2013 Apr;66(4):350-8. doi: 10.1007/s00284-012-0277-2. Epub 2012 Dec 9

106. Krüger M, Shehata AA, Schrödl W, Rodloff A. Glyphosate suppresses the antagonistic effect of Enterococcus spp. on Clostridium botulinum Anaerobe. Anaerobe, 2013 Apr;20:74-8. doi: 0.1016/j.anaerobe.2013.01.005. Epub 2013 Feb 6

107. US Patent 7771736: "Glyphosate formulations and their use for the inhibition of 5-enolpyruvylshikimate-3-phosphate synthase"

108. http://d3n8a8pro7vhmx.cloudfront.net/yesmaam/pages/774/attachments/original/1396803706/Glyphosate__Final__in_the_breast_milk_of_American_women_Draft6_.pdf?1396803706

109. http://feedtheworld.info/wp-content/uploads/2015/03/ehp0114-000260.pdf

110. http://cedb.asce.org/cgi/WWWdisplay.cgi?85599

111. http://www.cdc.gov/handwashing/show-me-the-science-hand-sanitizer.html

112. Triclosan, Wikipedia.org

113. FDA Taking Close Look at 'Antibacterial' Soap, FDA Consumer Health Information, December 2013

114. Reduction of Clostridium difficile Infection in a Community-based Hospital Using Hypochlorite Solution AJIC: June 2005, Volume 33, Issue 5, Pages e43-e44

115. Ozonated water for disinfection of MRSA and C difficile, J. Coulter, 11:30 AM-1:00 PM, Friday, September 12, 2008 Queen Elizabeth II Conference Centre Poster Hall 2

116. Swab study shows MRSA in pregnancy may not mean much, Carole Bartoo, Vanderbilt University Medical Center, 4/19/2012.

117. Arch Pediat Adoles Med. 2012; 166(6): 551-557

118. Pediatric 2002, 110:285-291

119. Acta Paediatrica Volume 92,s441:48–55

Credits

Cover
Bacteria ©iStockPhoto.com/Henrik5000
Vitruvian Man ©Luc Viatour/www.lucnix.be
Oil drop ©iStockPhoto.com/Synergee
Stethoscope ©iStockPhoto.com/bluestocking
Leaves ©iStockPhoto.com/robynmac
Plate ©iStockPhoto.com/Lindel
Mortar © iStockPhoto.com/Pears2295
Michelle Moore ©Lester Moore.

Front matter photos
Bacteria ©iStockPhoto.com/Henrik5000
Vitruvian Man ©Luc Viatour/www.lucnix.be
Oil drop ©iStockPhoto.com/Synergee.

Chapter 1
Action plan ©Lester Moore
Bacteria control ©Lester Moore
In, on, around ©Lester Moore
Medical support ©Lester Moore
Immune defense ©Lester Moore

Chapter 2
Staph bacteria ©PHIL/Arduino

Chapter 3
MRSA images 1-5 ©iStockPhoto.com/JodiJacobson

Chapter 4
Pills ©iStockPhoto.com/mcfields
Doctor ©Fotolia.com/18percentgrey
Culture plate ©iStockPhoto.com/Lindel
Susceptibility test ©PHIL/Stalons

Chapter 5
Operation ©iStockPhoto.com/Platinus

Chapter 6
Stethoscope ©iStockPhoto.com/bluestocking
Basil leaves ©iStockPhoto.com/robynmac

Chapter 7

Biofilm ©Lester Moore

Chapter 8
Alternative medicine ©Lester Moore

Chapter 9
Olive leaves ©Fotolia.com/joanna wnuk
Garlic ©iStockPhoto.com/galdzer

Chapter 10
Essential oil drop ©iStockPhoto.com/Synergee
Oregano ©Fotolia.com/margo555

Chapter 11
Essential oil bottle cap ©Lester Moore
Filling a capsule ©Lester Moore

Chapter 12
In, on, around ©Lester Moore

Chapter 15
Sinus rinse aid ©Lester Moore

Chapter 16
Unhealthy intestines ©Lester Moore
healthy intestines ©Lester Moore

Chapter 18
pH scale ©Lester Moore

Chapter 20
Greens ©PHIL/James Gathany
Smoothies ©iStockPhoto.com/loooby

Chapter 21
Spraying garden ©PHIL/Dawn Arlotta

Chapter 22
Hand sanitizer ©PHIL/Amanda Mills
Antimicrobial soap ©Fotolia.com/Marina Lohrbach

Chapter 23
Cleaning sink ©Fotolia.com/diego cervo
Bleach bottle ©Fotolia.com/Beth Van Trees

Chapter 25
Personal items ©Lester Moore

Chapter 26

Baby ©Fotolia.com/Silroby

Appendix D

EFT tapping 1-9 ©Lester Moore

EFT positions ©Lester Moore